PREVENTION.
FROM MOTHI

The word is out: The Am...
And if you're one of the nearly 50% of American who take vitamins regularly, or one of the 34% who have tried alternative medicine, you're on the cutting edge. More and more of us are turning to holistic, drug-free remedies to stay healthy, reduce the risk of serious disease, and treat illnesses from depression to heart disease.

This empowering, authoritative reference, backed by the latest proven scientific research provides comprehensive information on using natural remedies—including break-through antioxidants, powerful mineral combinations, potent herbs, and nutritional supplements—to prevent and treat a vast array of health problems, including:

* Allergies and asthma * Anxiety * Arthritis *
Cancer * Cold and flu * Diabetes * Digestive
disorders * Fertility problems * Heart
disease * Insomnia * Liver problems
* Menopause and PMS * Osteoporosis * Prostate
problems * Varicose veins
* AND MANY MORE

PLUS: Important information on new research, potential side effects, tips for achieving optimum effectiveness—everything you need to know about nature's best-kept secrets!

**THE CORINNE T. NETZER BIG BOOK OF
MIRACLE CURES**

Books by Corinne T. Netzer

THE CORINNE T. NETZER ANNUAL CALORIE COUNTER
THE CORINNE T. NETZER BRAND-NAME CALORIE COUNTER
THE COMPLETE BOOK OF FOOD COUNTS
THE CORINNE T. NETZER CHOLESTEROL COUNTER
THE CORINNE T. NETZER CARBOHYDRATE COUNTER
THE CARBOHYDRATE DIETER'S DIARY
THE CORINNE T. NETZER DIETER'S DIARY
THE CORINNE T. NETZER ENCYCLOPEDIA OF FOOD VALUES
THE CORINNE T. NETZER FAT COUNTER
THE CORINNE T. NETZER FIBER COUNTER
THE CORINNE T. NETZER LOW FAT DIARY
THE DIETER'S CALORIE COUNTER
THE COMPLETE BOOK OF VITAMIN & MINERAL COUNTS
CORINNE T. NETZER'S BIG BOOK OF MIRACLE CURES

THE COMPLETE BOOK OF FOOD COUNTS COOKBOOK SERIES:

100 LOW FAT SMALL MEAL AND SALAD RECIPES
100 LOW FAT VEGETABLE AND LEGUME RECIPES
100 LOW FAT SOUP AND STEW RECIPES
100 LOW FAT PASTA AND GRAIN RECIPES
100 LOW FAT FISH AND SHELLFISH RECIPES
100 LOW FAT CHICKEN AND TURKEY RECIPES

CORINNE T. NETZER'S
BIG BOOK OF
MIRACLE
CURES

■

CORINNE T. NETZER

A DELL BOOK

Published by
Dell Publishing
a division of
Random House, Inc.
1540 Broadway
New York, New York 10036

This book is not intended to take the place of medical advice from a trained medical professional. Readers are advised to consult a physician or other qualified health professional regarding treatment of their medical problems. Neither the publisher nor the author take any responsibility for any possible consequences from any treatment, action, or application of medicine, herb or preparation to any person reading or following the information in this book.

ISBN: 0-440-22609-0

Printed in the United States of America

Published simultaneously in Canada

March 1999

10 9 8 7 6 5 4 3 2 1
OPM

ACKNOWLEDGMENTS

To Susan Waggoner, lead researcher, and Peggy Webb,
associate: for service above and beyond the call
Without their dedication and tireless effort this book
would not have been possible

To Elaine Wittman Chaback: editor and friend

To Glenn S. Rothfeld, M.D.:
for his overview of the manuscript and excellent
comments.

To Jacqueline Miller: keeper of the flame

CONTENTS

INTRODUCTION

*Medicine is an enormous achievement, but
what it will achieve practically for humanity,
and what those who hold the power will allow it
to do, remain open questions.*
                    —Roy Porter
                    The Greatest Benefit to Mankind

Almost everyone would like to be healthier and take
steps to prevent serious diseases such as cancer, heart
failure, arthritis. The question is *how*? We live in a world
where there are many choices but few concrete answers.

Even though we often hear that Americans are drown-
ing in information, there's one type of information that
can be frustratingly difficult to come by—sound, accurate data about nutritional supplements and their ability
to forestall and clear up health problems.

That's what this book is about. We've studied the research and discarded the dubious and inconclusive to
bring you news about *proven, scientifically sound*
cures—cures that you can buy immediately, without
waiting for a doctor's appointment or a prescription.

If you read even one chapter of this book, you'll be
solidly informed about an important aspect of your

health. And after you read the entire book you will have acquired knowledge that even today many doctors don't possess.

IF THESE REMEDIES WORK, WHY HAVEN'T WE HEARD MORE ABOUT THEM?

Without a doubt Western medicine is one of mankind's greatest achievements. It has stopped plagues and turned once-common killers such as diphtheria and smallpox into rare and isolated occurrences.

But the high-tech, white-coat approach to medicine, practiced and envied throughout the world, does have a few blind spots. It can be impersonal and, because of that, frightening. It can be so absorbed with fixing the body it ignores the patient inside that body. It can become so enamored of chemically synthesized drugs that it overlooks remedies that have worked for centuries.

These shortcomings are especially true in America. While our system of for-profit medicine has given us one of the finest medical systems in the world, it has allowed important research to remain undone.

All research, even research on inexpensive nutritional supplements, costs money. Pharmaceutical companies fund an enormous amount of research in hopes that their investment will result in medicines that can ultimately be patented and marketed. But in America no one can patent or own vitamins, minerals, herbs, or other nutrients. This is good for consumers, of course, since it keeps costs low. The down side is that without a profit incentive pharmaceutical companies have no reason to fund research.

Insurance companies, which fund studies on many aspects of life and health, are also uninterested in this type of research. To date, they have been required to cover only "officially approved" treatments, and this has not included vitamins, herbs, or other supplements. Without a financial stake in discovering what works and what doesn't, it's hard for corporations to justify expensive studies and trials.

For the most part, this kind of research has been left to hospitals and universities. The work they have accomplished is invaluable. The problem is that there is simply too much research to be done, competing with too many other urgent and pressing projects, to assure a steady flow of information.

Even when research is conducted, even when the findings are quite impressive, many of us never learn about them. Consider the rapidity with which "Prozac" and "Viagra" became household words. In both cases a pharmaceutical public-relations effort blended seamlessly with the media eager to embrace the newest high-tech cure-all.

For a complex, technically written study to enter the information mainstream, someone must write about it in ordinary terms, and get his or her article published in an ordinary magazine or newspaper. This doesn't happen as frequently as it should. Too often the media hop on the Prozac or Viagra bandwagon, and other important work goes unnoticed.

WELCOME TO THE PEOPLE'S REVOLUTION

The American medical scene *is* changing. And it's changing by popular demand.

If you're one of the nearly 50 percent of Americans

who take vitamins regularly, or one of the 34 percent of Americans who have tried alternative medicine, you're on the cutting edge. Your actions have been duly noted. And changes are being made.

Not too long ago, nutritional supplements were only available in health food stores, and health food stores were few and far between. Today health food stores can be found everywhere. Nutritional supplements of all sorts can be purchased in drugstores, national chain stores, and even some grocery stores.

And today the word "supplements" means far more than vitamins and minerals. Sales of herbal remedies are increasing at a rate of 12 percent to 15 percent each year, and more than two hundred companies in the United States produce herbal remedies of one form or another.

However belatedly, the American medical establishment is bending to consumer wishes. It is acknowledging that traditionally used herbs form the basis of many modern medicines, including quinine and digitalis. It is also acknowledging that more recent discoveries—such as the cancer-fighting drugs derived from the Pacific yew tree—justify continued research in this area.

In 1992 the government-sponsored National Institutes of Mental Health created an Office of Alternative Medicine. Its mission is to fund research into the safety, effectiveness, and potential usefulness of remedies that fall outside traditional boundaries.

HOW DO WE KNOW WHAT WORKS?

If research is just starting to be done on nutritional supplements, is it possible to know what works and what doesn't? Yes, it is!

Research may be just beginning in the United States, but this is one area in which we definitely are not a world leader. When it comes to studying and using natural remedies, much of the rest of the world is way, way ahead of us.

Germany and France, especially, have done a good deal of pioneering research, and doctors in both countries frequently prescribe nutritional supplements for patients. Such prescriptions are not mere placebos, and the curative effects of many supplements are supported by convincing research. In fact the German government funds a highly respected body known as Commission E, whose sole mission is to review current research and approve various herbal supplements for use.

A good deal of sound, reliable research has also been done in England, Sweden, Finland, Japan, and China. Fortunately, more of these studies are now available in the English language than ever before. And, as information flows out, more and more of these miraculous cures are becoming available for use in the United States.

HOW WE CHOSE THE CURES IN THIS BOOK

Today you can go into any drugstore or health food store and find literally hundreds of nutritional supplements for sale. You can read mountains of newsletters and magazines packed with advertisements, testimonials, and miraculous case studies. If you have a computer and an Internet connection, you can surf your way to dozens of sites that sell thousands of products.

Amazing life-saving cure! the ads shout. *Proven effective in dozens of studies!*

Are all of these products as effective as their manufacturers claim? In a word, No.

This book discusses over sixty healing nutrients. As the References section shows, we've included hundreds of studies. What that section doesn't reveal are the many supplements and thousands of studies we reviewed but didn't include because they didn't meet our tough criteria.

In planning this book, a commitment was made to include only the most effective, best-researched supplements on the market. This meant looking not only at the quantity of supportive research but evaluating its quality as well. The purpose of this book is not to jump on the bandwagon of the latest fad nutrient.

It probably won't surprise you to learn that when it comes to the winning but vague phrase *Studies prove,* many manufacturers, and even a few writers, bend the findings to fit their own agenda. For example, studies may prove that a nutrient kills harmful microorganisms in a petri dish—but that doesn't mean the nutrient will kill the same microorganisms in living creatures. Many miraculous "cures" (including innumerable antidotes for cancer), have been discovered in petri dishes, only to prove disappointingly ineffective when tried on lab animals and humans.

One of our more surprising findings in this vein concerned ginseng, touted everywhere as a universal energizer. Ginseng *does* boost your energy—if you're a lab rodent. Seldom publicized is the fact that when tried on human beings ginseng has not lived up to this claim. (Ironically ginseng has a far more dramatic effect on humans as a cancer preventative, which we discuss in chapter 6.)

We also ruled out another strategy of eager marketers: personal testimonies and individual case studies. There are a few problems with these. First, we don't doubt that most people who offer testimonies are sincere and honest. But individuals suffering from a health problem have such a strong wish to be well that even ineffective treatment may make them feel well.

In science this is known as the placebo effect. Symptoms such as pain, fatigue, and discomfort are especially likely to be influenced by the placebo effect. In fact, about 30 percent of patients with these complaints will claim to improve even if the pill they were given contains nothing but sugar and a bit of food coloring.

Another problem with testimonials and single case studies is that sometimes patients get better for reasons even doctors don't understand. Life-threatening tumors seem to dissolve of their own accord, allergies vanish, diabetes goes away. The patient fully recovers and goes on with his or her life. But that doesn't mean the drugs, nutrients, or other remedies the patient took will work for others.

Individual case studies *do* have a place in medical literature, and they can be quite useful in suggesting avenues of research to explore. But, like personal testimonies, such cases have too many unknowns to be taken as proof of a particular method of treatment.

To validate claims made for various nutrients, we looked for carefully controlled clinical trials that tested the nutrient in question on groups of humans. When a study's findings were positive, we looked for other studies that confirmed these findings.

Needless to say, not all studies are equal. When we say "carefully controlled" study, we mean a trial that has been constructed to eliminate as many errors as possible. One way to guard against the placebo effect, for example, is to divide volunteers into two groups, giving one group the active nutrient and the other a harmless placebo.

A well-designed study of this type will take pains to make the two groups as equal as possible in terms of age, general health, and other variables. It may also ask volunteers to follow certain guidelines during the test period (such as refraining from taking other nutrients or over-the-counter remedies) in order to preserve the integrity of the results.

When you read ads or promotional materials for various nutrients and find yourself wondering if the favorite phrase *studies prove* means all it seems to, your skepticism is often justified. You needn't have such concerns in this book. If convincing research wasn't available on a nutrient, we left it out.

HOW TO USE THIS BOOK

We have arranged this book alphabetically by disorder or problem. If you are wondering about a specific problem and don't see it listed on the contents page, please refer to the index at the back of the book. If you are wondering whether a particular nutrient is discussed and where to find information on it in the book, the index is also your best guide.

Here are some pointers that will help you make the most of this information:

- **Don't dispense with your doctor.** Nothing in this book is meant to take the place of traditional medical diagnosis and treatment measures. We don't advise that you act as your own doctor or prescribe your own remedies for conditions and problems. This book is meant to be used in addition to—never instead of—regular medical care.

- **Read sections on nutrients thoroughly.** Warning: The information in this book causes excitement! You may be tempted to skim just enough to find out what nutrients to take without finding out how to take them. We urge you to take the few additional minutes needed to read the entire entry that's of interest to you, including our instructions for use.

  The nutrients in this book are safe and effective if taken according to the guidelines set forth. If these guidelines are ignored, the nutrient you take may be neither safe nor effective. We want to make sure you get the health benefits you deserve from each and every nutrient, so do take time to learn about dosages, tips for use, and possible cautions.

- **Read the "major" and the "minor" listings in chapters of interest to you.** You'll notice that in addition to in-depth discussions of various nutrients, many chapters conclude with a "What Else Can You Do?" section. This section includes shorter discussions of additional nutrients.

  Why do some nutrients get more attention and some less? Does it mean that nutrients in the "What Else Can You Do?" section are unproven? There are a few answers to these questions.

  Nutrients chosen for in-depth discussion are those that have been proven most effective for the problem at hand. This means the research was the most convincing and clearly demonstrated that the nutrient worked for *most* of the people *most* of the time.

This does not mean that nutrients given less discussion space are speculative or untested. They may simply have worked for a smaller number of people. It's important to remember that even in the case of the "most effective" prescription drugs ever developed not everything works for everyone. A nutrient placed in the "What Else Can You Do Section?"— because it didn't help as many people as one of the nutrients given more attention—may be a true miracle for you, and well worth trying.

Nutrients were also placed in the "What Else Can You Do?" section for other important reasons. One was that the nutrient in question may play a supporting—rather than a key—role in dealing with the problem at hand. Very often this same nutrient *does* play a major role in another health concern, and is given a full discussion elsewhere in the book. To learn more about a nutrient, always consult the index.

Finally, lack of research caused some very promising remedies to be given shorter rather than longer discussions. More studies may need to be done to confirm early but still unsubstantiated findings. Or "rave reviews" from individual users may need to be proven by scientific studies.

In no case did we include a nutrient, even for short discussion, based solely on manufacturers' claims or offers of proof. And we have tried, in each case, to provide you with only responsible and verified information.

- **Know that you may be a special case.** The guidelines for the use of various nutrients in this book are safe and effective for most people. However, you may have a condition that makes you a special case. The guidelines in this book do not apply to children or to pregnant or breast-feeding women. And if you have a disease for which you are being treated, or are taking medication, you must, to be safe, get your doctor's advice before beginning a supplement program.

SUPPLEMENTS: HOW TO GET YOUR MONEY'S WORTH

Throughout this book we avoid using brand names and making recommendations regarding specific manufacturers. Not because there aren't good companies out there. That's one of the problems. There are many very good manufacturers, and naming only a few of them might give you the idea that companies we did not name turn out substandard products.

There's another reason we do not name specific manufacturers. We don't want to give you the idea that certain companies have spoon-fed us research or promotional information. As we mentioned above, in no case did we rely on anything but exhaustive research for the preparation of this manuscript.

That said, there are some things you should keep in mind when shopping for and using nutritional supplements. Here are three simple rules to follow to make sure you always get your money's worth:

- **Always buy from a reputable manufacturer.** Some people assume that these products, like medications, are regulated by the government and must meet certain standards. This is not true. And, unfortunately, some companies have taken advantage of the lack of regulation to increase their profit margins. There have been instances of highly adulterated products being sold. Varo Tyler, a noted authority on herbs as medicine, has noted that an analysis of fifty-four ginseng products found that 25 percent of them contained no ginseng at all. To avoid wasting your money, buy from reputable manufacturers who are willing to guarantee the quality of their products.

- **Look for standardized products.** Products you buy should be guaranteed to contain a specific amount of active substances. This is important for two reasons. First, untrustworthy manufacturers may include a lot of filler and very little of the product itself. Second, herbal products are subject to many variations. Plants vary in chemical composition from plant to plant, crop to crop, and season to season. A good manufacturer has found a way to overcome all of these obstacles and is able to guarantee that each and every dose you take contains the same amount of the desirable ingredient. Where possible, we have included guidelines for these substances in this book.

- **Read and follow the manufacturer's package instructions.** Just as you should take time to read the guidelines for each nutrient given in this book, you should take time to read the manufacturer's own guidelines. Since products may vary in strength and quantity of active ingredients, it wasn't always possible for us to give you hard-and-fast instructions.

When in doubt about how much of a nutrient to take, follow the manufacturer's package directions.

Following these three simple rules will help you get the most for your money. But there is one final word of caution. Unfortunately, a few people have fallen prey to a particular myth. The myth goes something like this: "If it's natural, it's safe in any quantity, and more is better than less."

This is not true at all. Some nutrients *can* be toxic, and overdoing it can be harmful. Too much vitamin E, for example, can cause blood to become so thin it fails to clot properly. And, as you'll discover in the chapter on colds, licorice that has not been deglycyrrhizinated is so potent it can only be used for short periods of time. Remember, the nutrients included in this book were chosen because they have a significant action on the body. Their power should not be underestimated.

THE FUTURE OF MIRACLE CURES

The remedies in this book are indeed miraculous. Not in the clouds-and-angels sense of the word but in its hard, scientific sense. It is indeed a miracle that inexpensive, readily available nutrients can spare us the ravages of life-threatening diseases such as cancer, heart attack, and stroke. Just as it is miraculous that these same nutrients can outperform many far more expensive prescription medications.

Even in Europe, where study is more advanced than it is here, we are still very much at the beginning of the journey. There is much that remains to be discovered.

And, in time, science may find a way to bioengineer certain nutrients to make them even safer and more effective. In time, nutrient-based medicines may come to replace many synthetic drugs in use today.

CHAPTER ONE

Overcome Your

Anxiety

Tense? Think of the warm sun, gentle breezes, and fragrant flowers of the South Pacific islands. If that isn't enough to take away your tension, there's one more gift from the tropics you should know about, a miraculous stress-buster that's been around for thousands of years!

Anxiety, along with depression, is one of the most common complaints of our era. A hallmark of modern life, anxiety is so common many accept it as a given. Others go to doctors or psychiatrists for prescription medications, most of which are expensive and a few of which can be habit-forming. If neither of these alternatives is appealing to you, why not try soothing anxiety the natural way?

THE PROBLEM

In many ways, "anxiety" is just another way of saying "worry, worry, worry." When you suffer from anxiety, your mind cannot seem to stop running over a constant list of problems both real and imagined. Some people become so paralyzed thinking of all they have to do that their productivity actually decreases. Others worry about unlikely possibilities that will never come to pass. Still others carry such a burden of concerns that they can never fully relax and enjoy themselves, causing them to become exhausted and more tense than ever before.

WHO GETS ANXIETY?

Everyone can (and probably will, at some point in life) suffer from anxiety. From the first moment we draw breath, we are susceptible to this universal ill. In this vein, "anxiety" has become a broad-based term that can have more than one meaning.

The kind of anxiety most of us suffer from is temporary and nonclinical. It does not meet the criteria for clinical anxiety disorders, which can be long lasting and stubborn enough to require professional treatment (see "What You Need To Know," page 20).

Unlike clinical anxiety, the ordinary anxiety from which many of us suffer is not a permanent feature of our personalities but arises from the everyday circumstances of our lives. Some of the most common circumstances that produce feelings of anxiety and tension are:

- **Changes.** You don't need to be a rocket scientist to figure out that unwelcome changes bring about anxiety. But most people don't realize that positive changes—such as moving into the house of your dreams or receiving a big promotion at work—are almost as likely to produce tension. As humans, we're creatures of habit, and alterations in our little corner of the world challenge us to readjust. In most cases this kind of anxiety diminishes as we master our new circumstances.

- **Losses.** Losing friends, family members, jobs, or pets, can undermine our sense of security and make us feel vulnerable. People who have endured important losses often feel as if they are "holding their breath," waiting for the other shoe to drop.
- **Work.** For some people, their job is literally their worst enemy. In a postdownsizing world, people may find themselves working longer and harder, with less job security and less staff support than ever. Ironically, anxiety may be higher at lower levels of the corporate ladder than at higher ones. Workplace studies have shown that bosses feel less stressed than their secretaries. The reason: Both people work hard, but managers have much greater control than workers who have little input in the carrying out of tasks assigned by others.
- **Marriage or family disruptions.** It makes sense that conflicts with spouses and children will produce their share of tension, but so can situations that aren't necessarily conflict-based. Having a new baby, deciding that Mom should work outside the home, taking in an elderly parent, living in a blended family, and helping children grow into adults—all of these ordinary circumstances can produce extraordinary levels of anxiety.
- **Financial woes.** Worry and tension about the future of your bank account is an obvious cause of anxiety.
- **Illness or accident.** People who make it through serious illnesses and accidents often find themselves hamstrung with anxiety after the danger has passed. Sometimes the anxiety is tied specifically to the event, as in the case of heart attack survivors

being afraid to engage in even mild forms of exercise. In other cases, the anxiety is free-floating and pervasive, and the person feels a vague, general, and continual sense of anxiety for some time.

- **Lack of balance in life.** Work, play, love, and sleep are all necessary ingredients for a calm and productive human being. The problem is that many of us are living lives that are out of balance. Overwork and lack of sleep, the usual culprits, can produce high levels of anxiety.

WHAT ARE THE SYMPTOMS?

You need not be told that the key symptom of anxiety is excessive worry. But here are some other symptoms you may not be quite as aware of:

- **Irritability.** Your patience is at an all-time low and it doesn't take much to lose your temper.
- **Feeling overwhelmed.** Your duties, cares, and worries seem so numerous and complex that you feel you will never gain control over them.
- **Procrastination.** You are so aware of how much you have to do or how many problems you must resolve that you find it difficult to do anything at all. You feel your efforts will barely make a dent in things, yet you feel guilty for not "doing it all."
- **Runaway thoughts.** Your worries and fears crowd into your thoughts, unbidden, when you are trying to focus on other things. Once the worry train gets rolling, it's hard to bring it to a halt. You may even imagine things getting much worse than they are. For example, "I can't get this job finished, I'm go-

ing to get fired, I'll never find another job and my family and I will end up living in the street.''

- **Being unable to let go of your worries.** Your problems are always with you, and you find it impossible to set them aside completely, even for short periods of time.
- **You can't relax and enjoy life.** Things you ordinarily find pleasure in fail to bring you pleasure. You can't remember when you last ''let go'' and enjoyed yourself. You never feel completely relaxed, and almost always feel on edge.
- **Insomnia.** Being unable to fall asleep at night, waking too early, or waking in the middle of the night and having difficulty falling asleep again are all typical symptoms of tension and anxiety.
- **Eating too much or too little.** Do you find yourself compelled to eat when you're not hungry, or consuming quantities of food almost without tasting it? Or do you forget to eat or feel too nervous to sit down and enjoy a meal? Disrupted eating habits are a common consequence of anxiety.
- **Drinking, using drugs, and other self-destructive behaviors.** Activities people think of as ''addictive'' may actually be attempts to quell anxiety. Problems such as overspending, compulsive sexual relationships, gambling, and overeating (mentioned above) fall into this category as well.
- **Physical symptoms.** Tension often finds expression through the body, in the form of stiff muscles, headaches, racing pulse, nervous stomach, vague aches and pains, and so on.

WHAT'S THE OUTLOOK?

For most people, anxiety is nonclinical and temporary, clearing up and dissipating gradually over a period of time. Unfortunately, anxiety can become a habit if you don't learn how to deal with it, and it may return anytime you are under stress or challenged by the ordinary speed bumps of life. For a few people, anxiety is clinical and may require professional help to resolve.

WHAT YOU NEED TO KNOW

If you suffer from anxiety, you should know whether your stress is ordinary and temporary or a form of clinical anxiety. There are several types of clinical anxiety, including phobia, agoraphobia, panic, post-traumatic stress syndrome, and obsessive-compulsive disorder. If you have one of these forms of anxiety, you may want to seek professional help from a psychologist or psychiatrist—not because you can't "cope" on your own, but because clinical anxiety can become deep-rooted and stubborn over time, significantly impairing your ability to live a productive and enjoyable life. Also, there's substantial research to indicate that clinical anxiety has a strong biological underpinning and can best be addressed by therapy and medication.

How can you tell what kind of anxiety you have? You can't for sure. But if the checklist below seems to describe you a little too well, you might consider talking to a therapist about your problem.

CLINICAL ANXIETY CHECKLIST

Although only a professional can correctly diagnose clinical anxiety, here's a checklist of things to watch for:

- **No obvious cause.** Your anxiety hasn't been triggered by a specific event or situation, such as those listed above (see pages 16–18).
- **Duration.** Your anxiety doesn't abate on its own but becomes a more or less permanent feature of life.
- **Interferes with work or academic performance.** Anxiety keeps you from meeting deadlines, performing up to your abilities, or fulfilling other tasks at work or school.
- **Limitation and avoidance.** Your anxiety is severe enough to prevent you from doing things you would ordinarily do or going places you would ordinarily go.
- **Magical thinking, repetitions, or rituals.** You find there are certain acts you *must* perform—such as compulsive washing, hoarding, etc.—or you are obsessed with beliefs your rational mind tells you are untrue, such as the idea that touching a doorknob will flood you with fatal germs.

PROVEN MIRACLES

KAVA

WHAT IS KAVA?

Kava (also known as kava-kava), a native plant of the South Pacific region, certainly sounds exotic. Actually, it's a member of the pepper family and closely related to the same plant that gives us the black pepper we sprinkle on food.

Although kava has no food uses, extract from the root of the plant has long been revered for its potent ability to relax both the mind and the body. Recently, science has established that kava's reputation is well deserved. Locked within the root of this otherwise ordinary shrub are substances that have a proven, significant effect on the central nervous system!

THE MIRACLE EFFECT

For centuries, kava's effectiveness as a tension-soother was attributed to its ability to soothe muscles. Early researchers were on the right track, and numerous studies have now proven that kava contains substances, called kavalactones, that work to relax skeletal muscles throughout the body. But it turns out that kavalactone isn't the only active ingredient that makes kava potent. Recent research has discovered that kava also possesses substances that work on the brain itself to reduce stress and anxiety.

What most of us refer to as "mood" is influenced not only by the events in our lives but by the processes that go on within the brain. Substances called neurotransmitters act as chemical messengers in an extremely complex relay system, and the disruption of this system has been linked to depression, anxiety, and other problems. Synthetic drugs such as Prozac are designed to work on the neurotransmitter system. In the 1990s researchers discovered that substances in kava, called pyrones, have significant effects on neurotransmitters, including nor-adrenaline, which regulates feelings of anxiety.

Is kava better than synthetic drugs now on the market? Very possibly. Studies show that kava has some big advantages over many of these drugs. Not only is kava not habit forming, it sedates without making you drowsy or interfering with mental alertness.

HAS KAVA BEEN USED BEFORE?

When the British explorer, Captain Cook, arrived in the South Pacific islands in 1770, he was offered a beverage made of scraped, pulverized kava root and coconut milk. The ceremonial beverage was valued throughout the region for its ability to instill a sense of happiness and calm. The root was brought back to Europe and soon gained popularity as a relaxant and antidote for a wide range of nervous conditions.

RESEARCH FINDINGS

In the past decade, new research has emerged to support the use of kava as an effective alternative to synthetic drugs for anxiety. Two European studies are especially noteworthy.

In one, conducted by researchers in Düsseldorf, fifty-eight patients with anxiety were divided into two groups and studied over a four-week period. One group received a special preparation of kava extract, while the other received a harmless placebo. Neither doctors nor patients knew who received the real medication and who did not. Anxiety was measured by giving a standardized test at several points before, during, and after the study. Patients who received kava extract began to improve after week one, and continued to improve markedly throughout the next three weeks. At the end of the study, researchers concluded that kava had a significant and positive effect on anxiety.

A second report, published in 1997, was conducted by researchers in the psychiatry department of Jena University. This study involved 101 patients who suffered from a diagnosable anxiety disorder (according to standards set by the American Psychiatric Association), and lasted twenty-five weeks. This research supported the findings of the earlier work and noted that kava became even more effective from the eighth week of use on. They also noted that kava had fewer side effects than synthetic medications commonly prescribed for depression and anxiety.

Germany's Commission E has endorsed kava as an effective and safe aid for stress, nervous anxiety, and restlessness when used as directed.

OTHER WAYS KAVA CAN HELP

Because of its effectiveness as a muscle relaxant, kava has often been recommended for easing menstrual cramps. More recently it has been proven to be effective for anxiety associated with menopause (see chapter 20, page 340).

Another fascinating study suggests kava may have usefulness in another area of medicine as well. Researchers at the University of Marburg in Germany have discovered that kava may work to protect the brain from damage from traumas such as accident or stroke. When mice were fed an oral dose of kava an hour before receiving artificially induced damage to a cerebral artery, less of the brain was damaged than in mice who did not receive kava. More research may suggest practical ways in which this miracle plant can protect the human brain as well.

HOW TO TAKE KAVA

What form does it come in? Kava comes in many forms, including tablets and capsules, liquid, and concentrated drops. The dried root can also be purchased in powdered form and brewed into tea.

What's an effective dose? In the human studies mentioned in Research Findings on pages 23–24, subjects received 100 milligrams of kava extract (containing 70 milligrams of kavalactones) three times a day. Since strengths of the product can vary, you are best advised to follow the manufacturer's package instruction.

Since overuse of kava can have negative side effects (see below), it's important never to exceed the manufacturer's recommended dose.

Tips for use. Though kava is considered safe, it's important to remember that it *is* a plant, and a few people may be allergic to it. To be safe, try a small amount first to make sure you won't have an allergic reaction. It has also been noted that because kava is a member of the pepper family, it can irritate the skin. Taking kava in tablets or capsules can eliminate the risk of irritation to your lips, tongue, or oral tissues.

Are there side effects? For short-term use in small recommended doses, kava does not appear to produce side effects in most people. Remember, however, that a few people *are* allergic to kava and may have a reaction to even small doses. Also, adverse reactions have been noted in people who take kava with other drugs that work on the central nervous system.

Finally, kava does produce significant and harmful side effects in heavy users. A 1988 study found that people who routinely used more than 310 grams (3,100 milligrams) of kava a week were likely to suffer from a scaly rash and more likely to complain of overall poor health than occasional users. At greatest risk were people who habitually used more than 440 (4,400 milligrams) grams weekly. These people were underweight, showed imbalances in their blood and urine, had abnormal heart rhythms, and suffered from shortness of breath.

Bottom line: Used when needed in moderate doses, kava can be a true friend. Used in heavy doses as a way of life, it can be truly hazardous to one's health.

Caution! According to Germany's Commission E, kava should not be used with alcohol, barbiturates, antidepressants, anti-anxiety agents, or any other substances that act on the central nervous system. You should also avoid kava if you are pregnant or nursing. While kava is not addicting, numerous instances of kava abuse have been noted among peoples of the South Pacific. Therefore, only take kava when you need it.

CHAMOMILE

WHAT IS CHAMOMILE?

Chamomile (also spelled *camomile*) is a plant whose dried flowers have long been used in herbal medicine. There are actually two species of chamomile used by herbalists: German (also known as Hungarian) and Roman (also known as English). The German type is more common in continental Europe and is used almost exclusively in the United States, while the Roman type is more common in Great Britain. Although the two types are not chemically identical, they are similar and are used for similar purposes.

THE MIRACLE EFFECT

If chamomile appeared as a new substance today, it would undoubtedly create a buzz in the scientific community and become the subject of any number of research studies. The fact is, chamomile has been used throughout the Western world for so long that its effectiveness is no longer in great dispute. For this reason, little research has been done to establish *why* chamomile works so well at soothing nervous anxiety.

Animal studies suggest a double action. Orally administered chamomile oil has been shown to lower blood pressure and slow the pulse and breathing rates in dogs and cats. Chamomile also contains flavonoids, which have been shown to have an antispasmodic effect, especially on the tissues of the gastrointestinal tract.

HAS CHAMOMILE BEEN USED BEFORE?

Chamomile has been used for centuries, and has been especially venerated in Europe, where it achieved status as an all-purpose medicinal. The great Irish poet Thomas Moore even sang its praises in a poem, suggesting that physicians should wear wreaths of chamomile. Chamomile is still popular throughout the world. In 1986 alone, the world consumed more than four thousand tons of chamomile!

RESEARCH FINDINGS

Most contemporary research on chamomile focuses on newly discovered benefits, such as its healing properties. However, human studies documenting chamomile's soothing and sedating qualities have been done. One study, in which patients undergoing a cardiac procedure were given oral doses of chamomile extract, suggests that chamomile may even be an effective sleep-inducer!

OTHER WAYS CHAMOMILE CAN HELP

The ability of chamomile to stop spasms in the gastrointestinal tract makes it ideal as a remedy for nervous indigestion, upset stomach, and even nausea. Studies show that chamomile also has a healing effect when applied to skin wounds, abrasions, and infections. This, along with its antispasmodic effect, may explain why chamomile has traditionally been used for gastric ulcers.

HOW TO TAKE CHAMOMILE

What form does it come in? Chamomile comes in a variety of forms, including concentrated oil, dried flowers, and tea. Of these, tea is the most common form, especially in the United States.

What's an effective dose? A cup of brewed tea should help lower your anxiety level and is safe to take before bedtime. If you take chamomile in a different form, follow the manufacturer's packaged directions regarding dosage.

Tips for use. Varo Tyler, one of America's leading authorities on phytomedicines, delivers an important warning to consumers who want to try chamomile in oil form. Because this highly concentrated product is expensive, some untrustworthy manufacturers adulterate the product. In fact, a German study done in 1987 found that 75 percent of products on the market contained adulterations or synthetic additives. Therefore, make sure you purchase standardized products from reputable manufacturers who have a real interest in providing quality products to consumers.

Are there side effects? For most people, chamomile is extremely safe. Chamomile is not considered toxic or habit forming and does not produce side effects when taken in moderate amounts. However, some people have reported allergic reactions.

Caution! In researching this book, we found many sources that insisted that allergic reactions to chamomile were "rare"—and just as many sources that said allergic reactions were "common." The controversy may be due to the fact that chamomile comes in different preparations and strengths and use of a more concentrated product may trigger allergic reactions in some people. Also, as mentioned above, users of chamomile oil may unwittingly be using a product containing synthetic adulterations, and it may be these substances that are the cause of the problem.

That said, even mild doses of chamomile seem to trigger an allergic response in some people. This isn't too surprising as the part of the plant that is most useful—the flower—contains pollen as well as petals. Moreover, chamomile belongs to the same family as ragweed, asters, and chrysanthemums. If you are allergic to any of these, you may be allergic to chamomile as well, and you should avoid using *all* forms of this miracle herb. If you aren't sure whether you're allergic or not, try a cup of weak chamomile tea, or dab a bit on a small area of skin to check your reaction.

Excessive use of chamomile should also be avoided by pregnant and lactating women, as animal studies have suggested that there is some risk to the health of the fetus.

WHAT ELSE CAN YOU DO?

Even miracle workers, like kava and chamomile, can't make anxiety go away if other factors in your life are out of balance. To make sure you get all the calm that's coming to you, ask yourself these simple but important questions.

ARE YOU GETTING ENOUGH SLEEP?

Nothing can fray nerves like being short on sleep. In fact, chronic and severe sleep deprivation can even bring about temporary psychosis. If you don't have enough time to sleep, try to make time. It's more important to be rested and calm than tired and too keyed up to work efficiently.

ARE YOU GETTING PROPER NUTRITION?

Notice that we didn't ask "Are you eating enough?" Most people do eat enough, but it's possible to overeat and still not get the food you really need. If you're anxiety-ridden, it's worthwhile to jot down what you're taking in each day and see whether or not your diet meets the minimum daily requirements for vitamins, minerals, and other nutrients.

If you're dieting to lose weight, do it gradually. Drastic measures—such as eliminating *all* fat for long periods of time—can result in anxiety, anger, and agitation. Remember, too, that drugs, caffeine, alcohol, and tobacco also affect mood, both temporarily and over extended periods of time.

CHAPTER TWO

Get Relief From Painful
Arthritis

What's the remedy of choice for the most common form of arthritis? If you answered "aspirin," you're wrong. Today's first lines of defense are natural nutrients—substances that ease the pain by taking aim at the disease process itself!

What can you do about arthritis? Until recently, the answer was "not much." If you had arthritis, the most you could hope for was alleviating some of your pain with analgesics and, when things got bad enough, surgery. Today the picture is different. For the first time, there's real hope of doing more than just treating the pain.

Studies done over the past few decades suggest that damage done by the two most common forms of arthritis, osteoarthritis and rheumatoid arthritis, may well be reversible. The good news is that the miracle workers aren't drugs with harmful side effects but natural nutrients—nutrients that are safe, readily available, and inexpensive to use.

THE PROBLEM

Each joint in your body comes equipped with its own set of shock absorbers. In a healthy joint the ends of the bones are capped with cartilage—a cushion of smooth, white, resilient, extremely tough material that prevents the bones from grinding against each other. Another shock absorber is the moist, flexible, sinewy connective tissue that holds the joint together. Synovial fluid, which resembles raw egg white, lubricates the joint and provides additional cushioning. Arthritis occurs when these natural shock absorbers deteriorate or become inflamed, causing pain and swelling and preventing the joint from working properly.

There are actually numerous forms of arthritis. By far the most common form is *osteoarthritis,* also known as DJD, short for Degenerative Joint Disease. Osteoarthritis affects over sixteen million people in America alone and is especially common among people over the age of fifty-five. You've probably also heard of *rheumatoid arthritis,* the second most common form of this condition. If you have either of these two common forms of arthritis, the answer to your problems might lie in this chapter.

WHO GETS ARTHRITIS?

Even osteoarthritis, one of the most common diseases known to man, doesn't affect everyone. Nor is there a simple test to determine who will and who won't be affected. Like many diseases, it doesn't come down to one gene or one lifestyle choice but to a combination of culprits that tip the scales one way or another. If you're concerned about arthritis, here are some factors to be aware of:

- **Age.** In the case of osteoarthritis, the older you are, the more likely you are to develop the problem. Whereas osteoarthritis is increasingly more common *past* midlife, rheumatoid arthritis generally shows up *before* midlife.
- **Being a woman.** Most forms of this disease—including osteoarthritis and rheumatoid arthritis—are far more common in women than men.
- **Heredity.** If your parents, grandparents, or siblings developed arthritis, you have an increased chance of developing arthritis yourself.
- **Overweight.** Being overweight is considered a risk factor for osteoarthritis. The theory is that added weight increases stress on the joints and makes cartilage and connective tissues less able to adequately replenish themselves.
- **Injury.** If the cartilage and connective tissue in a joint is damaged or injured, it is not able to replenish itself as effectively as before. This may explain why the finger you fractured ten years ago now feels stiff and arthritic, while the other joints in your body are fine.
- **Occupational stress.** People whose jobs make unusual physical demands may be more likely to develop arthritis. This is true for people with jobs that are obviously demanding—such as athletes and dancers—as well as for people whose jobs seem less demanding. The woman who uses her wrist to turn over items on an assembly line, for example, may be fine after her first year of work, but many more years of this simple, repetitive motion may speed the deterioration of the overused wrist joint.

- **High heels.** It has long been noted that twice as many women as men suffer from osteoarthritis of the knee. In 1998 researchers at the Harvard Medical School and the Spaulding Rehabilitation Hospital in Boston published a study suggesting that wearing high heels (defined as 2.5″) may be a strong contributory factor, because they force the joints of the leg—and the knee joint in particular—to compensate for the changed position of the ankle.

WHAT ARE THE SYMPTOMS?

The chief symptom of arthritis is joint discomfort. This can range from occasional stiffness and mild twinges of pain to continual severe pain, swollen joints, and loss of mobility. In addition to the joint pain and stiffness, people with rheumatoid arthritis can experience a number of other symptoms, including fatigue, loss of appetite, low-grade fever, and anemia.

WHAT'S THE OUTLOOK?

The bad news is that arthritis gets worse over time. Unlike an infection the body can fight and overcome, arthritis is a chronic disease that progressively deforms and ultimately destroys joints. The good news is that there are steps you can take that may help you reverse or significantly slow the damage, improving your mobility and putting an end to crippling pain!

WHAT YOU NEED TO KNOW

If you are experiencing pain and stiffness in your joints, you *must* see your doctor for a professional diagnosis. Although arthritis is a common disease, joint discomfort can be caused by a number of other disorders, including—to name just a few—infections, injuries, tumors, and fibrocystic disorders.

Before you can take advantage of the discoveries in this chapter, you also need to determine what type of arthritis you have. This is a necessary step in determining which specific nutrients will be helpful to you—nutrients that work for osteoarthritis aren't useful for rheumatoid arthritis, and nutrients helpful for rheumatoid patients have no proven effect on people with osteoarthritis.

Finally, only your doctor can tell you how advanced your arthritis may be, and whether or not additional medical treatment is needed. One of the interesting quirks of this disease is that symptoms do not necessarily reflect the intensity of disease itself. While people with mild cases can experience mild and fleeting pain, they can also experience substantial pain, and vice versa.

PROVEN MIRACLES

GLUCOSAMINE AND CHONDROITIN
FOR OSTEOARTHRITIS

WHAT ARE GLUCOSAMINE AND CHONDROITIN?

Glucosamine and chondroitin are not drugs but common natural substances. Not only have you eaten small amounts of them in food, your body produces them on a daily basis. Both play key roles in the health and repair of the body's joints.

Glucosamine, an amino sugar, is a building block that must be present if the body is to replenish the shock-absorbing materials of the joint. One of the substances glucosamine helps make is chondroitin (also referred to as chondroitin sulfate). When cartilage deteriorates, it becomes dry and brittle. Chondroitin is crucial in preventing this fluid loss, helping cartilage stay spongy and maintain its ability to cushion and protect the bones of the joint.

THE MIRACLE EFFECT

What if you could take a pill that didn't just ease the pain of osteoarthritis but stopped the disease itself? Throughout most of human history, this question has been looked on as nothing more than wishful thinking. People with osteoarthritis had to resign themselves to a lifetime of pain-killing medications, limited mobility, and, as a last resort, surgery. Arthritis was thought to be incurable, as inevitable as aging.

For a number of researchers, this outlook just wasn't good enough—they wanted to stop the crippling process of osteoarthritis itself. In 1956 Dr. Lennart Roden of Sweden's Karolinska Institute, discovered that when glucosamine was added to a laboratory sample of joint tissue, it stimulated production of several joint-nourishing substances, including chondroitin.

Roden's experiment was a breakthrough in osteoarthritis research. For the first time, a way had been found to reverse the ravages of this "incurable" disorder. As Dr. Roden and his colleagues demonstrated, a glucosamine supplement could speed up the body's natural repair process, acting as effectively as glucosamine produced within the body to stimulate the production of the very substances needed to build and maintain vital cartilage and connective tissues.

Building on Roden's strategy, later researchers experimented with other nutrients vital to joint health. They discovered that chondroitin, when taken as a supplement, also showed amazing results. Whereas glucosamine works by accelerating the repair process, chondroitin works by *slowing down* the damage. By blocking the action of nutrient-robbing enzymes, it retards the breakdown of cartilage and keeps tissue moist and well nourished.

Studies show that both glucosamine and chondroitin can be beneficial on their own. However, as Dr. Jason Theodosakis has pointed out in his book, *The Arthritis Cure,* glucosamine and chondroitin have a synergistic effect when taken together. In combined form, these two substances produce an effect that is greater than the sum of both parts.

HAVE GLUCOSAMINE AND CHONDROITIN
BEEN USED BEFORE?

Although both of these nutrients are present in foods, they occur in such small amounts that man could not access them in substantial amounts until modern lab techniques came into practice. Now that glucosamine and chondroitin are widely available, they are widely used. First in Europe and now, belatedly, in America, millions of people are using them to safely reverse the effects of osteoarthritis. Doctors have recommended them to hundreds of patients. Writing in the October 1997 issue of the *International Journal of Alternative and Complementary Medicine,* London-based physician Dr. John Briffa concluded that, "It is clear that glucosamine sulfate represents the agent of choice in the treatment of osteoarthritis."

RESEARCH FINDINGS

How did Dr. Roden know that glucosamine would work as well on real people as it did on tissue in a petri dish? He didn't, but other researchers soon took up the challenge. In 1980 an Italian pharmaceutical company sponsored a series of studies to determine whether or not glucosamine would help patients with osteoarthritis. The results were more than promising—they were overwhelming. Of an estimated 2,500 people who received a daily oral dose of 1,500 milligrams of glucosamine supplement, more than 80 percent reported less pain and improved joint mobility after four to six weeks. In other words this ordinary and unremarkable little substance helped four out of every five people who tried it—a far higher rating than over-the-counter pain relievers, and without any of the unpleasant side effects.

OTHER WAYS GLUCOSAMINE AND CHONDROITIN CAN HELP

Can glucosamine and chondroitin help with health problems other than arthritis? It's very possible. Nearly thirty years ago, a sample of forty-six patients with constricted blood vessels was given chondroitin sulfate as a supplement. Testing showed that chondroitin lowered cholesterol and triglyceride levels in these people and further helped by reducing the blood's tendency to clot inside the vessels. To date, this promising research has not been followed up on.

More recently it's been suggested that glucosamine, taken the first few days after injury or surgery, may promote healing. The theory behind this is that higher levels of glucosamine may increase production of hyaluronic acid, which promotes healing and reduces scarring.

HOW TO TAKE GLUCOSAMINE AND CHONDROITIN

What form does it come in? Both glucosamine and chondroitin are effective taken orally, and you should be able to find them in combined form without too much trouble.

People are sometimes confused by the fact that more than one type of glucosamine is sold. Although the original studies were done on glucosamine sulfate, other types of glucosamine have since been found effective, including glucosamine hydrochloride and N-acetyl-D-glucosamine.

What's an effective dose? In one study patients began with a dosage of 400 milligrams of glucosamine sulfate three times a day for seven days, then increased to a dosage of 500 milligrams. In other studies patients started at 500 milligrams three times a day. Patients in both studies benefited, and neither group reported side effects.

It's important to remember that there are several different formulations of glucosamine. For example, glucosamine sulfate is not quite the same as glucosamine hydrochloride, and some formulations are combined with chondroitin or other nutrients. Because of this, you should follow the manufacturer's label instructions, rather than prescribe your own dosage level.

Tips for use. Because it's important to provide your body with a steady, reliable supply of this nutrient, take glucosamine according to manufacturer's directions, and try to stay on schedule.

Remember that glucosamine and chondroitin are not analgesics and do not provide instant relief. They work by helping the joint maintain and repair itself, and these kinds of results take time. Don't give up if you don't feel better in a few days or even in a few weeks. Studies showed that many people who had seen little change after the first few weeks reported dramatic improvements at the six-to-eight-week mark.

Are there side effects? No significant side effects have been associated with either of these nutrients. Studies show that glucosamine is gentler on the stomach than most analgesics, including ibuprofen. Where stomach upsets did occur, they were more likely to be caused by preexisting stomach disorders or by other medications, such as diuretics. However, as with any preparations (even natural ones), it's important to consult your doctor before going ahead.

Caution! Although glucosamine and chondroitin are both regarded as safe, it's important to remember that glucosamine is a form of glucose, or sugar. If you are diabetic, do not consider taking this without your doctor's knowledge and advice.

Another factor to take into consideration is salt. If you have high blood pressure or are watching your sodium intake for other reasons, taking 500 milligrams of glucosamine sulfate three times a day can add from 375 to 450 or more milligrams of sodium to your daily intake. For these reasons, you might want to consider taking a different form of this nutrient.

OMEGA-3
FOR RHEUMATOID ARTHRITIS

WHAT IS OMEGA-3 OIL?

Omega-3 oil is one of several essential fatty acids (EFAs) needed by the body to do its work. Since the body cannot make its own EFAs, the only way to get them is through the foods you eat or through dietary supplements.

Omega-3 oils contain one or more types of omega-3 fatty acids. EPA (short for eicosapentaenoic acid) is an important omega-3 fatty acid and is common in most fish oil supplements. DHA (docosahexaenoic acid) usually occurs with EPA and has a similar effect on the body. The best sources of EPA are high-fat cold water fish, such as salmon. The diet eaten by the average American, high in red meats and low in fish, leaves most people undersupplied with this essential nutrient.

THE MIRACLE EFFECT

You've probably already heard of omega-3 oil as a wonder-worker for lowering cholesterol and reducing the risk of heart attack. Claims you've heard on that score are true. Omega-3 *is* an amazing heart helper. But did you know omega-3 also has a natural anti-inflammatory effect? If you suffer from rheumatoid arthritis, the form of arthritis that leaves membranes and tissues in the joints continually inflamed, omega-3 may be your best over-the-counter friend.

Double-blind, placebo-controlled studies have consistently shown that patients who receive omega-3 oil supplements experience an improvement in joint pain, tenderness, and stiffness while patients who receive a placebo do not. In at least one study, people were even able to stop taking anti-inflammatory pain relievers without experiencing a recurrence of pain!

How is this miracle substance helping people find relief? Researchers have demonstrated that omega-3 oil reduces levels of leukotrienes and other substances found in body tissues. Although these substances are natural, they have an inflammatory effect, and may be overabundant in people with rheumatoid arthritis.

HAS OMEGA-3 OIL BEEN USED BEFORE?

Many people think omega-3 is a new discovery. Actually, what's "new" is our discovery that we aren't getting enough of it. Humans evolved on a diet that was much higher in omega-3 than today's modern diet, and medical researchers have suggested that a lack of omega-3 plays a role in rheumatoid arthritis and several other diseases.

The concept of fish oil as a health protector goes way back. You may remember old movies and books in which children revolted against doses of cod liver oil. The link goes back even farther, as researcher and consultant to the National Marine Fisheries Services in Seattle, Maurice Stansby, recently discovered. While sifting through documents from a hospital in Manchester, England, he found that doctors of the late 1700s routinely prescribed cod liver oil for patients with arthritic joints.

RESEARCH FINDINGS

Omega-3's healing effect on rheumatoid arthritis has too often been overlooked. Studies done on patients with the disease lay buried in journals, and the press has focused instead on the astounding benefits this substance has on the heart and circulatory system.

In 1995 a group of researchers decided to review the evidence to see if omega-3 really did have an effect on rheumatoid arthritis. Their standards were demanding. To be included in the review, studies had to meet several qualifications. They had to be done on actual patients with rheumatoid arthritis and they had to use standardized evaluative procedures. Most important, they had to be double-blind and placebo-controlled—in other words, some patients had to receive real treatment while others received a harmless substitute, and both patients and administrators were kept in the dark throughout the study. Ten studies were found that met these tough standards and when the analysis was complete, the results were startling. In each study, patients who received omega-3 oil reported a significant improvement of their symptoms, while those receiving an ineffective placebo did not.

Close review of individual studies yields another amazing fact: If you have rheumatoid arthritis, you may be able to substantially reduce—and in some cases eliminate—the amount of analgesics you take.

OTHER WAYS OMEGA-3 CAN HELP

Omega-3 is a truly amazing nutrient that has an astounding ability to fight disease on several fronts at once. It's been estimated that more than two thousand studies have been done on this nutrient, yielding a treasure trove of findings. Among other things, studies have shown that omega-3 can cut heart attack risk, discourage arterial clotting, regulate blood pressure, and lower cholesterol (see chapter 7, pages 138–140).

HOW TO TAKE OMEGA-3

What forms does it come in? Capsules containing omega-3 oil are readily available, and for reasons of taste, most people prefer them to taking oil by the spoonful. Some people think fish oils are the only way to get omega-3. This isn't the case. Fish oils are the richest source of omega-3, but certain types of vegetable oils also contain omega-3 factors. These include flaxseed oil, canola oil, and walnut oil.

If you decide to try a fish oil supplement, beware of cod liver oil. Although cod liver oil is a good source of omega-3, it is also rich in vitamins A and D, and you cannot fulfill your need for omega-3 without overdosing on these two vitamins. Oil from salmon, mackerel, and other cold water fish is a better choice. In addition to preparations that are free of vitamins A and D, you should also look for products that have no cholesterol and no cetoleic acid, which can damage the heart muscle.

What's an effective dose? No recommended dosage has been established for this nutrient. Some have suggested that fish oils should account for one-sixth of our total fat intake.

In one of the studies conducted by Dr. Kremer and colleagues, people with rheumatoid arthritis received a dose of 130 milligrams per kilogram (2.2 pounds) of body weight per day. This is a large dose—over 9,000 milligrams daily for a 160-pound man—and could be hazardous to health. Moreover, massive doses don't appear to be necessary. According to Dr. Kremer, much smaller doses of 2,500 to 5,000 milligrams a day, given in previous studies, were equally effective.

As with any nutrient, be sure to read labels carefully to see exactly what you're getting. As we mentioned above, cod liver oil, a potential source of omega-3, has levels of vitamins A and D that make it inappropriate for use as an arthritis-fighter.

Tips for use. If you have rheumatoid arthritis and are currently on medication, *do not stop*. Studies with patients already under medical treatment showed positive results when omega-3 was added as a supplement. No study we looked at recommended switching to omega-3 as a *replacement*. Only after patients felt an improvement did doctors work closely with them to taper their medication. Under no circumstances should you reduce medication without your doctor's approval.

If you want to try an omega-3 supplement, be prepared to stick with it. All of the studies we looked at were long-term, lasting from three to six months. This suggests that omega-3 is most useful as an ongoing daily supplement.

Are there side effects? When taken in moderate amounts, there are no significant side effects associated with omega-3.

Caution! If a little omega-3 helps a little, will more help a lot? No! Too much of this wonderful nutrient can do more harm than good. Omega-3 is a good natural blood thinner, but too much can lead to anemia or excessive bleeding from a wound. If you already have blood clotting problems, you should not take this nutrient. As we mentioned above, you should also avoid formulations that contain vitamins A and D, cholesterol, and cetoleic acid.

CAPSAICIN CREAM
FOR RHEUMATOID AND OSTEOARTHRITIS

WHAT IS CAPSAICIN?

Capsaicin is the active ingredient in cayenne, the powder derived from dried red chili peppers.

THE MIRACLE EFFECT

Numerous studies done over the years have confirmed that creams and rubs prepared from cayenne can cut pain and boost joint flexibility in people with arthritis. The reason why seemed fairly obvious. If you've ever tasted very hot salsa, you're probably familiar with the burning and tingling sensation produced by pepper products. You may even have felt slightly flushed or fevered, the result of cayenne's ability to dilate blood vessels.

Researchers assumed that capsaicin cream worked the same way. When the ointment was rubbed into the skin over the joint, blood vessels dilated, increasing the flow of blood and stepping up the supply of nutrients to the affected joint. However, new research shows that capsaicin acts in a more complex way. Not only does it help pain, it can retard the degenerative process itself! People with osteoarthritis have elevated levels of something called *decapeptide substance P* (DSP for short) in their blood and in the fluid in their joints. Increased DSP causes joints to deteriorate faster than usual and causes people to feel pain more acutely. Researchers have found that capsaicin works by retarding the action of DSP. When capsaicin ointment is massaged into the skin, it penetrates to the joint below where it slows the destruction and buffers the pain signal.

HAS CAPSAICIN BEEN USED BEFORE?

Although the active ingredient, capsaicin, has only been identified in this century, the medicinal use of hot chili peppers stretches back over centuries. There are references to chili peppers not only in western folkloric medicine but in the traditional medicines of Asia and India. In addition to being used as a pain relieving salve, chili pepper preparations have also been used orally, usually as a tonic or fever-breaker.

Capsaicin is proving extremely popular with present-day users. For example, according to a study published in the *Journal of Physical Medicine & Rehabilitation* in 1995, 75 percent of twenty-two chronic neck-pain patients who completed a five-week study at Walter Reed Army Medical Center in Washington, D.C., said they would choose to use the cream for future bouts of pain.

RESEARCH FINDINGS

Over the past decade, more than one thousand scientific studies of capsaicin have been published in various medical journals around the world. In 1994 Dr. Roy Altman of the University of Miami Medical School conducted a well-constructed study of ninety-six patients with arthritic knees. In addition to asking patients whether or not they felt an improvement, Dr. Altman and his colleagues actually measured patients' physical movements. At the end of the twelve-week study, 81 percent of patients had less pain, less stiffness in the morning, and greater flexibility in their knees.

A shorter study, which evaluated patients after just four weeks of use, found that a smaller but still significant number—26 percent—improved in this relatively short time.

HOW TO USE CAPSAICIN

What forms does it come in? Capsaicin comes in a cream, ointment, or salve that can be rubbed into the skin. If you want to try one of these products, note that some manufacturers use the name "hot pepper" instead of capsaicin.

What's an effective dose? Since capsaicin cream comes in different potencies, be sure to read the product label before you buy. The two most common strengths are .025 percent and .075 percent. Dr. Deal, of the Case Western Reserve University School of Medicine, strongly recommends starting with the .025 percent preparation and trying the more concentrated cream *only* if the first proves ineffective. In all probability, the lower-strength cream will work for you—patients in all of the studies cited in this chapter improved on the .025 percent preparation.

How often you use the cream is probably more important than the strength. In some studies, patients applied the cream four times a day, in others only twice. Although patients in the second group benefited, those who used the cream more often saw faster and more dramatic results.

Tips for use. To use capsaicin cream effectively, only a small amount is necessary—a dab the size of a pea is enough for an entire knee joint. Dot small amounts in a circle around the joint, then take time to massage the cream in until none is left on the skin's surface. Although some people feel relief in a few days, many others don't see results until a few weeks have passed, so be patient.

Are there side effects? Many people reported a burning or tingling sensation during the first few weeks of use, but most said this side effect diminished over time and was not a significant problem.

Caution! Some people can have an adverse skin reaction to capsaicin. If at any time your skin becomes red and irritated, you should discontinue use immediately.

WHAT ELSE CAN YOU DO?

Do you think you've tried everything for your pain and stiffness? Not likely. Ongoing research suggests a number of strategies to try.

THE POWER OF PANTOTHENIC ACID

It has long been noted that people with rheumatoid arthritis have significantly lower blood levels of pantothenic acid (vitamin B5) than people who don't suffer from the disease. In an experiment, researchers injected twenty rheumatoid arthritis patients with 50 milligrams of calcium pantothenate daily, enough to bring blood levels up to normal. Patients reported relief from many of their symptoms, but those symptoms returned when the injections were stopped.

This intriguing lead lay dormant until 1980, when the U.S. General Practitioner Research Group conducted a study of orally administered calcium pantothenate. Patients began on a dosage of 500 milligrams of pantothenate once a day, and by day ten were taking 500 milligrams four times a day. These patients reported an improvement in pain and stiffness, while patients who received a placebo reported no change. Promising though this study is, follow-up studies are needed to determine the long-term safety and effectiveness of use.

THE "C" CONNECTION

Studies have shown that people who suffer from arthritis, asthma, and a number of other diseases have lower blood levels of vitamin C than healthy people. Based on this finding, researchers theorized that people suffering from these disorders might benefit from large doses of supplemental vitamin C (1,000 to 2,000 milligrams daily), which may relieve the symptoms of arthritis. Support for the idea comes from a long-term tracking study conducted by the Boston University Arthritis Center. Patients with osteoarthritis of the knee were first examined in 1983–85, then again in 1992–93. Researchers found that what the patients ate had a dramatic effect on their disease. Compared to those who consumed low levels of vitamin C, those with high vitamin C intake were three times less likely to show disease progression or experience knee pain.

"E" CAN BE EFFECTIVE

The Boston University study mentioned above also found that people who consumed more vitamin E in their diets experienced less pain and slower disease progression. This backs up studies done by German researchers, who found that patients taking 400 IUs (International Units) of vitamin E a day had less pain and used fewer analgesics than people who didn't take supplemental vitamin E. Another study, published in November 1997, confirmed the pain-killing effect of vitamin E. Of thirty-nine patients with rheumatoid arthritis, 60 percent reported a marked decrease in pain while taking vitamin E supplement daily. When they stopped taking the vitamin, pain increased, leading researchers to conclude that vitamin E plays a central role in reducing pain in arthritis patients.

THE PROMISE OF GINGER

In 1989 a provocative study appeared suggesting that ginger may offer significant benefits to people with rheumatoid arthritis. In the study, as little as 100 to 1,000 milligrams of powdered ginger daily improved mobility while reducing joint pain. Unfortunately, much research remains to be done in this area. One potential problem may be that medications for rheumatoid patients often include a blood thinner, and ginger—which also inhibits clotting—may be incompatible with this. For more about ginger, see chapter 11, pages 199–202.

QUERCETIN: A RECENT DISCOVERY

In September 1997, researchers at Japan's Nagoya University published results of a lab study that could have far-reaching consequences for people with rheumatoid arthritis. They treated human cells from the synovial fluid that lubricates the joints with quercetin, a natural substance with strong anti-inflammatory capabilities. Researchers then exposed these cells to substances known to promote inflammation. The presence of quercetin significantly reduced inflammation in the cells, suggesting that quercetin supplement may be extremely helpful to people with rheumatoid arthritis. Although querciten has been established as safe and effective for other uses, studies need to be done on this promising front.

CUT DOWN ON OMEGA-6 OILS

Earlier in this chapter, you read about the miraculous effect omega-3 oils can have on rheumatoid arthritis. Some researchers contend that another type of essential fatty acid—omega-6—can have a negative effect on people with rheumatoid arthritis, if eaten in large proportions.

Researchers at the Royal Adelaide Hospital in Australia argue that humans evolved on a diet whose ratio of omega-6 to omega-3 essential fatty acids was approximately 2:1. The modern diet is drastically out of proportion compared to this. Not only do we consume low amounts of foods rich in omega-3, we consume vast quantities of foods high in omega-6 nutrients. Instead of a balance of 2:1, the modern diet is a decidedly *un*balanced 25:1. Since omega-6 fatty acids promote inflammation, ridding the diet of excess sources of omega-6 may improve the outlook for rheumatoid arthritis sufferers. Avoid foods rich in omega-6 essential fatty acids, such as:

- Raw nuts
- Seeds
- Legumes
- Oils such as corn oil, safflower oil, cottonseed oil, sunflower oil, sesame oil, soybean oil, borage seed oil, grape seed oil, and primrose oil.

Instead of using oils high in omega-6, enjoy oils high in omega-3 essential fatty acids, such as canola, flaxseed, and walnut oils.

WATCH FOR MORE NEWS ON STINGING NETTLE

At least two studies have found evidence that taking extract of stinging nettle leaf boosts the effectiveness of anti-inflammatory drugs. For patients this means more relief with less medication. Researchers are not yet ready to recommend this as a course of treatment, but say results to date are promising. In addition, they have called for further research to investigate whether stinging nettle alone might provide relief.

LIFT WEIGHTS

It isn't a nutrient, but weight training for arthritis was named by the medical journal *Hippocrates* as one of the top ten medical advances of 1996. According to Ronenn Roubenoff, a rheumatologist at Tufts University, lifting weights can help even those with severe rheumatoid arthritis. In a study published in March 1996, Roubenoff and his colleagues reported that a modest weight training program diminished pain, improved mobility, and helped people increase their strength by as much as 60 percent.

CHAPTER THREE

Reduce Your Susceptibility to
Asthma and Allergies

Asthma and allergies are on the rise, but these nutrients can put a dent in the trend.

Allergies used to be a spring discomfort, just as asthma used to be uncommon. No longer. Allergies have become a year-round phenomenon, and people who never had so much as a tickle in their throats are becoming first-time allergy sufferers. The picture is even more alarming when it comes to asthma, and pediatricians are especially concerned about increases among children.

If you've ever put up with itchy, watery eyes or a runny nose, or if you or someone you know experiences frightening bouts of asthma, you're not as helpless as you may think. Researchers are finding that a simple, natural nutrient may help people with both these conditions.

THE PROBLEM

Allergies and asthma aren't the same disease. However, there is a strong link, not only in symptoms and remedies, but in the fact that people with asthma often suffer from allergies. Asthma, in fact, is one of the ways that allergies (food allergies as well as allergies to airborne substances) make themselves known. However, it's important to remember that not all people who have asthma have allergies.

The big difference between asthma and most allergies is severity. While a few allergies (such as to bee stings) are serious enough to require a trip to the emergency room, most allergies are merely uncomfortable and annoying. Asthma, on the other hand, is a serious chronic disorder, and can be life-threatening.

WHO SUFFERS FROM ALLERGIES
AND ASTHMA?

Allergies and asthma have always been with us, and some people are burdened with sensitivities that cause these conditions. However, that doesn't explain why the number of people who suffer from these conditions has risen dramatically over the past few decades, especially in industrialized countries.

Causes ranging from physical to lifestyle to psychological have been proposed. A leading theory, which has some scientific support, is that certain people who profess to have the allergy-of-the-moment aren't truly allergic but are unconsciously expressing feelings of stress, anxiety, fear, or depression. This explanation doesn't account for the very many people whose symptoms can be authenticated or the fact that asthma is especially on the rise among children, who are generally unaware of trend-setting ailments.

In attempting to understand why these breathing problems are on the rise, investigators have focused on two major areas of risk: the air we take into our lungs and the food we take into our bodies.

Environment

It's hard to look at a city overhung with smog and not feel your lungs begin to close up—for good reason. Each day our lungs and airways take in thousands of substances nature never intended them to. From easy-to-see cigarette smoke and air pollutants to invisible particles from fabrics, upholstery, aerosol sprays, and other modern inventions, our respiratory systems are stressed and challenged.

Despite the bad publicity pollution gets, the most common allergens are natural ones. Heading the list are dust mites (found in even the cleanest homes), microscopic molds (also found in clean environments), pollen (which has increased as we've planted gardens and lawns coast to coast and cultivated other previously fallow areas), and pet dander. When you add up the natural and synthetic, and realize that the modern world presents people with tens of thousands of diverse substances each and every day, it's no wonder that we're finding more to react to.

Diet

Obviously, some people are allergic to some of the foods they eat—or, as is often the case, the *additives* in the foods they eat. Sulfites (used to keep fresh fruits from discoloring) are common causes of asthma attacks. It's also a well-documented fact that people with asthma and hay fever are far more likely to have food sensitivities than others.

But diet seems to have a far greater impact. Over the past years, a research trail has been steadily growing. When it comes to food, what you *don't* eat might be as important as what you do eat. As early as 1985, doctors began to notice that children with asthma had lower levels of vitamin C in their blood than children without asthma. Numerous studies have supported this finding, not only among children but in adults as well. Low blood levels of vitamin E have also been noted in asthmatic adults.

In a 1996 report, British researchers Soutar, Seaton, and Brown suggested that it might not be industrialization but the modern, industrialized diet that fosters asthma and allergies. In particular, they wondered whether a twenty-five-year decrease in intake of certain dietary vitamins and minerals correlated with a rise in asthma and allergies. Their findings? Those who had the lowest intake of vitamin C and manganese were more than five times as likely to have allergies or asthma.

WHAT ARE THE SYMPTOMS?

The most common symptoms of allergies are:
- Runny nose (fluid is clear—opaque yellow or greenish fluid indicates a cold or sinus infection)
- Stuffiness
- Sneezing
- Itchy nose and/or eyes
- Watery, runny, or gummy eyes

- Asthma (see below)
- Temporary skin blotches, bumps, or rashes

Unlike allergic reactions, an asthma attack doesn't involve the nose or eyes, although morning coughing is a common symptom. Asthma is a disease of the airways in the lungs, which become inflamed and irritated. During an attack, the muscles around the bronchial tubes contract and narrow, causing asthma's chief symptoms:

- Wheezing
- Gasping
- Difficulty taking in or breathing out enough air
- Rapid and shallow breathing

WHAT'S THE OUTLOOK?

Both asthma and allergies are chronic conditions. Unlike viruses and other illnesses, they don't clear up and go away on their own. Moreover, these conditions don't necessarily show up in childhood. As an adult, you can develop either one of these conditions seemingly out of the blue. Although asthma is on the rise among children, adult-onset asthma is also increasing. As for allergies, as illogical as it seems it *is* possible to develop an allergy to something you were not previously sensitive to.

WHAT YOU NEED TO KNOW

Asthma is a serious, life-threatening condition that requires medical attention. None of the research findings in this chapter should be considered as an alternative to medical treatment, but as an addition to it. As always, keep your doctor informed, and don't make any changes without his or her approval.

PROVEN MIRACLES

VITAMIN C

WHAT IS VITAMIN C?

Humans are one of the few species that must consume a steady supply of vitamin C to remain healthy. We cannot manufacture this essential nutrient, nor can we store it. Dietary sources of vitamin C are fresh fruits and vegetables, but as Soutar and colleagues pointed out, the modern diet no longer assures an abundant supply of C, and low levels of this and other vitamins seems to be a risk factor for asthma and allergies.

THE MIRACLE EFFECT

Vitamin C has a two-fold implication for asthma and allergy sufferers. First, low intake of vitamin C has been identified as a risk factor for bronchial sensitivity. Beyond that, taking extra C offers a definite protective benefit. One thousand milligrams of vitamin C each day produces an antihistamine effect, and a review of several studies shows that it especially helps to:

- Improve overall lung functioning.
- Decrease bronchial and airway sensitivity to histamines, smog, cold, pollen, hay, and other irritants.
- Decrease chances of an asthma attack triggered by exercise.

Part of vitamin C's amazing ability lies in its activity as an antioxidant. Exposure to environmental oxidants (which promote the formation of free radicals) is one cause of asthma. Oxidants are also produced within the body. Some people's bodies produce so many oxidants that an asthma attack is triggered.

Not only is vitamin C a powerful antioxidant, it is the *key* antioxidant as far as the lung is concerned. According to experts, it protects the airways by neutralizing both the inhaled oxidants and those produced within the body.

Vitamin C may work in another way as well. Even when asthma sufferers aren't experiencing an attack, their condition is affecting them. People with this condition have chronic lung inflammation. The membranes that line the walls of the airways become swollen and produce excess mucus. Excess mucus forces the lungs to work harder and may reduce their ability to exchange carbon dioxide for fresh air. Since vitamin C plays a key role in tissue replacement and repair throughout the body, it may facilitate healing here as well, and reduce the inflammation that ultimately triggers an attack.

HAS VITAMIN C BEEN USED BEFORE?

People have always valued fruits high in vitamin C, and Nobel prize-winner Linus Pauling put this nutrient on the map for good in the 1970s. According to Pauling, if a little C is good, a lot is much, much better. These days, supplemental forms of this vitamin are taken by millions of people, making C one of the world's most popular nutrients.

HARD EVIDENCE

Numerous studies have demonstrated the benefits of vitamin C for asthma and allergy sufferers. Here are just a few of the startling results:

- In an Italian study by Bucca and colleagues, allergy sufferers were divided into two groups and given either a placebo or 2,000 milligrams of vitamin C. They then inhaled allergy-triggering histamines. The study was repeated the next day, this time with the placebo-takers receiving vitamin C. Neither the administrators nor the people in the study knew who received the vitamin on which day until the results were in. The findings were conclusive: Vitamin C had a significant histamine-blocking effect compared to the placebo, which had no effect at all.

- Exercise frequently triggers attacks in asthma sufferers. To assess the possible effect of vitamin C on these people, Cohen and colleagues conducted a study on twenty asthma sufferers ages seven to twenty-eight. Half the group received 2,000 milligrams of vitamin C one hour before exercising on a treadmill for seven minutes, and half received a placebo. A week later, the test was repeated with each person taking the alternative pills. No one involved in the study knew who received the placebo during which session. It was found that, for nine of the twenty people, taking vitamin C before exercise provided significant protection. Four of these people continued to take vitamin C at a reduced dose of 500 milligrams a day and enjoyed the same protective benefits.

• In another study on the protective effects of vitamin C during exercise, Miric and Haxiu measured the airways of asthma sufferers before and after exercise and found that vitamin C prevented the constriction of airways that is the hallmark of an asthma attack.

OTHER WAYS VITAMIN C CAN HELP

If you have asthma or allergies, you may have a supersensitive respiratory system. Does it seem you have far more colds, coughs, and upper respiratory infections than other people do? If so, C can help you on that front as well. It stimulates the immune system and acts as a powerful infection fighter, allowing for quicker recovery from colds and other upper respiratory illnesses (see chapter 8, pages 155–159).

Beyond this, vitamin C plays a key defensive role in the two major killers of our time—heart attack and cancer. Vitamin C cuts the chances of heart attack by promoting health in coronary arteries (see chapter 13, pages 240–246). As a potent antioxidant it blocks the formation of the free radicals that promote cancer, and studies have found that people with high vitamin C intake have lower chances of developing several types of cancer (see chapter 6, pages 105–110).

HOW TO TAKE VITAMIN C

What form does it come in? Vitamin C comes in several forms, but the most common are tablets and chewable tablets.

What's an effective dose? Most of the studies we reviewed relied on daily dosages in the range of 1,000 to 2,000 milligrams. This was especially true for studies that administered vitamin C in a single dose before exercise. When vitamin C is taken on a regular basis the same protective effect was achieved with a dose of just 500 milligrams a day.

Tips for use. Because vitamin C can't be stored by the body and because large doses can cause stomach upset, it's best to divide your daily intake into several smaller doses to take throughout the day, preferably with meals. If you haven't taken this vitamin recently it's advisable to begin with a small dosage and build up over a period of time.

Are there side effects? While vitamin C is considered safe and nontoxic, it can cause stomach irritation and diarrhea. Following Tips for use, above, will help minimize these discomforts.

Caution! Some doctors warn against taking high doses of vitamin C during pregnancy, so be sure to consult your obstetrician if you want to take supplemental doses.

WHAT ELSE CAN YOU DO?

HOW VITAMIN E CAN HELP

Like vitamin C, vitamin E is an important antioxidant and many nutritionally oriented practitioners recommend it for people with asthma and allergies. At least one study has found that vitamin E supplements helped asthma patients by stimulating depressed immune functioning. Another study, by Troisi and colleagues, suggested that dietary vitamin E had a mild protective effect on asthma.

QUERCETIN POWER

Perhaps the best known of the flavonoids (also called bioflavonoids), quercetin is emerging as a new aid for people with allergies. Like all flavonoids, it's a naturally occurring plant pigment and is found in high concentrations in such foods as green tea, tomatoes, apples, and green peppers. Isolated and used as a supplement, studies suggest, it has both an anti-allergin and anti-inflammatory effect. Leading nutritionally oriented physician Robert Atkins, who recommends quercetin to his patients with allergies, suggests 600 to 1,200 milligrams divided in small doses daily on an empty stomach.

MAGNESIUM: TOMORROW'S RESEARCH

Cutting edge research on asthma and bronchial sensitivity is currently focused on magnesium, a common and abundant mineral found in the body. Magnesium is known to influence muscle contraction and relaxation within the lungs. It is also known that people who have asthma attacks often have lower than normal blood levels of magnesium.

In particular, low intake of dietary magnesium has been linked to wheezing, poor lung function, and heightened sensitivity in bronchial tubes. Given by intravenous injection or in the form of an aerosol spray, magnesium suppresses asthma attack or makes symptoms less severe.

If you have asthma or allergies, you want to make sure you're getting at least the recommended daily amount of magnesium.

CHAPTER FOUR

Ward Off
Bladder Infections

Today, doctors are discovering that this painful and all too common disorder may be largely preventable—not with costly antibiotics but with inexpensive everyday nutrients.

Bladder infections, known in the medical field as urinary tract infections (or UTIs for short), aren't considered life threatening—but that doesn't mean they can be ignored.

Once a bladder infection sets in it should be medically treated as soon as possible. If the infection is a common UTI, it will respond quickly to treatment, and pain and discomfort will soon begin to diminish. That's the good news. The bad news is that if you've suffered from a bladder infection once, you're likely to suffer again. Some people are prone to developing this condition while others will go a whole lifetime without a flare-up. If you're unlucky enough to fall into the risk pool, you want to do everything you can to cut down your chances of a repeat performance.

Is there anything you can do? Yes! Researchers have discovered that miracles of nature, not medicine, are our key allies in forestalling that age-old nemesis, the common urinary tract infection.

THE PROBLEM

Common urinary tract infections begin when bacteria enter the urethra, the passage that carries urine away from the bladder for excretion. Although the body is naturally resistant to these bacteria, the defense mechanism can fail for a number of reasons, including individual body chemistry, decreased immune function, and a variety of other problems.

Once the bacteria have entered the urethra from the outside, they multiply and climb the walls of the urethra to the bladder, where they settle in and could start a raging infection. A bladder infection, even a mild one, requires prompt medical attention and treatment with an antibiotic. If the infection is not treated, it may progress to the kidneys and become quite serious.

Although a variety of bacteria can cause UTI infections, the most common culprit by far is Escherichia coli. E. coli, present in the human intestinal tract, is regularly excreted with solid waste products. Even if one has the best hygienic habits in the world, these ever-present bacteria can easily make their way to the opening of the urethra, giving infection an opportunity to begin.

WHO GETS BLADDER INFECTIONS?

Although some people are prone to these infections throughout their lives, others who've never had a problem may find themselves suddenly susceptible. Risk fac-

tors frequently associated with common urinary tract
infections include:

- **Being a woman.** Although men can get urinary
  tract infections, women get them far more often. At
  least part of the explanation lies in anatomy. Not
  only is the opening of the male urethra located farther from the rectum (source of E. coli bacteria), the
  male urethra is much longer than its female coun-
  terpart. The short, straight female urethra poses little challenge to invading bacteria, and its location
  further increases exposure to irritants of all sorts.
- **Using a diaphragm or spermicidal jelly.** Women
  who use diaphragms are more than twice as likely
  to suffer from bladder infections as women who
  don't, probably because diaphragms irritate the vaginal surface, giving bacteria a chance to adhere,
  multiply, and migrate to the urethra. Spermicidal
  jellies can also cause problems, because they interfere with the helpful bacteria that attack infection-
  causing bacteria.
- **Being postmenopausal.** Older women have greater
  rates of recurrent common UTIs than do younger
  women. Doctors believe this is related to changed
  pH levels and the breakdown of the vaginal lining
  that begins after menopause.
- **Suffering from other bladder problems.** Some
  people have medical problems that prevent them
  from completely emptying the bladder during urination. Other people suffer from incontinence and use
  absorbent pads to manage the problem. Both of
  these conditions create ideal opportunities for bacteria to grow.

Attention men! Although urinary tract infections are far less common in men than in women, they can be far more serious when they appear, because they may be linked to an underlying prostate problem.

WHAT ARE THE SYMPTOMS?

To anyone who has ever had a urinary tract infection, the symptoms are unmistakable. They include:

- A burning or stinging sensation during urination.
- A persistent urge to urinate, even though you have just gone to the bathroom.
- Frequent urination that produces only small amounts of urine.
- Change in urine: it may be cloudy, foul smelling, or even tinged with blood.

WHAT'S THE OUTLOOK?

While bladder infections can be treated, the chance of recurrence is great. In some cases the infection recurs almost immediately. This happens because the lining of the bladder, injured during the initial infection, has not completely healed and is susceptible to new waves of bacteria. In other cases, bladder infections are chronic because the underlying conditions that favor them—such as being a woman—are "givens." Fortunately, there is a natural miracle that can help you overcome your natural vulnerabilities. If you've been plagued with bladder infections, you may never have to suffer from their pain or discomfort again!

WHAT YOU NEED TO KNOW

While most urinary tract infections are caused by common bacteria, a few are not. Infections can also be caused by viruses transmitted during sex, and these require a different treatment approach. You should also know that some bladder problems are not due to infections but are caused by other conditions. If you have symptoms and/or discomfort, see your doctor for proper diagnosis and treatment.

PROVEN MIRACLES

CRANBERRY

WHAT IS CRANBERRY?

Cranberries are the fruit of a small evergreen shrub that grows throughout much of the world. It belongs to the same family as the blueberry, which may share some of cranberry's remarkable powers to prevent recurrent bacterial urinary tract infections.

THE MIRACLE EFFECT

If you've suffered from recurrent urinary tract infections, the nutrients in a tart little red berry could keep you from ever suffering again! Cranberry juice has long been thought of as a curative for bladder problems, and many thought it was effective because it caused the urine to be more acidic. That theory was disproved, and only in the last few years has the source of cranberry's real power been discovered.

To understand cranberry's miracle effect, a little background is needed. Scientists have already noted that people with high urinary levels of a natural substance called Tamms-Horsfall glycoprotein have very little risk of developing urinary tract infections. The reason: The glycoprotein attaches to E. coli bacteria and prevents them from sticking to the bladder wall.

The breakthrough in learning came in the late 1980s, when researchers in Ohio, in Israel, and at Utah's Weber State University discovered a substance in cranberry that works just like Tamms-Horsfall glycoprotein. Like the body's own glycoprotein, it attaches to E. coli bacteria and keeps them from clinging to the bladder wall. Instead of lingering to start an infection, they are flushed out with other waste products. In fact, the team of researchers at Tel Aviv University concluded that cranberry juice might well contain not one but "at least two" of these astounding inhibitors.

Although numerous other fruit juices (including grapefruit, orange, and pineapple) have been analyzed for the presence of this compound, it has thus far been found only in the juice of cranberry and its cousin blueberry. As Mark Monane and Jerry Avorn concluded in the August 1994 issue of *Healthline*, "Mom was right when she recommended it for these infections."

HAS CRANBERRY BEEN USED BEFORE?

Cranberry has a revered place in folk medicine and has long been a popular home remedy for relief from urinary tract infections. In fact, cranberry was so popular in nineteenth-century Europe that German scientists began to study its relationship to bladder health more than 150 years ago.

A wave of clinical studies was conducted in America in the 1960s, but when researchers failed to find a clinical reason for cranberry's purported effectiveness, scientific interest waned. The scientific cause behind cranberry's miraculous effect has only recently been unlocked—but millions of proponents didn't need proof from the experts. Their own experience was more than enough to convince them that cranberry works!

RESEARCH FINDINGS

The definitive modern study of cranberry was headed by Drs. Mark Monane and Jerry Avorn of the Harvard Medical School. In the study, 153 elderly women with a history of recurrent common urinary tract infections were divided into two groups. One group was given ten ounces of authentic cranberry juice cocktail each day while the other group drank a similar amount of a beverage that looked and tasted like cranberry juice but was an artificial placebo beverage. The study lasted six months, and neither the women nor those conducting the study knew which group received the placebo beverage. Urine samples showed that bacteria levels in the urine of women who received authentic cranberry declined markedly after the first month and remained low throughout the remainder of the study. During the study, only 15 percent of the women experienced UTIs, compared with 28 percent in the placebo group.

Other findings led researchers to conclude that cranberry not only prevented urinary tract infections but also helped cure mild existing infections.

OTHER WAYS CRANBERRY CAN HELP

Among its other virtues, cranberry is high in vitamin C, which may explain its reputation as an all-round infection fighter. Research suggests it has some effect against yeast activity, though definitive studies have yet to be done in this area.

A particularly exciting study, carried out by researchers at the University of Illinois, evaluated the anti-cancer potential of cranberry, blueberry, and lingonberry. This complex study, which may well become a catalyst for future researchers, concluded that chemical compounds found in cranberry, blueberry, and lingonberry showed strong potential to inhibit the growth and spread of cancerous tumors.

HOW TO TAKE CRANBERRY

What form does it come in? Can you get enough cranberry in its natural form to help? Not by eating the berries; but their juice, as studies have shown, can be effective *if* you are scrupulous about drinking a specified amount every day. Cranberry also comes in dried, powdered form in convenient capsules, available over the counter in your local health food store.

What's an effective dose? At present, there is no established recommended dosage of cranberry. In the landmark study of elderly women done by Monane and Avorn, participants drank ten ounces of cranberry juice cocktail daily.

Dehydrated cranberry in capsule form is far more potent, and should be taken according to the manufacturer's package directions.

Tips for use. If you decide to use cranberry to prevent chronic UTIs, think of it as an ongoing regimen—if you stop taking this miracle nutrient, chances are you'll be right back where you started. If you prefer to get your cranberry boost in a beverage rather than capsules, know what you're buying. Products we surveyed in the grocery store ranged from 100 percent juice right down to 10 percent or less. If you're dieting, remember that pure cranberry is extremely tart, and most beverages contain added sugar. Capsules are not only far more potent but can be taken without adding calories.

Are there side effects? No significant side effects have been reported to date, and cranberry is rated as very safe.

Caution! If you're diabetic, remember that most cranberry beverages contain some form of sweetener. Take cranberry in capsule form or look for artificially sweetened beverages.

WHAT ELSE CAN YOU DO?

If you're prone to bladder and urinary tract infections, here are a few other steps you can take to cut your risk of recurrent infections:

DRINK WATER

Pure, inexpensive, and dynamite when it comes to overall urinary tract health, nothing beats water. The more water that flushes through your system the less chance bacteria have to remain in the body and start an infection.

URINATE FREQUENTLY AND COMPLETELY

Don't put off going to the bathroom until you can't wait another minute. Instead, urinate often, and when you do, take time to empty your bladder completely. Urinating before and after sex also helps flush out bacteria that might otherwise work their way into the urethra.

BE CAREFUL ABOUT VAGINAL PRODUCTS

Diaphragms, spermicidal gels, and other products can irritate the vaginal lining and upset its natural pH balance. This gives bacteria a chance to multiply and possibly migrate to the urethra, triggering a urinary tract infection. If use of these products causes even mild inflammation, consider switching to another form of birth control.

CHAPTER FIVE

Strengthen and Protect Your
Blood Vessels

Healthy blood vessels are a key ingredient in living a long life. Fortunately, there's an off the shelf answer for your needs.

Lines in the face and gray hairs are obvious signs of age. Blood vessels age too, but we often don't notice until the process is well under way. Fortunately, there's a nutrient that not only keeps our vessels "younger" longer, it may even help reverse the damage done by diet, age, lack of exercise, and other bad habits.

THE PROBLEM

Healthy arteries, veins, and capillaries are tough yet elastic. They're also more or less impenetrable, and pass the blood along smoothly. Vessels that aren't healthy lose this toughness and elasticity. They become weak, flaccid, and somewhat porous. They tear and rupture easily, causing small and insignificant or large and life-threatening hemorrhages.

WHO SUFFERS FROM DAMAGED
BLOOD VESSELS?

Some of the factors that contribute to blood vessel fragility include:

- **Age.** The aging process is probably the number one cause of blood vessel problems. As we get older, cells don't replace themselves as often as they once did. Tissues, including the tissues of the blood vessels, become less resilient.

- **Diabetes and other diseases.** Diabetes takes an especially high toll on the body's blood vessels, making them weaker and less able to carry oxygen and nutrients to the tissues that need nourishment. Inflammation, infections, and other conditions can also damage blood vessels.

- **Exposure to free radicals.** Free radicals are both produced within the body and enter it through such common processes as breathing. These damaging molecules contribute to many degenerative diseases by taking over healthy cells and converting them to mutant cells. Free radicals attack many different kinds of cells, including the cells that line our blood vessels. This sets the stage for atherosclerosis (hardening of the arteries), coronary artery disease, heart disease, and stroke.

- **Lifestyle.** Innumerable factors in our daily lives affect the health of our blood vessels. Some, such as smoking, not getting enough exercise, or eating a diet high in saturated fats, are within our control. Others, such as living in an area where the air is polluted or having a job that requires us to stand for long periods of time (which slows down circulation) aren't as easy to control.

WHAT ARE THE SYMPTOMS?

Blood vessels that are weak or damaged don't necessarily give off warning signals. By the time they do, the problem may have become advanced. Here are a few things to watch for:

- Easy bruising
- Small capillaries that rupture easily and frequently, often visible in the skin or the whites of eyes
- Varicose veins (discussed in chapter 24)
- Swollen feet, ankles, or legs
- Sharp and severe cramps in the legs during exercise
- Angina (see chapter 13)
- Throbbing or pain during mild exertion, especially in the main artery of the neck

WHAT'S THE OUTLOOK?

Sometimes blood vessels are weakened as a result of temporary conditions such as illness. More often, the condition is due to aging, lifestyle, diet, and other long-term factors. Because of this, poor blood vessel health is seen as chronic and degenerative, a condition that does not reverse itself without deliberate effort.

WHAT YOU SHOULD KNOW

Some of the symptoms of damaged, diseased blood vessels can signal that you are at risk for a heart attack or stroke, or that you may be suffering from some other health problem that needs attention. If you have any of the symptoms described above, be sure to report them to your doctor.

PROVEN MIRACLES

> ### OPC
> ### (FOUND IN PYCNOGENOLS, GRAPE SEED EXTRACT, AND OTHER SOURCES)

WHAT IS OPC?

OPCs, pycnogenols, pine bark extract, grape seed extract—what are these substances anyway? Let's set the record straight right now. OPCs (short for oligomeric proanthocytanidins) are antioxidant flavonoids. Like other flavonoids, OPCs are found in a variety of plants. Two plant sources are especially rich in OPCs—pine bark extracts (marketed as pycnogenols) and grape seed extract.

In other words, if you take pine bark extract (pycnogenols) or grape seed extract, you will be taking OPCs in each case, but in a different mix, because they are derived from different sources. In Europe, OPCs have been found so effective they are available as patented medication.

THE MIRACLE EFFECT

OPCs are powerful antioxidants, but their helpfulness goes far beyond that. When it comes to the body's system of blood vessels, they have a threefold action. As antioxidants, they help mop up the harmful free radicals that attack the cells of the vessels. They also have a strong anti-inflammatory effect. But the action that makes OPCs the nutrient of choice for arteries, capillaries, and veins is their unique ability to strengthen the specialized tissues of the blood vessels.

Weak, diseased blood vessels are abnormally permeable because the collagen and elastin that make them tough and resilient has deteriorated.

The ability of flavonoids to reduce permeability in capillaries was first noticed in the 1930s by the Nobel prize–winning doctor and researcher, Albert Szent-Gyorgyi. His work with citrus extracts prompted further research, and flavonoids were soon dubbed vitamin P. Over the years, one class of flavonoids, the OPCs, were found to be especially effective for fixing leaky blood vessels, and today are used in preference to all others.

OPCs such as those found in grape seed and pycnogenols bind with the collagens and elastins that make up arteries, veins, and capillaries, protecting and strengthening them by fighting off the enzymes that attack and destroy these materials. The result, as dozens upon dozens of European studies have shown, is that previously weak vessels become stronger and less likely to rupture. No other nutrients have quite this effect, not even antioxidant powerhouses like vitamins C and E.

HAVE THESE SUBSTANCES BEEN USED BEFORE?

The first people to have discovered the benefits of pine bark may have been native North Americans, who chewed it in the winter to prevent scurvy when fruits and vegetables were unavailable. Modern use of these miraculous nutrients was pioneered in Europe, especially in

France. As early as 1950, researchers discovered the strengthening effect OPCs had on capillaries.

It took a few decades more for these nutrients to become generally available, but OPC-based products are now being used by millions of people throughout Europe, South America, Australia, New Zealand, and Asia. In the United States, pycnogenols and grape seed extract, leading sources of OPCs, are rapidly gaining recognition as the superstar protectors of blood vessels.

RESEARCH FINDINGS

Numerous studies have confirmed the effectiveness of OPCs for reducing permeability in blood vessels. One of the earliest studies was done by Jacques Mesquelier, who pioneered use of the nutrient in France. He gave forty-five people suffering various forms of blood vessel impairment a single 100-milligram dose of pycynogenols (standardized to 85 percent OPCs).

Seventy-two hours later, the patients were examined and capillary resistance had soared by an average 140 percent. Though other studies have not always found this high rate of improvement, all have confirmed the benefits of OPCs in improving capillary resistence. These findings include OPCs derived from pine bark as well as grape seed extracts.

OTHER WAYS OPC CAN HELP

OPCs are terrific, but their success in strengthening blood vessels threatens to be their undoing. Unfortunately, their introduction to the United States has been accompanied by a mountain of unfounded claims. According to some manufacturers, OPCs can "cure" everything from Alzheimer's disease to attention deficit disorder to aging. Many of these claims have yet to be proven and should be taken with a healthy dose of skepticism.

Solid research does exist, however, for OPCs' benefits on several health fronts, including:

- **Varicose veins.** As the name implies, this disorder afflicts only the veins, not the whole circulatory vessel system. While horse chestnut has been found specifically effective for varicosities, OPCs also help. In one study, nearly 80 percent of varicose vein sufferers treated with OPCs experienced some degree of improvement. (For more on horse chestnut and varicose veins, see chapter 24.)

- **Vision problems related to diabetes.** Diabetes is notoriously hard on blood vessels. When small capillaries in the retina hemorrhage (a condition known as diabetic retinopathy), vision loss is a real possibility. When patients with this problem were given daily dosages of an OPC product, capillary hemorrhaging declined markedly. In fact, this strategy was found so effective that OPC products are now officially approved in France for the treatment of diabetic retinopathy. OPCs can help other diabetes-related problems as well (for more information, see chapter 10, pages 180–184).

- **Cardiovascular problems.** OPCs' ability to strengthen blood vessels, the pathways on which the heart depends, makes them essential for anyone with heart disease.

HOW TO TAKE OPC

What form does it come in? OPC products come in tablets and capsules. Depending on the source of the OPCs they contain, you may find them under a variety of different names, such as grape seed extract, pycnogenols, and so on.

What's an effective dose? Studies have found that a daily dose of 50 to 100 milligrams of OPCs (standardized to 85 percent active substance) is sufficient to strengthen blood vessels. Since the product you buy may be standardized to a different level, be sure to follow the manufacturer's package instructions.

Tips for use. When purchasing a product, be sure to check the standardization to see the percent of active OPCs it contains. The level should be quite high—80 percent or above. If it isn't, you either won't get an adequate amount of the nutrient or will have to take so many pills your "bargain" find will become quite expensive. Another thing to remember is that the active ingredients are water soluble and can't be stored by the body. Continued use is necessary to get the full benefits of these nutrients.

Are there side effects? In human trials, OPC products have been extremely well tolerated. However, there is always the possibility that an individual will have an adverse reaction. If you experience discomfort or rash, discontinue at once.

WHAT ELSE CAN YOU DO?

There's no doubt that right now OPCs are the most effective nutrients we have for strengthening blood vessels. However, that doesn't mean they're the only ones. There are a few other substances you should know about as well.

CARNITINE: THE CRAMP RELIEVER

Long known as an amino acid essential to heart health, conventional wisdom held that it benefited this organ by releasing fats the heart needs for energy. New research suggests that carnitine may benefit the heart by improving its blood supply and strengthening the body's entire blood vessel system.

Severe leg cramps during walking or exertion can be the result of atherosclerosis (hardening of the arteries).

A 1996 report in the journal *Circulation* found that carnitine dramatically improved the walking ability of patients with this problem. In the study, carried out by Brevetti and colleagues, participants received 500 milligrams of carnitine intravenously, then were monitored during exercise. While this study was extremely promising, more testing needs to be done to confirm these results.

GINKGO FOR BETTER BLOOD FLOW

Ginkgo biloba extract, made from the green leaves of the ginkgo tree, is a proven vasodilator. In other words, it helps arteries and capillaries expand, promoting the flow of the blood that nourishes every part of the body. Placebo-controlled double-blind studies have found it effective for the leg cramps that accompany impaired circulation.

More recent studies show that ginkgo is especially effective for the arteries that feed the brain. For that reason, you'll find a full discussion of ginkgo in chapter 19 on Memory and Mental Alertness.

CHAPTER SIX

Build Your Defenses Against

Cancer

The next new wave in cancer prevention may not come from a chemical laboratory but from nature's own supplements.

It seems that every week—and sometimes every day—there's a cancer headline in the news. Researchers have discovered a new gene, habit, or other risk factor, and suddenly the things you thought you knew are thrown into question. And what's worse, the findings often seem contradictory. With so much research being done, and so much information available, it sometimes seems the answer is nowhere in sight.

This chapter will eliminate some of the confusion and explain how researchers are enlisting nutrients to help in the war against cancer.

THE PROBLEM

Although some older myths about cancer are finally waning, such as the notion that cancer is contagious, other mistaken ideas persist. Test your knowledge on our myth-o-meter, below:

- *Myth #1: Cancer is one disease.* No. Cancer is a general term for several distinctly different problems, all involving the abnormal proliferation of cells and the destruction of normal cells and tissues.
- *Myth #2: Cancer happens overnight, when a single cell turns malignant.* Not necessarily. Many forms of cancer take years to develop, with cells passing through many evolutions before becoming outright malignant. Detecting and interrupting this process can help lower mortality rates in several types of cancers.
- *Myth #3: We're losing the war on cancer.* The media have made much of the fact that we haven't won the war against cancer. However, we are in the process of winning, not losing. In practical terms, that means we know more about how to prevent and treat various forms of cancer than we ever have before.
- *Myth #4: Eventually science will find a single cure for cancer.* The chances that science will find a single "magic bullet" solution to the myriad forms of cancer is almost inconceivable, and cancer is far more likely to leave the scene through a series of small steps rather than one big one. Many well-respected researchers do not even believe we will "cure" cancer. Instead, they believe cancer in the future will become much like diabetes is today—a chronic but controllable disorder that can be managed over the course of a lifetime.
- *Myth #6: If you get cancer, you'll probably die from it.* Not anymore. With a more than 50 percent over-

all survival rate (and much higher in some types of cancer) the chances are that you probably *won't* die of your disease. According to the National Cancer Institute, 7.4 million Americans have been medically determined to be cancer survivors.

WHO SUFFERS FROM CANCER?

Our study of the research proved one thing beyond a doubt: There are almost as many alleged risk factors for cancer as there are forms of cancer. From cell phones to power lines to talcum powder, almost everything in our environment has fallen under suspicion—often with surprisingly incriminating results. Some of these factors have been or will be proven erroneous, but so many substantiated ones remain that it's safe to assume *most* of us have some degree of risk. However, three of the biggest risk factors are ones you can control:

- **Smoking.** Smoking cigarettes is like building your very own toxic waste dump in your chest, next to your lung cells, where it's guaranteed to do the most damage. The proof? Tobacco (including cigarettes, cigars, and chewing tobacco) is linked to approximately one-third of all cancer-related deaths in America.
- **Diet and nutrition.** Another one-third of cancer deaths in America are linked to dietary habits, and diet can literally hurt as well as help. A high-fiber diet that includes lots of grains, fresh fruits, and vegetables definitely has a positive effect, while a diet high in red meat, sugar, and alcohol consumption promotes cancer.

- **Alcohol.** According to the American Cancer Society, heavy use of alcohol accounts for approximately 20,000 cancer deaths in America per year.

Other Risk Factors

In addition to the "big three" above, there are several other factors that contribute to one or more types of cancer, including:

- **Obesity and lack of exercise.** In time, according to the American Cancer Society, these two interrelated factors may creep up the list to join smoking, diet, and alcohol. Obesity is a risk because fat cells are estrogen-rich, and excess estrogen is a factor in breast, ovarian, and other common cancers. One antidote to obesity can be exercise. Exercise is more than just a means to control weight—even people who aren't obese can reduce their risk of cancer by exercising regularly.

- **Genetic inheritance.** There has been so much recent publicity regarding genes that "cause" cancers that many people actually overestimate this factor. Inheriting a faulty gene doesn't mean you will get cancer. You inherit two sets of genes, one from each parent, and in most cases, a healthy gene compensates for a defective gene. Moreover, it's not completely accurate to say that a single gene causes cancer. In addition to defective genes that switch on runaway cell reproduction, there are genes whose mission it is to switch it off again, requiring at least a two-stage process for cancer to take hold.

- **Environmental and occupational exposure.** Ever since the nineteenth century, when soot was linked to the astonishingly high rate of testicular cancer among chimney sweeps, researchers have known that exposure to high concentrations of certain chemicals and toxins can cause cancer. In addition to chemicals, overexposure to natural factors such as sunlight can also promote cancer.

WHAT ARE THE SYMPTOMS?

A cancerous tumor has no nerve endings of its own. For this reason, cancer may not be noticed or felt until it begins to push against nearby tissues. Cancers that don't involve tumors, such as leukemia, may also be present for a while before they are detected.

Even when symptoms are noticeable, each cancer has a different set of symptoms, and it would be impossible to cover all the bases here. A few general things you should watch for include:

- An unusual lump or thickening anywhere in the body, but especially in areas such as the breast or scrotum
- A cough that will not go away
- Any change in a mole, or the appearance of irregularly shaped molelike or scablike patches on the skin
- Any unusual bleeding or discharge
- Unexplained changes in vision, balance, or coordination

Before you get too worried, we want to assure you that all of these symptoms are extremely common ones, and usually the cause is not cancer. However, because cancer is so serious and because so much can now be done to treat it, a little vigilance on your part will pay off.

If you have any of the above symptoms, don't live in fear—see your doctor.

WHAT'S THE OUTLOOK?

Undiagnosed and untreated, most cancers result in pain, suffering, and early death. At one time, medical treatment didn't improve on that grim progression with much success. This is not true today. Cancer, of course, remains a leading cause of death. In the next year, more than 500,000 Americans will die from it. But that's less than half the 1.3 million Americans who will be diagnosed.

The best approach to cancer prevention is to use knowledge about nutrition and nutritional supplements to cut your risk as much as possible.

WHAT YOU SHOULD KNOW

Research makes a powerful argument for the protective powers of the nutrients presented in this chapter. That doesn't mean that we believe they are a replacement for regular medical checkups. Nor are they a replacement for established cancer therapy. The nutrients discussed in this chapter are intended to be used in addition to—not instead of—appropriate care and treatment.

Your best plan is to take care of yourself on all fronts and, if you are being treated for cancer, work with your doctor toward a complete recovery.

PROVEN MIRACLES

THE ANTIOXIDANT POWERHOUSES

Each day of our lives, our cells are exposed to free radicals, harmful chemical molecules that get into our bodies through breathing, through the pores of our skin, as by-products of the foods we eat, and by other means. Free radicals target healthy cells and do something much worse than just killing them off. They damage the healthy cell, causing mutations that can ultimately result in cancer.

Antioxidants interrupt this process by latching on to free radicals and neutralizing them. Research has proven that several nutrients act as antioxidants. Unfortunately, there are hundreds of types of free radicals, and no one nutrient is effective against all of them. That's why researchers keep discovering that a combination of antioxidants—especially selenium, vitamins C and E, and the carotenes—are far better than any one alone.

SELENIUM

WHAT IS SELENIUM?

Selenium, a trace element, is essential for health. According to many experts, dietary intake of selenium is falling, at least in the Western world. And that, experts agree, increases cancer risk.

THE MIRACLE EFFECT

Selenium's protective role against cancer is just beginning to be fully understood. Current thinking holds that selenium deficiency is extremely common, even among people who have a healthy diet. Adding selenium appears to guard against deficiency and protect against several types of cancer. In lab studies, selenium dramatically slows the growth of tumor cells. It also seems to protect against these specific cancers:

- Breast (in both men and women)
- Lung
- Liver
- Gastrointestinal
- Colorectal
- Urogenital
- Prostate
- Ovarian
- Cervical

To explain selenium's cancer-protective effect, researchers have focused on its role in the antioxidant process. Selenium forms enzymes that remove two especially harmful free radical substances (lipids and hydroperoxides) from the body. Without selenium, those enzymes can't form and the body's defense shield is faulty. A low level of selenium in your body may do more than just fail to protect you. It may actually help the enemy, cancer.

In a fascinating study, living cells were taken from three different human colon cancers and isolated in vitro. Different amounts of selenium were applied to each of the three cell clusters. As the researchers hoped, high concentrations of selenium greatly slowed reproduction of the cancerous cells. But the researchers also discovered something they weren't looking for. To their shock, low concentrations of selenium actually *speeded up* cell reproduction. And, as everyone knows, uncontrolled cell growth is what makes cancer lethal.

HAS SELENIUM BEEN USED BEFORE?

As early as 1976, researchers began to discover that declining dietary selenium meant rising health problems. That year, an article in the *Archives of Environmental Health* drew a connection between selenium-depleted soil and high rates of cancer in certain areas of the United States. Studies from other areas of the world noticed the same pattern.

These and other findings, with all their disastrous implications, have prompted countries such as Finland to take safeguard measures such as adding selenium supplements to soil fertilizer, flour, salt, and other items.

RESEARCH FINDINGS

Can something as simple as selenium really cut your risk of cancer? Yes, according to the studies—by as much as 50 percent for some people.

In the early 1990s, solid proof began to emerge showing that selenium supplements *can* ward off many types of cancer. One of the earliest large-scale studies came out of China in 1992. In the study, more than 4,000 people at high genetic risk for liver cancer were divided into two groups. Individuals in one group received a daily selenium supplement, while the people in the other group received a daily yeast tablet. The study lasted four years. At the end of the test, twice as many new cancers had developed in the control group as in the group taking selenium, and the authors concluded that selenium had a strong protective effect against liver cancer.

The same research team decided to test selenium's effect on the general population. Participants included more than 130,000 residents from five towns in an area whose soil is low in selenium. Half of the group used table salt with added selenium, while the other group used ordinary salt. At the end of eight years, the group using selenium-treated salt had 35 percent fewer cases of liver cancer than the other group.

In the United States, a study was begun in 1983 to see if taking selenium could guard against skin cancer. The study lasted until 1991, and included a total of 1,312 people who had all been treated for skin cancer. Half of these received selenium supplement, while the other half received a placebo. To the dismay of the researchers, selenium did not prevent new outbreaks of skin cancer. But it did prevent other types of cancers. While there were 119 cases of cancer in the placebo group, there were only 77 in the group that took selenium. Most important, selenium saved lives. Only 29 people in the selenium group died of cancer, compared to almost double that—57 deaths—in the group that didn't get selenium.

In the past, skeptics have argued that low levels of selenium are the result of cancer, not the cause. Studies like the two above challenge this idea head-on and make a powerful argument for the benefits of selenium supplements.

OTHER WAYS SELENIUM CAN HELP

Selenium's ability to guard against cancer is enough to earn it a place of honor. But the fact is, selenium does more. The same lipids and hydroperoxides that damage cells also contribute to heart disease and hardening of the arteries. When selenium-dependent enzymes mop up these substances, they lower the risk of these diseases.

Another new report finds quite a different use for selenium. When men with low fertility took selenium supplement, they doubled the count of viable sperm. For more on this, see chapter 18, pages 309–310.

HOW TO TAKE SELENIUM

What form does it come in? Selenium comes in tablet or capsule form. Many experts feel the best way to take selenium is in organic preparations, such as selenized yeast or garlic that has been specially grown in selenium-rich soil, which are better absorbed by the body. Selenium is also included in many good multivitamins.

What's an effective dose? There are no established government guidelines for selenium. The studies referred to in this chapter found that 200 micrograms a day was effective for preventing cancer. This is considered the maximum nontoxic daily dose.

Tips for use. Remember that selenium is only *one* of several important antioxidants. Studies show that when levels of selenium are low, cancer risk increases. But when levels of selenium and vitamin E are both low, the risk of cancer is even greater.

Are there side effects? Selenium is safe when taken at recommended doses, and no side effects have been reported.

Caution! Do not take more than 200 micrograms of selenium daily.

GINSENG

WHAT IS GINSENG?

There are several types of ginseng, and it pays to know which you're purchasing. Although one variety of the plant is grown in America, most American ginseng is exported. In this chapter, we're referring to red panax ginseng, which is grown primarily in Asia and is often labeled Chinese or Korean ginseng.

THE MIRACLE EFFECT

News of ginseng's ability to protect against certain types of cancer comes to us from Asia, where most of the research has been done.

In comparing health histories of people who took ginseng to those of people who didn't, researchers noted that ginseng users had far lower rates of cancer. While various forms of ginseng offered some protection, one type of ginseng—red panax ginseng—offered the best protection by far. In particular, this type of ginseng appears to protect against cancer of the:

• Lip
• Mouth

- Esophagus
- Voice box
- Lung
- Stomach
- Colon and rectum
- Liver
- Pancreas
- Ovary

In laboratory and animal studies, extract of this herb has been shown to have a powerful effect. It decreases the number of tumors formed in response to various carcinogens and slows the growth rate of tumors that do develop.

A number of reasons have been put forth to explain ginseng's cancer-fighting capabilities. First, it appears to boost immunity in individual cells and make them less susceptible to mutation. Ginseng also increases the activity of the specialized cells, known as NK cells, responsible for stopping tumor growth.

Researchers also note that ginseng has an antioxidant effect and may work to neutralize specific chemicals that promote cancer.

HAS GINSENG BEEN USED BEFORE?

Use of ginseng dates far back in time. It was used by Native Americans and has long been a staple of Chinese medicine. Although millions of people around the world now use ginseng as an overall tonic, its importance as a cancer-fighter is still not well known outside of Asia.

RESEARCH FINDINGS

One of the largest studies of ginseng's effect on humans, by Yun and Choi, compared rates of cancer in four thousand ginseng and non-ginseng takers, all of whom were smokers.

As a whole, ginseng takers had only half as much incidence of cancer as those who didn't take ginseng. Within the former group, some types of ginseng were found to be far more effective than others. For example, drinking ginseng tea offered no protective benefits at all. At the other end of the spectrum, offering far more protection than either fresh ginseng or white ginseng preparations, was red panax ginseng.

According to the report, those who had a long-standing history of taking red panax ginseng cut their odds of getting cancer by as much as 80 percent.

The report noted that people who took red panax ginseng on a regular basis, and took it consistently for years, enjoyed greater protection than those whose use was sporadic.

Compared to patients who didn't take ginseng, users of red panax ginseng cut their risk considerably. Researchers found that the ginseng takers had:

- **85% less** ovarian cancer
- **78% less** cancer of the pancreas
- **64% less** cancer of the stomach
- **58% less** colorectal cancer
- **53% less** cancer of the lip, mouth, or voice box
- **52% less** liver cancer
- **45% less** lung cancer

Numerous lab and animal studies have backed up these findings. In addition, numerous lab and animal studies have shown that red panax ginseng may well prove effective against several other types of the disease, including melanoma, breast, cervical, and vaginal cancers.

OTHER WAYS GINSENG CAN HELP

Although ginseng has been widely touted as an energy tonic, it is actually more effective for increasing sexual function and fertility in men (see chapter 18, pages 301–305).

Another promising use for ginseng is as an aid to mental alertness. It has been shown to improve mental capabilities under stress. It also works as a memory aid and helps buffer the effects of aging on the brain (see chapter 19, page 324).

HOW TO TAKE GINSENG

What form does it come in? Ginseng comes in a variety of forms, including tea and bottled tonics. The most reliable way to get a guaranteed amount of ginseng's active ingredients is to buy standardized capsules. Make sure you buy only red panax ginseng, as other varieties haven't been proven effective when it comes to protecting against cancer.

What's an effective dose? Ginseng root is expensive, and studies have shown that some manufacturers, at least in Europe, have adulterated their product. To get an effective dose, you must buy a standardized product from a reputable manufacturer. Because strength varies from product to product, follow the manufacturer's package directions for your product.

Tips for use. To protect against cancer, ginseng must be taken on a long-term basis, as part of your regular vitamin regimen. For best results, take it with food or water, and avoid taking it with stimulants such as caffeinated coffee, tea, or cola beverages.

Are there side effects? Although a few early studies suggested that ginseng could cause high blood pressure, later studies did not find this true. Most researchers now agree that ginseng is safe in moderate doses. However, some individuals may be allergic to ginseng. If you develop heart palpitations or chest pain, nausea, headache, agitation, or insomnia, discontinue at once.

Caution! Ginseng can be toxic in very large amounts. Do not take more than your package directions recommend. You should not take ginseng if you are taking antipsychotic medications or if you are receiving hormone treatment. You should also avoid ginseng if you are taking any of a class of antidepressant medications, MAO inhibitors (also referred to as MAOIs). If you are using this type of drug for depression or anxiety, your doctor will already have told you that you cannot eat certain foods, including aged meats, cheese, and red wine.

VITAMINS C AND E

WHAT ARE VITAMINS C AND E?

Vitamins C and E are powerful antioxidants. In the body, they neutralize free radicals, the harmful chemicals that promote cancer by transforming healthy cells.

Low dietary intake of both has been linked to several forms of cancer. We are discussing them together here not only because they have a similar role in cancer prevention but because they seem to be more effective when taken together than either would be taken alone. One reason for this may be that when a vitamin E molecule is damaged by interacting with a free radical, C lends support by converting it back to its original form.

THE MIRACLE EFFECT

Vitamins C and E are such powerful antioxidants that some researchers have dubbed them antimutagens—meaning that they can protect against the cell mutations that give rise to cancer. Several studies offer proof that these vitamins more than deserve this label. In one instance, cell cultures treated with vitamin C showed far less DNA damage when exposed to damaging X rays than did untreated cells.

Researchers believe that vitamins C and E protect against cancer by mopping up the various free radicals that trigger specific types of cancer. For example, among the free radicals vitamin C has been shown to neutralize is one produced in the stomach, which seems to explain why people who take in high levels of C have low levels of stomach cancer. Low intake of vitamin C may meet government guidelines but has also been linked to abnormal pap smears and may be a risk factor for cervical cancer.

Low levels of vitamin E may also play a role in cervical cancer. And, along with beta-carotene, vitamin E has been shown to have a protective effect on cells in the mouth.

These vitamins may also hold promise for people who already have cancer. When applied to certain types of cancer cells, vitamin C has a lethal effect, killing off cells and stopping their runaway growth. In patients with bladder cancer, a vitamin cocktail that included both C and E reduced the rate of recurrence by 50 percent.

HAVE VITAMINS C AND E BEEN USED BEFORE?

Interest in these vitamins as protectors against disease dates back to the 1930s. Canadian Dr. Evan Shute prescribed vitamin E to his patients with heart disease. Thirty years after that, Nobel prize–winner Linus Pauling gained public attention when he asserted that very large doses of vitamin C could ward off colds.

Today, as proof mounts that these nutrients can indeed cut cancer risk, more and more people are going out of their way to make sure they get an adequate supply of each, either through diet or in supplement form.

While these two vitamins have always been part of the human diet, not all of us eat the way we should. To make matters worse, exposure to cancer-causing agents seems to be an inescapable part of modern civilization.

RESEARCH FINDINGS

In the course of our research, we found many articles that questioned the usefulness of these supplements. The main concern: adding nutrient supplements is not the same as improving diet, and might not offer the same protection. Fair enough. And, indeed, several early studies have been inconclusive.

First, as we've already mentioned, antioxidants are far more effective when taken in combination, so testing any one nutrient alone may be misleading. More important, short-term studies aren't likely to be very helpful. The damage done by cancer-causing agents takes a long time to make itself known. It isn't surprising that the protective benefits of nutritional supplements would take an equally long time to become noticeable.

Fortunately, some long-term studies have been undertaken and reveal a more complex picture. We think it best to let the results speak for themselves. Antioxidants can:

- **Cut overall cancer death rates, reduce cancer of the esophagus.** One of the largest investigations to date, the Linxian studies, involved 29,584 adults in a region of China noted for extremely high rates of stomach cancer and cancer of the esophagus. Participants took one of four different combinations of antioxidants for a five-year period. Those who took a combination of vitamin E, beta-carotene, and selenium had the lowest death rates from all types of cancer, and an amazing 42 percent fewer cases of cancer of the esophagus.

  Studies conducted in the U.S. have backed up

this finding and concluded that vitamin E also protects against cancers of the mouth and pharynx.

- **Slash colon cancer risk by 57 percent.** Researchers closely examined vitamin supplement use in two groups of people—444 patients diagnosed with colon cancer and 427 people without colon cancer. For both groups, research went back ten years prior to diagnosis. People who took 200 IUs or more of vitamin E daily had a 57 percent lower rate of colon cancer than people who didn't.
- **Reduce prostate cancer deaths by more than 40 percent.** A group of 29,133 male smokers in Finland were given either vitamin E supplement, vitamin E plus beta-carotene, or a harmless placebo for a period of five to eight years. Vitamin E, either alone or combined with beta-carotene, proved to be a life-saver for those who took it. It reduced cases of prostate cancer by 32 percent. More important, it drove down deaths from prostate cancer by 41 percent.
- **Cut recurring bladder cancer by half.** Sixty-five patients diagnosed with bladder cancer all got vitamin supplements. The difference? One group received large doses of vitamins C, E, B6, A, and zinc, while the other group received only the recommended daily allowances. Over a ten-month period, cancer returned in 80 percent of the patients who received the recommended daily allowance. But only 40 percent of patients who took large doses of vitamins had recurrences.

OTHER WAYS VITAMINS C AND E CAN HELP

Until today you probably thought of vitamin C as a weapon against colds and sore throats rather than against cancer. And for good reason. If you turn to chapter 8 (Colds, Coughs, and Other Upper Respiratory Infections), you'll see why this vitamin is indispensable for such minor illnesses. And both vitamins C and E play an important role in protecting against heart attack and stroke. Vitamin C is especially important for strengthening the heart and the heart's arteries (see chapter 13), while vitamin E pitches in to help lower cholesterol and triglycerides (see chapter 7).

HOW TO TAKE VITAMINS C AND E

What form do they come in?   Vitamin C comes in tablets, including chewable tablets. Vitamin E comes in capsules, tablets, and drops.

What's an effective dose?   Studies we looked at used between 200 and 400 IUs of vitamin E, and 2,000 milligrams of vitamin C. Since these doses are substantially higher than those recommended by the government, you may want to check with your doctor first.

Tips for use. Vitamins C and E have a special synergistic effect and should be taken together. They should also be taken with food and water. If you want to take large doses of vitamin C, don't shock your system—start at a low dose and build up.

Are there side effects?   Both vitamins C and E can cause diarrhea and stomach upset.

Caution! People with anemia, poorly clotting blood, liver disease, or overactive thyroid should not take vitamin E supplements without consulting a doctor.

Pregnant women should not take megadoses of any vitamin unless their doctor specifically recommends it.

QUERCETIN AND OTHER FLAVONOIDS

WHAT ARE FLAVONOIDS?

Flavonoids (also referred to as bioflavonoids) are a huge group of vitaminlike substances found in plants. There are hundreds of flavonoids, and very few of them are known by their technical names. More often, we talk about the magical benefits of the substances that contain them. The real health secret of red wine, green tea, grape seed extract, and pine bark extract is that they are especially rich in flavonoids.

THE MIRACLE EFFECT

Studies show that flavonoids regulate the body's use of vitamin C, boosting its beneficial effect. But flavonoids also have powers that are all their own.

As a group, flavonoids are powerful antioxidants. In addition to this, individual flavonoids seem to be especially potent against specific types of cancer. Researchers are just beginning to learn which flavonoids have the strongest anti-cancer potential. To date, only a few have been identified. Leaders of the flavonoid pack include:

- **Quercetin.** One of the first flavonoids to gain name recognition, quercetin is found in such ordinary food items as onions, broccoli, and apples. *Protects against:* cancer in general, lung cancer in particular.

- **Gallate compounds found in green tea.** Green tea isn't the only source of gallates. Grape seed extract also has them. However, green tea or green tea extract is the richest source. More than 30 percent of green tea's flavonoids are gallate compounds. *Protects against:* cancer in general, cancers specific to women in particular.

- **Genistein and daidzein found in soy products.** High consumption of these flavonoids seems to explain why cultures that eat a lot of tofu and other soy products have extremely low rates of some cancers. *Protects against:* prostate cancer and breast cancer in men and women.

- **Tangeretin found in citrus.** Researchers now believe that while vitamin C has gotten all the credit for the health benefits of a diet high in citrus fruits, at least some of the credit really belongs to this flavonoid. *Protects against:* cancer in general.

According to breaking research, flavonoids actually fight cancer in two ways. In addition to protecting us from this dread disease, flavonoids can also help us recover! By dramatically slowing the runaway reproduction of cancer cells, they act as a kind of natural chemotherapy, with one big advantage: They don't harm normal cells. While they can't take the place of traditional medical treatment, they can help the body's overall recovery. In time, science may even use them to make better and safer chemotherapeutic drugs.

HAVE FLAVONOIDS BEEN USED BEFORE?

Cultures with a diet high in fruits and vegetables naturally ingest a large variety of flavonoids. The use of flavonoid supplements is relatively recent. However, numerous flavonoid-rich herbal medicines—including horse chestnut, used for varicose veins (see chapter 24), and hawthorn, used for the heart (see chapter 13)—have been widely used throughout Europe, Japan, and China for decades.

RESEARCH FINDINGS

Remember when your mother told you to eat an apple a day? A twenty-four-year-long Finnish study found that ten thousand people who took this advice and ate a diet high in apples cut their overall risk of cancer by 20 percent. The risk reduction for lung cancer was even greater. Flavonoid-eaters had 46 percent less risk of lung cancer, while flavonoid-eaters who were also non-smokers cut their risk by an astonishing 87 percent. The reason, according to researchers, is that apples are particularly rich in the flavonoid quercetin.

In Japan, researchers found a similar protective effect from the flavonoids in green tea. After studying the eating and drinking habits of people age forty and over, Imai and colleagues concluded that women who drank ten or more cups of green tea daily cut their chances of getting cancer by 43 percent. Even when women who drank large amounts of tea did develop cancer, they contracted it an average of nine years later than women who drank less tea. Writing in *Preventive Medicine,* the authors of the study concluded that the ''Strong potency of green tea in preventing cancers . . . points us toward a new strategy of cancer chemoprevention without toxic effects."

So far, numerous studies like the ones above show that dietary flavonoids form a powerful cancer shield. But what about flavonoid supplements? Since use of these is relatively recent, it will take some time for long-term studies to be completed.

One measure of the potency of these nutrients comes from quite a different type of challenge—applying flavonoids directly to cancer cells. And the results have been astounding. For example:

- **Quercetin and genistein,** applied separately, both slowed the reproduction of colon cancer cells.
- **Quercetin** slowed the growth of cells taken from head and neck tumors.
- **Tangeretin,** the citrus flavonoid, was applied to several types of leukemia cells. It was not effective for all cell lines. But for one specific kind of leukemia, tangeretin reignited the important natural process in which faulty cells "commit suicide."
- **Green tea flavonoids** were fed to half of a group of rats with induced breast tumors. Although the flavonoids did not cure the cancers, they dramatically increased survival. Tumors were smaller and softer, and 93.8 percent of the flavonoid-treated rats were alive at the end of the thirty-four-week study, versus only 33.3 percent of the rats who did not receive flavonoids.

  In another study, green tea flavonoids were capable of triggering "suicide" in several types of cancer cells, including skin cancer and prostate cancer cells.

In each case, flavonoids were effective in doses that did not harm normal cells.

OTHER WAYS FLAVONOIDS CAN HELP

Science is just getting a handle on the potential uses of flavonoid supplements. As we've said before, there are hundreds—and some say thousands—of important flavonoids, and only a few have been studied in any detail.

We know that, in addition to helping win the war on cancer, quercetin benefits people with arthritis (see chapter 2). You'll also find a class of flavonoids known as OPCs as the focus of our chapter on blood vessel health (see chapter 5). Over the next decade, as researchers examine more and more of these miracle nutrients, the list of disease-blasting flavonoids will undoubtedly grow.

HOW TO TAKE FLAVONOIDS

What form do flavonoids come in? Flavonoids come in capsules and tablets. A few well-known flavonoids, such as quercetin and pycnogenols, are plainly labeled that way. More often, they are sold under the name of the plants they are derived from, such as green tea extract and grape seed extract.

What's an effective dose? There is no recommended daily allowance for flavonoids. Although these nutrients do not appear to be toxic, you should follow the manufacturer's package instructions.

Tips for use. Since research is still discovering which flavonoids are the best protectors against cancer, you might want to take a flavonoid complex product, ensuring that you will get a mix of these important nutrients.

Are there side effects? No known side effects have been reported when flavonoids are used according to the manufacturer's package directions. However, since these are plant products, there is always the possibility of an allergic reaction.

BETA-CAROTENE, LYCOPENE, AND THE CAROTENOIDS

WHAT ARE CAROTENOIDS?

Carotenoids are the color-giving plant pigments found in red, yellow, and orange fruits and vegetables. Beta-carotene is by far the best known of the carotenoids, but in the 1990s a new member of the carotenoid family leaped onto newspaper pages across the country. Lycopene, found in concentrated tomato products, such as tomato sauce and paste, was heralded as a new and effective ally in the war on cancer.

THE MIRACLE EFFECT

Although there are more than six hundred known carotenoids, not all of them are equally useful. About thirty to fifty of them are converted to vitamin A, an anti-cancer vitamin, in the body and a few carotenoids have cancer-fighting abilities all their own.

Diets rich in carotenoids have been associated with

low overall rates of cancer and lower rates of several individual types of cancer, including:

- Breast
- Colon
- Lung
- Mouth
- Prostate
- Stomach
- Thyroid

Much like the flavonoid family of nutrients described above, several carotenoids have been shown to do double duty against cancer. First, they act as antioxidants, knocking out various free radicals that promote the cell changes that can lead to cancer.

Carotenoids that act against free radicals associated with cancer include alpha-carotein, beta-carotene, lycopene, lutein, cryptoxanthin, and zeaxanthin.

Research is now focusing on a second line of defense provided by carotenoids. Studies show that several of them have the ability to slow or stop the reproduction of cancer cells. This is extremely important, since one of the traits that makes cancer lethal is the rapid, uncontrolled multiplication of cells. To date, the most potent carotenoid in this group is lycopene, but beta-carotene and other carotenoids have also shown this ability in lab studies.

HAVE CAROTENOIDS BEEN USED BEFORE?

The role of carotenoids in cancer prevention came to the attention of the health community when researchers began to study just where and how people used various carotenoids. Study after study has shown that people who eat a diet high in carotenoid-rich foods have dramatically lower rates of several types of cancers than people whose diets are lacking in carotenoids.

Lycopene is just one example of the fact that carotenoids don't have to be eaten fresh. While fresh tomatoes contain little lycopene, cooked and concentrated tomato products—such as tomato puree, paste, and sauce—are rich in lycopene. And, as studies have shown, it's the use of these cooked and concentrated products—the more concentrated the better—rather than consumption of fresh tomatoes or even tomato juice, that lowers the risk of cancer.

RESEARCH FINDINGS

While a few long-term studies have been done on carotenoids and cancer, they haven't taken other factors—such as smoking and drinking habits—into consideration. For this reason, their results probably don't reflect the true contribution of these miracle nutrients. For a fair evaluation, long-term, carefully controlled studies must be completed. Until those become available, findings from other studies have found that carotenoids can:

- **Help lower overall cancer death rate, cut rates of cancer of the esophagus.** One of the largest tests of supplements to date, the Linxian studies discussed earlier in this chapter, involved 29,584 adults in a region of China noted for extremely high rates of stomach cancer and cancer of the esophagus. Participants took one of four different combinations of antioxidants for a five-year period. At the end of the study, the group that received a combination of beta-carotene, vitamin E, and selenium had signifi-

cantly lower death rates from cancer than the other
groups, and 42 percent fewer cases of cancer of the
esophagus.

- **Cut risk of prostate cancer.** The ongoing Physicians' Health Study monitors the dietary and vita-
min-taking habits of more than 22,000 U.S. doctors.
Beta-carotene supplements have not made a difference for those with already high levels of beta-carotene (due to dietary intake), but men with the lowest
levels who took supplements had 19 percent fewer
cases of prostate cancer than expected over a
twelve-year period.
- **Slow reproduction of endometrial and breast
cancer cells.** Cancer of the uterine lining (endome-
trium) is a common form of the disease among
women. To test the effect of various carotenoids,
Levy and colleagues prepared cultures of both endometrial and breast cancer cells. Lycopene proved
to be a superstar inhibitor of cancer growth. It
slowed cell reproduction within twenty-four hours
and the effect remained for three whole days. An
even more amazing finding was the effect it had on
normal cells: almost none. Despite its lethal effect
on cancer, reproduction of normal cells was slowed
only slightly, and the effect was shorter lasting.
Also effective in slowing growth in these cancers
were the beta-carotene and alpha-carotene, although
higher concentrations were needed to get the same
results.
- **Slow reproduction of prostate cancer cells.** Researchers applied a variety of carotenoids to individual cultures of prostate cancer cells. Several
carotenoids significantly slowed the growth of these

cancer clusters. The most effective carotenoids proved to be beta-carotene and canthaxanthin, which reduced growth by 56 percent and 45 percent, respectively. Lycopene, lutein, and several other carotenoids also inhibited growth, but were not as dramatically effective.

• **Protect against ultraviolet light damage.** Exposure to the sun's ultraviolet rays is considered a leading cause of skin cancer. To see what role carotenoids might play in protecting us from the sun, researchers pretreated female volunteers with both beta-carotene and lycopene, then exposed a small area on the forearm of each woman to ultraviolet light.

Later, they compared carotenoid concentrations in the exposed skin to the concentrations in unexposed areas. There was no difference in amounts of beta-carotene, but lycopene levels in exposed skin tissue was depleted. The meaning of this? Researchers concluded that the missing lycopene had been used up neutralizing the damaging chemicals released by the ultraviolet rays.

What About Negative Findings?

A few years ago, enthusiasm for beta-carotene hit a brick wall when large-scale studies showed the supplement might actually *increase* rates of lung cancer. Unfortunately, many people began to avoid this nutrient without ever finding out the facts behind the headlines.

An important four-year study, known as the Beta Carotene and Retinol Efficacy Trial (CARET), examined 18,314 heavy smokers, former smokers, and former asbestos workers. Half of the group received a placebo while the other half received a daily supplement of 30 milligrams of synthetic beta-carotene combined with a megadose (25,000 IUs) of vitamin A. Alarmingly, those in the supplement group developed more lung cancers than those in the control group, and the study was stopped early.

A study of thirty thousand Finnish male smokers age fifty to sixty-nine had similar findings. Men who received 20 milligrams of beta-carotene daily had 18 percent more new cases of lung cancer than men who didn't.

What's the story behind these findings? Should we all throw our supplements down a sink? The answer, for most of us, is *No*.

There are a few reasons that may explain the study findings. First of all, these studies used synthetically prepared beta-carotene supplements. Synthetic beta-carotene is chemically different from beta-carotene extracted from natural sources. When researchers gave one group of volunteers a synthetic supplement and another group a supplement derived from natural sources, it was clear that the natural supplement was far more effective.

Another problem was that these studies used only one type of carotenoid, beta-carotene. By not using a complex of mixed carotenoids, they eliminated other important members of this family, including alpha-carotene, lycopene, and other anti-cancer carotenes.

The most important factor, though, seems to be *who* the supplements were tested on. Both of the studies in which rates increased involved people who are at extremely high risk for cancer: smokers, former smokers, and asbestos workers. And the increase was only for one type of cancer, cancer of the lung.

The people in these studies had already been exposing their lungs to carcinogens for quite some time, and it's likely that cell changes were already under way. Several researchers have speculated that the precancerous changes in lung cells make the lung unable to properly use beta-carotene or vitamin A. Instead of helping, the supplements can actually do harm, especially when megadoses of vitamin A are given in addition to beta-carotene. Finally, most of those who developed lung cancer carried an additional risk factor. They were heavy alcohol users.

These studies have caused researchers to caution against supplementation for people already at high risk for lung cancer. But the real health issue here is to stop smoking.

OTHER WAYS CAROTENOIDS CAN HELP

Because of their antioxidant activity and their ability to disarm free radicals, carotenoids may play a role in protecting the heart and the arteries that feed the heart and brain.

Carotenoids may be especially helpful for women. One study showed that when cows were fed a diet low in beta-carotene, they developed ovarian cysts and became infertile. Another study suggested beta-carotene might help women fight off vaginal yeast infections.

HOW TO TAKE CAROTENOIDS

What form do they come in? Carotenoids come in tablets and capsules. You can buy individual carotenoids, such as beta-carotene and lycopene, or you can buy carotene complex, a blend of carotenes. Based on our research, we recommend you use carotenoids derived from natural sources.

What's an effective dose? This will depend on what preparation you buy, so follow the manufacturer's package instructions.

Tips for use. To maximize your protection, take carotenoids as part of an overall supplement program that also includes other antioxidants (such as selenium and vitamins C and E.)

Are there side effects? Carotenoids are considered nontoxic when taken in moderate amounts, and no side effects have been reported.

Caution! Based on their research, the authors of the CARET study (mentioned above), have recommended that, ''Individuals at high risk of developing lung cancer, i.e., current smokers and asbestos-exposed workers, should be discouraged from taking supplemental beta-carotene (and the combination of beta-carotene with vitamin A).''

WHAT ELSE CAN YOU DO?

In addition to the anti-cancer supplements we've already discussed, there are a few other nutrients that show promise.

DON'T FORGET VITAMIN A

Beta-carotene and other carotenoids help form vitamin A, but you also get this vitamin from other sources. Vitamin A is important for overall health, and you should make sure you get the government's recommended allowance of 5,000 IUs per day.

Studies indicate that this vitamin may have a protective effect against cancer and, like several other nutrients, may play a role in squelching tumor growth. It may eventually prove especially useful in the prevention and treatment of melanoma, the rarest but most serious form of skin cancer.

Don't go overboard, because vitamin A can be toxic in large doses. But if you have specific risk factors (such as sun-damaged skin or large, irregular moles), make sure you get as much as government guidelines suggest.

CALCIUM + VITAMIN D = REDUCED RECTAL CANCER

The relationship between rectal cancer and dietary habits was studied in 34,702 postmenopausal women living in Iowa. The study lasted nine years. Although high consumption of several vitamins (including A, beta-carotene, and C) had a slight protective effect, the biggest protector proved to be the combination of calcium and vitamin D. Women who had the highest intake of these two nutrients cut their risk of rectal cancer by nearly half (47 percent), compared to women who got the least amount of these nutrients.

COENZYME Q-10: A NEW AID
IN CANCER TREATMENT?

Most people think of coenzyme Q-10 as the heart-protecting antioxidant, but in the late 1970s and early 1980s, reports appeared suggesting a whole new avenue of usefulness. In rodents exposed to chemotherapeutic chemicals, it significantly buffered the medicine's toxic effects. Unfortunately, these trials never resulted in guidelines for human use.

Coenzyme Q-10 holds another tantalizing hope as well. Isolated case reports and a few small studies suggest that in megadoses coenzyme Q-10 may shrink tumors of the breast and liver. To date it has helped only a fraction of the patients who have tried it, and researchers aren't yet recommending it as beneficial. Large-scale studies need to be done, and long-term testing is necessary to determine if coenzyme Q-10 is toxic in the very large amounts (ten to thirteen times the average daily dose) needed. More research should certainly be done on this promising possibility.

PROBIOTICS: THE COLON'S BEST FRIEND

Probiotics are friendly bacteria that protect the digestive tract from numerous harmful bacteria (see chapter 11). For a variety of reasons, many of us don't have enough of these helpful microorganisms. Fortunately, we can take them in capsule form. In addition to helping us fight intestinal infections, they may also help us fight cancer.

Recently, one of the most common probiotics was shown to have a profound effect on colon cancer in rats. When rats fed these probiotics were injected with tumor-promoting substances, they fared far better than rats that didn't receive probiotics. In the treated group, fewer rats developed tumors; in those that did, tumors were fewer and smaller.

SILYMARIN AND THE SUN

As you may already know, skin cancer is on the rise. Even our most potent sun protectors may not be effective enough. But researchers at Cleveland's Case Western Reserve University may have found a surprising source of help. The name of this serious sun-protector is silymarin. Silymarin is the active substance in milk thistle, the amazing aid for the liver (see chapter 17 for a discussion of milk thistle).

When silymarin was applied to the skin of mice before and after exposure to ultraviolet light, only one in four mice developed tumors. In a group of untreated mice exposed to the same light, 100 percent developed skin tumors. The results were so encouraging that the authors of the study recommended human testing and speculated that adding silymarin to sunscreen might dramatically cut the rate of skin cancer.

ALPHA LIPOIC ACID

Often referred to simply as lipoic acid, this nutrient with the harsh-sounding name is actually good for your body. It's a powerful antioxidant that plays both offense and defense. On offense, it neutralizes free radicals and protects against cancer. On defense, it protects other antioxidants, including vitamins C and E and coenzyme Q-10, from harm. For more about alpha lipoic acid, see chapter 10.

SUPPLEMENTS AND CANCER THERAPY

Some physicians feel nutritional supplements like the ones discussed in this chapter interfere with chemotherapy, radiation, and other cancer therapies, and warn their patients against taking them.

Dr. Charles Simone, author of *Cancer and Nutrition,* has noted that many studies support the use of vitamins during cancer therapy. For example, vitamins A, beta-carotene, C, E, and selenium seem to protect the heart from some of the toxic effects of Adriamycin, a common chemotherapy drug. Megadoses of vitamin B6 may help people undergoing radiation.

If you're being treated for cancer, the first thing you should do is follow your doctor's advice. But the issue of supplements may be worth discussing.

CHAPTER SEVEN

What You Can Do to Lower
Cholesterol and Triglycerides

If changes in diet and exercise just aren't enough, let nature's miracle nutrients help you out.

Good cholesterol, bad cholesterol, triglycerides—it sometimes seems that components in our blood, and in our food, are out to get us and there's nothing we can do about it. To make matters worse, the things we're told to do, such as watch our diet and take cholesterol-lowering drugs, often yield skimpy benefits. Maybe that's why medical researchers are taking a further look at natural solutions and coming up with fresh strategies.

THE PROBLEM

Cholesterol, a nonsoluble waxy substance, is actually needed by the body to perform a number of tasks. But the body manufactures all the cholesterol it needs, and extra cholesterol from our food can become harmful. This wasn't a health problem for our ancestors, who were extremely active. But modern man is far less active and continues to consume a great deal of saturated fat and high-cholesterol foods.

You may have been confused by references to LDLs (low-density lipoproteins), the "bad" cholesterol, and HDLs (high-density lipoproteins), the "good" cholesterol. Both are found in the blood. To make matters as simple as possible, HDLs are cycled through the liver and removed from the body. LDLs remain in the blood, where they eventually convert to the plaque that clings to arterial walls. This promotes atherosclerosis (hardening of the arteries) and coronary artery disease, conditions that can cause heart attack and stroke.

When your total cholesterol reading is above 200 milligrams per deciliter, risk of heart disease begins to rise. When the reading is above 240 milligrams per deciliter, the risk of heart disease has doubled. If your doctor tells you that you have high cholesterol, he or she won't just try to lower the total reading, he will also want to see the level of HDLs rise while the level of LDLs fall.

Much like cholesterol, elevated triglyceride levels are also seen as a risk factor for heart attack, heart disease, and stroke. Triglycerides are fatty acids that aren't metabolized well and, as a result, accumulate in the blood.

WHO SUFFERS FROM HIGH CHOLESTEROL AND TRIGLYCERIDES?

Many factors contribute to high cholesterol and triglyceride levels, some controllable and some not. Risk factors associated with elevated blood levels of cholesterol and triglycerides include:

- **Diet.** Both cholesterol and triglyceride levels are influenced by what you eat. Eating a diet rich in meat, animal products, and saturated fats also raises cholesterol. A diet low in protein and high in carbohydrates is thought to raise triglyceride levels.
- **Family history.** Some people's bodies overproduce cholesterol, and high cholesterol appears to have a genetic link. Because of this and because poor eating habits are also passed along, cholesterol problems often run in families.
- **Age.** For both men and women, cholesterol and triglyceride levels creep upward with age.
- **Menopause.** Prior to menopause, women's cholesterol levels are usually lower than those of men of the same age. Menopause eliminates this advantage. Since estrogen tends to raise HDLs (good cholesterol) and lower LDLs (bad cholesterol), estrogen replacement therapy may help women with high cholesterol. Women also tend to have higher triglyceride levels than do men.
- **Overweight.** Being overweight tends to increase cholesterol and triglycerides, while shedding weight often brings these levels down. Whether this is an independent factor or the by-product of diet is not entirely clear.
- **Exercise.** It has been noted that increasing physical activity may help raise the levels of HDLs while lowering levels of harmful LDLs.
- **Alcohol consumption.** Much has been made of the benefits of wine for the heart. But too much alcohol actually increases levels of harmful cholesterol. The bottom line? A glass or two of wine with dinner can help, but much more isn't recommended. Heavy al-

cohol consumption is also a risk factor for elevated triglycerides.

- **Disease.** Certain diseases can raise cholesterol and triglyceride levels. Diabetes and hypothyroidism are two common conditions that raise these levels, although there are several other far less common disorders that can also play a role.

WHAT ARE THE SYMPTOMS?

There are no direct early symptoms of high cholesterol or high triglycerides. This is why it's important to have your reading taken by a doctor. By the time you begin to experience angina pains in your chest, discover you need a coronary bypass, or experience a stroke, you've had elevated levels of these substances for years.

WHAT'S THE OUTLOOK?

High cholesterol doesn't go away on its own. It requires a change of lifestyle on your part. But the effort does pay off. Changes in diet and exercise habits, and the miracle nutrients described in this chapter, can help reduce cholesterol and reverse the process that puts you at risk for heart disease, stroke, and other problems.

WHAT YOU SHOULD KNOW

The nutrients in this chapter aren't a license to eat an unregulated diet or to ignore other health risks, such as high blood pressure or smoking. To really lower your cholesterol, you'll also need to work on correcting the risk factors described above. It's also important to remember that controlling your cholesterol level isn't a be-all and end-all. Because many factors put you at risk for heart attack and stroke, you should also read chapter 13 (on Heart Disease and Coronary Artery Disease) and chapter 14 (on Homocysteine).

PROVEN MIRACLES

VITAMIN E

WHAT IS VITAMIN E?

Vitamin E is a powerful antioxidant. With vitamin C as a partner, it is essential to cardiovascular health. Although most of us take in enough vitamin E to meet the government's recommended daily allowances, recent research suggests that larger amounts play a key role in lowering cholesterol and preventing the harm usually done to arteries.

THE MIRACLE EFFECT

There's no doubt that vitamin E has shown an amazing ability to neutralize cholesterol and help unclog arteries. In fact, the British research team that conducted one of the largest studies to date concluded that this little vitamin is actually more potent than aspirin or cholesterol-lowering drugs. The reason for E's effectiveness, they feel, lies in its ability to knock out free radicals.

Most of us think of free radicals as catalysts for cancer, but few of us realize that these particles are also the underlying cause of arterial plaque and heart disease. And even fewer of us really know what a free radical is.

Free radicals are molecules that are present in oxygen and dozens of other substances; they are in our bodies as a result of the air we breathe and the foods we eat. There are numerous different types of free radicals, and some are more dangerous to certain body systems and organs than others.

The molecular structure of free radicals causes them to look for cells to attach themselves to. When this happens, the cell is forever transformed. The takeover process has been likened to the formation of rust. Particles of LDL cholesterol are inviting targets for free radicals. The new material formed by the binding process attacks the artery's endothelial cells, the specialized cells that allow the artery to expand to accommodate bits of debris in the blood. To make matters worse, the material becomes embedded in the artery walls. Over a period of years, the plaque accumulates and narrows the passageway while the artery becomes more and more scarred and rigid.

Exciting new studies suggest vitamin E helps stop this process in its initial stages. Researchers believe this vitamin acts as a kind of circuit breaker in the process, mopping up the free radicals by binding with them and rendering them inert. All antioxidants, including vitamin C, act in this manner, but vitamin E appears to have a special affinity for the free radicals that affect cholesterol. By neutralizing the free radical chain reaction, it helps keep arteries free and protects the endothelial cells from damage.

While researchers are convinced this is the vitamin's main activity, vitamin E may help in another way as well. Science has long identified it as a natural blood-thinner and anticoagulant. Since blockages are due not only to cholesterol but to blood clots as well, vitamin E may well act as a sort of all-purpose blood "detergent," eliminating the solid particles that cause millions of heart attacks and strokes every year.

HAS VITAMIN E BEEN USED BEFORE?

The widespread attention vitamin E is receiving may seem new but actually, E's use was pioneered in the early part of the twentieth century. In the 1930s Canadian Dr. Evan Shute prescribed the vitamin to patients with heart disease. His use of the vitamin was highly controversial and his efforts were ignored by mainstream medicine until the 1990s. Now, years after Shute's use of the vitamin, nutritionally oriented physicians are recommending it to their patients.

RESEARCH FINDINGS

Throughout the 1990s, animal studies attested to vitamin E's amazing effect on cholesterol. In one experiment two groups of primates, fed the same extremely high-fat diet, ended up with extremely different health profiles. The group that consumed vitamin E supplements along with their rich food had arteries that were far clearer than the clogged arteries in the other group. Moreover, when the primates whose arteries were clogged began to receive vitamin E as well, their condition began to improve. Arteries that had been one-third blocked had less than 8 percent blockage eight months later. In other words, vitamin E not only prevented the problem, it helped to correct it.

It now seems clear that the same claims can be made

for the vitamin's effect on humans. One of the largest studies of vitamin E's benefits, done by Stephens and colleagues of England's Cambridge University, tracked 2,002 patients over an eighteen-month period. In this double-blind study, the group that received a daily dose of vitamin E had 77 percent fewer nonfatal heart attacks than the group that received a placebo.

What made the findings even more remarkable was that the reduction occurred among a group at high risk for coronary disaster—all had some degree of coronary artery disease, and more than 37 percent had already been diagnosed as serious.

Another report, which attracted a good deal of attention when it broke in the headlines in 1997, dramatically demonstrated the immediate effects of vitamin E. In this study, men and women with normal cholesterol volunteered to test the effects of vitamin E on cholesterol by eating a particular breakfast once each week for three consecutive weeks.

The first breakfast contained more than 50 grams of fat, the second was extremely low in fat, and the third was identical to the first with one exception: Before eating, participants took 800 IUs (international units) of vitamin E and 1,000 milligrams of vitamin C. In each case, subjects were given ultrasound tests hourly for four hours after eating to monitor blood flow in the large artery of the upper arm.

Eating the high-fat meal significantly decreased blood flow in the artery, a sign that endothelial cells were being prevented from behaving normally. As researchers expected, eating a low-fat meal did not cause this problem. The surprise came when the effects of pretreatment with vitamins E and C were analyzed. Despite the very high levels of saturated fat, arterial flow was unrestricted. The vitamins had stepped in and protected the endothelial cells.

As the researchers were quick to point out, it would be a mistake to interpret the study as a license to consume large quantities of saturated fats. But it would be just as big a mistake to ignore the wonderful protective benefits of this heart-helping antioxidant.

OTHER WAYS VITAMIN E CAN HELP

Vitamin E's antioxidant abilities make it an effective all-purpose vitamin, ensuring the health of cells throughout the body. In particular, vitamin E has been shown to:

- **Help protect against cancer.** People with low levels of this vitamin have high rates of certain types of cancers, and research is now proving that adding E supplements can help bring the risk back down. (For more on this vitamin's cancer-fighting abilities, see chapter 6.)
- **Fight arthritis.** Several studies have shown that increasing vitamin E intake decreases pain for people with both osteoarthritis and rheumatoid arthritis and may even slow the progress of the disease itself (see chapter 2, page 53).
- **Relieve symptoms of menopause.** Taken in doses above 400 IUs per day, vitamin E induces fat cells to release estrogen contained within them, acting as a sort of naturally induced form of hormone therapy (see chapter 20, page 341).

HOW TO TAKE VITAMIN E

What form does it come in? Vitamin E comes in capsules, tablets, and drops.

What's an effective dose? Doses recommended for lowering cholesterol are considerably higher than government guidelines. Studies have shown that 400 IUs of vitamin E help lower cholesterol. Not all scientists think an effective dosage needs to be this high. German researchers Gey and colleagues feel that when taken with 140 milligrams of vitamin C, daily dosage of E can be lowered to just 100 IUs per day.

Tips for use. Studies have shown that vitamin E is even more effective when taken with vitamin C. The reason may be that when a vitamin E molecule is damaged by interacting with a free radical, C converts it back to its original form giving it, in effect, a second life.

Are there side effects? In some people vitamin E can cause nausea, diarrhea, and stomach discomfort. Taking it with food and water may help.

Caution! People with anemia, poorly clotting blood, liver disease, or overactive thyroid should not take vitamin E supplements without consulting a doctor. People taking blood-thinning medications should also avoid vitamin E.

OMEGA-3

WHAT IS OMEGA-3?

Most of us think of fat as bad because we generally eat far too much of it. But the fats known as essential fatty acids (EFAs for short) are actually necessary for the body. Of special interest are two types of EFAs, omega-3s and omega-6s. Although both are important, it's even more important to get the right balance of each. And if you eat a traditional American diet, you probably aren't getting enough omega-3s.

Because certain cold-water fish are rich in omega-3s, fish oil has become a popular supplement. In particular, fish oil contains two omega-3 fatty acids that are especially effective for keeping triglycerides low and cholesterol in balance. These are EPA (eicosapentaenoic acid) and DHA (docosahexaenoic acid).

THE MIRACLE EFFECT

Numerous studies have found an association between high intake of EPA- and DHA-rich fish products and low blood triglyceride levels. More important, adding these substances in supplement form has a triglyceride-lowering effect. In a world where mainstream medicine often looks harshly at natural remedies, this fact is no longer subject to even minor disputes. A survey of nearly seventy placebo-controlled studies found that adding fish oil supplements slashed triglyceride levels by 25 to 30 percent.

The reason for fish oil's effectiveness is still not completely known. Although researchers agree that EPA and DHA are the active substances, the complex chemical processes by which they work have yet to be traced.

HAS OMEGA-3 BEEN USED BEFORE?

As you can imagine, fish from cold waters has been a diet staple for people all over the world for thousands of years. It is only in recent times, when man has become wealthy enough to get more of his nourishment from red meat, cheese, and other dairy products, that fish intake has declined.

Its rediscovery began when Danish researcher Jorn Dyerberg noted that Greenland Eskimos had little heart disease despite their large consumption of rich, fatty fish. These findings inspired other researchers to examine isolated populations that also ate large quantities of EPA-rich fish. In each case, the findings were the same: more fish oil, less heart disease. Since then, millions of people have added fish oil or other omega-3-rich supplements to their daily regimen.

RESEARCH FINDINGS

As we noted above, dozens of studies attest to the ability of omega-3 and fish oil rich in omega-3 to dramatically lower triglycerides. In addition to innumerable animal studies, several studies have measured the effects of a diet rich in fish or fish oil supplements. The results have been overwhelmingly favorable. As one researcher concluded, for people with high triglycerides it is now "feasible to use fish oils as a drug of first choice."

The study that led to this conclusion compared the

effects of fish oil to those of a triglyceride-lowering medication widely used throughout Europe. Patients with high triglycerides and low HDL (good cholesterol) were divided into two groups. One group was treated with the traditional medication, the other group received 3,500 milligrams of omega-3 fatty acids a day. Although the prescription medication lowered triglycerides by 18 percent, omega-3 outperformed it, lowering levels by 23 percent. HDL levels increased in both groups.

In another study, patients with angina consumed 6,150 milligrams of omega-3s (in 4.4 ounces of canned sardines) each day for four weeks. Triglycerides plunged by 36.4 percent and LDLs (bad cholesterol) dropped by almost as much: 36 percent. Total cholesterol was lowered by 6.8 percent.

OTHER WAYS OMEGA-3 CAN HELP

In addition to lowering triglycerides, omega-3 works in several other ways to help guard against heart attack and stroke. It acts as a kind of natural blood thinner and keeps blood platelets from clumping together and forming dangerous blockages. It also strengthens the heart muscle, allowing it to contract more forcefully. Recent research suggests it may also help by reducing irregular heartbeat and lowering the chance of rapid, life-threatening, uncontrolled beating (known as ventricular fibrillation).

Omega-3s can help with other health problems as well. According to studies it can help people with rheumatoid arthritis (see chapter 2).

HOW TO TAKE OMEGA-3

What form does it come in? Omega-3 contained in fish oil comes in capsules. Omega-3s are also found in other oils, such as flaxseed oil, which are also sold in capsule form.

What's an effective dose? Since the mix and potency of omega-3 oils vary from product to product, be sure to follow the manufacturer's directions for the preparation you choose.

Tips for use. Omega-3 fatty acids can come from sources other than fish oil. However, fish oil has the richest concentration of EPA and DHA, the substances that are especially effective for lowering triglycerides.

Are there side effects? Omega-3 fish oil is considered generally safe when taken according to the manufacturer's package instructions. However, it may cause nausea in some people. To avoid this side effect, take with meals or divide your total daily intake into smaller doses taken throughout the day.

Caution! People taking blood-thinning medications, or people with blood that clots poorly, should not take these supplements without consulting a doctor.

GARLIC

WHAT IS GARLIC?

Garlic, the smelly but delicious little bulb used in cooking, turns out to have amazing health benefits. Eaten fresh, you'd have to consume more than might be socially acceptable to get all the benefits. Fortunately, you can also get garlic goodness in a tasteless, odorless supplement.

THE MIRACLE EFFECT

Garlic lowers the risk of heart attack and stroke by clearing the blood of cholesterol and other materials that can form blockages. Both fresh cloves of garlic and standardized preparations have been shown to:

- Lower overall serum cholesterol
- Increase HDL levels and lower levels of LDLs
- Work as antioxidants
- Act as natural blood thinners, helping to prevent clots by inhibiting the tendency of platelets to clump together

The substance thought to be responsible for most of these health benefits is allicin. There's just one catch. There's no allicin in garlic. Allicin is formed when two garlic substances, allin and allinase interact. Once formed, allicin has a very short life. Because of this, garlic supplements must be formulated so that allin and allinase are released and form allicin during the digestive process. If formulation is not done correctly, the garlic supplement may be inactive. For example, preparations that use heat or solvent extraction methods of processing contain no allinase and therefore have no allicin-releasing potential.

HAS GARLIC BEEN USED BEFORE?

Scientific interest in garlic dates back to the early 1930s, when a series of experiments revealed that artificially induced atherosclerosis (hardening of the arteries) in animals was significantly reversed when the animals were given fresh garlic juice or garlic extracts. Dozens of studies were undertaken as a result, and today garlic is used by millions. It is especially popular in Europe, where Germany's Commission E has officially approved it for use in lowering cholesterol.

RESEARCH FINDINGS

Numerous placebo-controlled double-blind human studies have found garlic extremely effective both for lowering total cholesterol and for improving the ratio of LDLs to HDLs. A few have also found it ineffective. What's behind these conflicting findings? One possibility is that the form of garlic used was ineffective. Another, more likely, explanation is that it takes garlic a good deal longer to work than some studies allow for.

The long time period needed for garlic's benefits to become evident was noted as far back as 1981. In a study published in the *American Journal of Clinical Nutrition,* garlic oil supplements were given to both healthy volunteers and patients with high cholesterol and heart disease. In both groups, the supplements lowered LDLs and raised HDLs—but this only became obvious after several months of use.

Another study found that a product containing both garlic and ginkgo extract lowered cholesterol in people with high readings by an average of 35 percent. The authors of this report concluded that garlic should be viewed as "continuous long-term therapy."

Studies showing that garlic works in shorter periods of time have often combined garlic with a cholesterol-lowering diet. This strategy would be expected to have a more-or-less immediate effect on cholesterol levels.

Another possibility for the conflicting findings is that garlic simply does not work for everyone. When study results are expressed as a group average, individual successes are overlooked. For example, in a study by Kenzelmann and Kade, forty-three patients with cholesterol levels ranging from 230 to 390 were enlisted to test the effectiveness of a garlic-ginkgo preparation. The two-month period surrounding the Christmas and New Year's period was chosen for the trial, and the patients were told to eat as they ordinarily would during the holiday season. Half of the patients received the active supplement and half received a placebo.

At the end of the trial, researchers found there were "no significant changes" in cholesterol levels of either group. However, when researchers looked at individual readings rather than the group average, they discovered that 35 percent of the people who received the active supplement *had* achieved a significant decrease in total cholesterol.

So many human studies have been done that we are not going to discuss the hundreds of animal studies here. However, one does bear mentioning because it provides an "inside view" of what garlic can accomplish. In 1996 Marquié and colleagues worked with obese rats that had high cholesterol and scarred arteries (similar to atherosclerosis). The rats were given a diet supplement of garlic combined with essential fatty acids. Not surprisingly, cholesterol rates fell. What *was* surprising was that the supplement had a healing effect, and the damaged arteries returned to normal.

OTHER WAYS GARLIC CAN HELP

Garlic's heart-helping powers work on a number of fronts. In addition to lowering cholesterol, garlic may help by:

- Inhibiting the release of a body chemical that causes blood vessels to constrict.
- Lowering blood pressure. Both prepared garlic supplement and fresh garlic have been shown to help reduce hypertension.

Garlic shows promise in other health areas as well. It fights microbes, which makes it useful for treating infection, colds, and flu (see chapter 8).

HOW TO TAKE GARLIC

What form does it come in? Garlic comes in tablets and capsules, both processed to eliminate odor.

What's an effective dose? The majority of studies have found garlic effective at doses of 900 milligrams a day, divided into three smaller doses. Be sure to look for a standardized product and to buy from a manufacturer you trust. Since standardization may vary, be sure to follow the manufacturer's package directions.

Tips for use. Garlic needs to be taken continuously to work. When garlic is withdrawn, cholesterol levels begin to rise. Some studies have shown that taking garlic and fish oil together is especially effective.

Are there side effects? Although garlic is considered quite safe, some people may experience a burning sensation in the mouth, throat, or gastric intestinal tract, and bouts of stomach upset and diarrhea have also been reported.

Caution! People whose blood is slow to clot, or who are taking blood-thinning medications should not take garlic.

WHAT ELSE CAN YOU DO?

The remedies in this chapter are not a license to ignore the dietary changes you know you should make. In addition to making these changes and incorporating the supplements we've already discussed, there are several more nutrients you should know about.

PANTETHINE

Since the 1980s, animal studies have been telling us that pantethine, a derivative of pantothenic acid (vitamin B5), can help lower cholesterol and triglyceride levels. Now human studies are backing that up. In one trial, women with high cholesterol readings were given 900 milligrams a day of pantethine. After four months, total cholesterol as well as LDL cholesterol were significantly reduced, while the ratio of LDLs to HDLs improved. Another study recommends that only 500 milligrams a day of pantethine are necessary for effective results.

GUGGUL

Also known as gugulipid, this nutrient is just beginning to be investigated by researchers in Europe and the United States. Guggul products are derived from the mukul, a small tree native to India and closely related to the tree that gives us myrrh (and myrrh, as you may remember, was the fragrant gift given by one of the three wise men).

In India, where almost all of the research has been done, guggul is widely used for lowering cholesterol and triglycerides. A 500-milligram daily dose of guggul has helped patients lower cholesterol by 11 percent and triglycerides by 16.8 percent.

When guggul is combined with dietary changes, the results are even more impressive, with 70 percent to 80 percent of patients achieving lower serum cholesterol (average 23.6 percent decline) and triglycerides (average 22.6 percent decline).

Although guggul is now available throughout the world, it hasn't yet become widely recommended for two reasons: Long-term studies have yet to prove that it's safe for continued use, and it hasn't been studied on patients whose Western diets are much different from the traditional Indian diet.

HAWTHORN

Hawthorn is known as weissdorn in Europe, where its popularity began. This number one heart-strengthening herb has a secondary benefit for those concerned with cardiovascular health—it appears to lower LDL cholesterol as well as triglycerides. For more about this outstanding herb, see chapter 13 on Heart Disease and Coronary Artery Disease.

VITAMIN C

Like hawthorn, vitamin C's main heart-helping activity is the strengthening, protective effect it has on cardiovascular tissues. Like hawthorn, it has a secondary benefit in helping to control serum levels of cholesterol and triglycerides. Vitamin C may help prevent heart attacks in another way as well. Excess iron, typical of a diet rich in animal proteins, has been linked to heart disease. Intake of vitamin C has been shown to lower the concentration of iron in the blood. For more on vitamin C's heart benefits, see chapter 13.

CHAPTER EIGHT

Rapid Recovery from
Colds, Cough, and Other Upper Respiratory Infections

Whether you want to stop a cold before it starts or recover quickly once the sniffles have started, nature has a solution for you.

Have you ever been told that the only thing you can do about a cold is to wait and let the virus run its course? Well, it's true that getting antibiotics from a doctor probably won't help much. But it's just as true that some natural aids can make symptoms milder and help you get back on your feet sooner.

THE PROBLEM

Medical science can give you a new hip, perform delicate surgery on infants before they're born, and look inside your genes—but after thousands of years of effort, it still can't cure the common cold. How come? Because there is really no such thing as *the* common cold—there are many. In fact, there are so many different strains of cold virus that by the time you've developed an immunity to one, you're likely to be exposed to another. In addition to colds, there are a host of other viruses that affect the upper respiratory tract, producing symptoms ranging from sore throat to laryngitis to aches and chills.

WHO GETS THESE INFECTIONS?

Everyone is susceptible to cold and upper respiratory tract viruses. Some people are more likely to become ill because their exposure is greater. For example, children in day care centers and schoolrooms pass colds along to each other, their teachers, and their families. People who ride crowded buses or trains have greater exposure than people who drive to work alone or work at home. Since the only way to safeguard yourself would be to retreat to a sterilized room and stay there, there's no practical way to cut your risks completely.

WHAT ARE THE SYMPTOMS?

A range of symptoms are associated with upper respiratory tract infections, including:

- Sneezing
- Runny nose
- Stuffiness
- Clogged sinuses
- Cough
- Sore throat
- Laryngitis
- Headache
- Earache
- General body achiness
- Fatigue

Not all upper respiratory infections are alike, and the symptoms depend on which strain of virus you've contracted.

WHAT'S THE OUTLOOK?

An upper respiratory tract virus should run its course in about five to seven days, although some symptoms may linger on for a few days.

WHAT YOU NEED TO KNOW

A common cold doesn't require a trip to the doctor. However, some of its symptoms are similar to symptoms of more serious ailments that do warrant medical attention. See your doctor if:

- Your symptoms are accompanied by high fever.
- You have pain in your chest (lungs) or shoulders.
- Some symptoms, such as cough, laryngitis, or sniffles, simply will not go away.

PROVEN MIRACLES

ECHINACEA

WHAT IS ECHINACEA?

Echinacea (also known as purple coneflower) is a member of the daisy family with attractive lavender or purple flowers. Several varieties of echinacea have been used by herbalists, including E. angustifolia, E. pallida, and E. purpurea. The miraculous powers of this plant come from its above-ground parts, although some studies suggest its roots and rhizomes may also be useful.

THE MIRACLE EFFECT

Some people think of echinacea as *the* remedy for colds. It is. But thinking of it in *only* that way is overlooking a lot. Echinacea doesn't act specifically on cold viruses. It's an all-purpose infection fighter that, research suggests, stimulates the body's immune system in a number of different ways.

Below are a few of the benefits that tests have shown echinacea to provide:

- Promotes the specialized process in which certain cells surround and devour harmful microorganisms.
- Encourages white blood cells to migrate to the site of infection.
- Boosts the activity of disease-fighting white blood cells and increases the production of antibodies and other helpful substances.
- Reduces inflammation, largely by inhibiting an enzyme that breaks down cells and allows them to be easily invaded.

Few herbs have been as chemically analyzed as echinacea, and hundreds of studies are available. While polysaccharides have most often been named as the source of the plant's beneficial effect, a number of other active substances have also been identified as active.

HAS ECHINACEA BEEN USED BEFORE?

The first Europeans who came to America found a hostile, inhospitable wilderness. But to Native Americans, this "wilderness" was a rich source of food, clothing, shelter, and even medicine. Remains of echinacea have been found by archaeologists investigating campsites of the Sioux, suggesting that this herb has been in use for hundreds (and perhaps thousands) of years. Newcomers learned about echinacea from these natives and began to discuss it in medical journals around the middle of the nineteenth century.

In the 1870s a Nebraskan doctor prepared a patent medicine of echinacea and later convinced a national pharmaceutical manufacturer to market the product. During the first two decades of the twentieth century, echinacea was extremely popular as an infection fighter throughout America. It fell into disuse when sulfa drugs came in in the 1930s. However, its use has continued in Europe, where contemporary research has continued to support the use of this drug.

Germany's Commission E has approved echinacea for supportive use in the treatment of respiratory and urinary tract infections, meaning it should be used in addition to (not instead of) other appropriate medications. The German habit of reaching for echinacea at the first sign of a cold is spreading, and over the past few years more and more Americans have come to swear by this native plant for dealing with the sniffles.

RESEARCH FINDINGS

Numerous studies have proven that echinacea is a highly effective infection fighter. The problem with these studies is that for the most part they evaluate echinacea given by injection rather than orally. This hasn't daunted consumer enthusiasm for the oral version of echinacea. It just means that at the moment more research needs to be done before oral echinacea can be declared effective for all the infections it works against when taken by injection. However, Bauer and Wagner, who have done a great deal of respected research on this herb, believe that oral preparations are at least comparable to (and perhaps even better than) injectable preparations.

Other recent studies conducted with oral preparations of echinacea uphold the conclusions of Bauer and Wagner. Consider these findings:

- In a double-blind placebo-controlled study, Braunig and colleagues found that echinacea drops, taken orally, outperformed placebo both in relieving upper respiratory symptoms and in shortening their duration.

- A 1992 article published in *Forum Immunologie* found that echinacea not only helped immediate symptoms, but helped ward off new infection. In a double-blind study, volunteers with a history of chronic upper respiratory tract infections (three or more in the past half-year) received either oral echinacea or a placebo. Not only did volunteers who received echinacea have milder symptoms of shorter duration, 36 percent of them suffered no recurrent infections during the two months of the trial.

- In a 1995 study, Melchart and colleagues found that an oral preparation of echinacea root extract "significantly enhanced" immune system activity as compared to placebo.

OTHER WAYS ECHINACEA CAN HELP

As we mentioned above, more studies need to be done to determine whether oral echinacea works as well as injectable echinacea against a range of infections. To date, we know that oral echinacea is a helpful addition to regular medical treatment for yeast infections, including vaginal yeast infections.

Researchers have also been able to prove the validity of another folkloric use of this herb—its potency as a topical application. Echinacea-based preparations designed for external use have been effective for a variety of skin problems, including cuts, abrasions, burns, and other inflammatory conditions.

HOW TO TAKE ECHINACEA

What form does it come in? Echinacea comes in a variety of forms, including capsules, tablets, extracts, drops, and even fresh juice.

What's an effective dose? Since dosage will vary depending on the form of echinacea you take and the potency of the individual product, be sure to follow the manufacturer's package directions.

Tips for use. For best results, start taking echinacea at the first sign of symptoms. Echinacea should not be taken for extended periods of time (see Caution, below).

Are there side effects? Side effects are not common when echinacea is taken in recommended doses. However, there have been a few reports of stomach upsets and diarrhea, both of which disappear when dosage is withdrawn.

Caution! Echinacea should not be taken for extended periods, and Commission E stipulates a maximum of eight weeks at a time. Because this is a plant product, some people may be allergic. If you develop skin irritation, rash, or itching, discontinue use at once. People with systemic illnesses (such as lupus, tuberculosis, and multiple sclerosis) should avoid echinacea.

VITAMIN C

WHAT IS VITAMIN C?

Vitamin C is a necessary, water-soluble nutrient. Because it cannot be stored by the body, it must be consumed on a regular basis. Although vitamin C is abundant in fruits and many vegetables, there is strong evidence to support taking extra C in supplemental form.

THE MIRACLE EFFECT

In 1971 Nobel prize–winner Linus Pauling put vitamin C on the map with the spectacular claim that the vitamin could, among other things, ward off colds. Whether this is true or not remains open to scientific debate. Many studies show that it wards off colds only in people who are deficient in this vitamin or under physical stress, such as athletes. Balanced against this are millions of users who swear by C, and one very interesting study using twins. In this test, pairs of twins were divided, and one of each pair was given vitamin C while the other was given a placebo. The group of twins taking vitamin C caught fewer colds than the group that received placebo pills.

Another claim of Pauling's, however, turned out to be unassailable—his assertion that, once a cold descends, taking vitamin C will make the symptoms fewer, milder, and shorter lasting. Research has found that vitamin C stimulates the immune system by stepping up production of the specialized cells that search out and destroy invaders. Vitamin C also stimulates the migration of these cells to the site of infection.

HAS VITAMIN C BEEN USED BEFORE?

You're probably familiar with one of the earliest uses of vitamin C to prevent illness—through the stories about sailors who, during the age of exploration, discovered that a supply of citrus fruit on board could forestall scurvy. These and other anecdotes led to early acceptance of this vitamin. However, vitamin C has also had supporters in modern times.

The big debate hasn't been whether or not to take vitamin C but how, and how much, to take. Some people contend that only "natural" forms of vitamin C are useful. Others insist that since vitamin C can't be stored in the body, taking more than one needs is a pointless waste of money. In the 1940s, for example, physician Fred Klenner helped polio victims with high dosages of C. Three decades later, Linus Pauling became a tireless spokesman for vitamin C, advocating it for a wide range of uses, including cancer prevention. Though Pauling was greeted with skepticism by many colleagues, the public listened and made vitamin C one of the best-selling supplements on the market.

As Pauling's research has been substantiated over the years, C's popularity has continued, and more and more former skeptics have come to recommend it as a supplement.

RESEARCH FINDINGS

Vitamin C may be the best known, most written about, and most researched vitamin in existence. Despite this, many people remain unsure about its benefits.

Can vitamin C really help stop colds and upper respiratory infections? Or is that claim, as some researchers have suggested, hyperbole? Until recently, both points of view could be backed up by research. However, a recent review of the literature found that the picture isn't as murky as once thought. Writing in the *Journal of the American College of Nutrition,* the authors of the review concluded that, "The current notion that vitamin C has no effect on the common cold seems to be based in large part on a faulty review written two decades ago." In fact, a review of twenty-one placebo-controlled studies done between 1971 and 1993 showed that all of these studies found vitamin C effective for shortening the length of colds as well as alleviating symptoms.

OTHER WAYS VITAMIN C CAN HELP

Because vitamin C stimulates the immune system, it can help battle a number of infectious conditions. Harri Hemila, a leading authority on vitamin C, has suggested that supplements may decrease susceptibility to pneumonia. Beyond that, vitamin C can play a role in:

- **Heart health.** Vitamin C promotes arterial health and flexibility, reducing the risk of blockage and constriction in the arteries that feed the heart (see chapter 13). It also helps lower LDL (harmful) cholesterol and raises (helpful) HDL (see chapter 7).

- **Cancer.** A diet high in vitamin C seems to lower the risk of several types of cancer. Other studies have shown that very large doses of this vitamin prolong life in some cancer sufferers (see chapter 6).
- **Asthma and allergies.** Vitamin C helps protect bronchial tubes and lung tissue, as well as acting to reduce inflammation (see chapter 3).
- **Wound healing.** Studies have shown that vitamin C promotes repair of skin wounds and sores, even in people not considered deficient in the vitamin (see chapter 23).

HOW TO TAKE VITAMIN C

What form does it come in? Most people take vitamin C supplements in capsules, tablets, or chewable tablets.

What's an effective dose? Most nutritionists believe that taking more vitamin C than the officially recommended daily values is beneficial. Studies showing vitamin C as effective for colds and cold symptoms deal with dosages of 600 to 2,000 milligrams a day. Harri Hemila's review of twenty-one studies found that 1,000 milligrams of vitamin C significantly reduced both symptoms and duration of symptoms in cold sufferers.

Tips for use. Since the body cannot store reserves of vitamin C, divide your daily intake into several smaller doses and take throughout the day.

Are there side effects? Even in large doses, vitamin C is considered safe and nontoxic. It does, however, have a very common side effect: bowel discomfort and diarrhea. Building up slowly to find your own tolerance level, taking the vitamin with meals, or trying a form that combines C with calcium or magnesium and has a buffering effect are good strategies for minimizing this problem.

Caution! Some obstetricians warn against taking high doses of vitamin C during pregnancy. If you've been taking this vitamin and become pregnant, or are pregnant and want to begin taking it, consult your doctor first.

ZINC

WHAT IS ZINC?

Zinc is a trace mineral distributed throughout the body. However, most of this zinc is locked away in bone and other tissues and is not available for use. To be healthy, we need a steady supply of zinc. Based on studies of the average American diet, many nutritionists now conclude that the average American diet is zinc-deficient.

THE MIRACLE EFFECT

We know that zinc is essential to cells, including the myriad cells that fight viruses and infections. This led researchers to test the idea that taking zinc supplements could help ease cold symptoms. The theory worked, and cold sufferers found that zinc was especially helpful for certain symptoms. The symptoms that zinc helps most include:

- Congestion
- Runny nose
- Cough
- Headache
- Sore throat
- Laryngitis

HAS ZINC BEEN USED BEFORE?

In the 1980s, zinc was suddenly all the rage for colds and coughs. Then, just as suddenly, the hype went away. Only in the late 1990s did new reports shed light on the confusion.

The fuss began when a 1984 report found zinc lozenges extremely helpful for cold symptoms. Subsequent studies done over the next few years failed to repeat the findings, and scientific enthusiasm for zinc subsided. Nevertheless, many users continued to insist that zinc worked for colds. The source of the confusion came to light when researchers Godfrey and colleagues did a careful review of the earlier studies. They found that several of the tests used an inactive form of zinc, or gave it in doses too small to be effective. In view of this, the people who have continued to rely on zinc may soon be joined by many more users.

RESEARCH FINDINGS

Although users insist zinc makes cold symptoms milder, "severity" is a matter of personal judgment, making assessment difficult. Easier to measure is the length of time it takes to recover, and here zinc has a clearly impressive record.

A double-blind placebo-controlled study done on young adults found that zinc lozenges significantly shortened the duration of colds, from 6.1 days in the placebo group to 4.9 days in the group that took zinc. A similar study found an even greater difference for zinc versus placebo groups.

SYMPTOM	DURATION IN PLACEBO GROUP VS. ZINC GROUP
Congestion	7.0 days vs. 4.0 days
Coughing	4.5 days vs. 2.0 days
Headache	3.0 days vs. 2.0 days
Hoarseness	3.0 days vs. 2.0 days
Sore throat	3.0 days vs. 1.0 days

OTHER WAYS ZINC CAN HELP

You don't need zinc just when you have a cold. You need it all the time. As we've already mentioned, nutritionally oriented practitioners are becoming increasingly concerned that modern diets leave even healthy, well-nourished people zinc-deficient. Zinc deficiency may contribute to macular degeneration, a common cause of blindness. Over one-third of people with Crohn's disease, a gastrointestinal disorder, are deficient in zinc.

HOW TO TAKE ZINC

What form does it come in? Zinc comes in capsules, tablets, chewable tablets, and liquid form. Zinc comes combined with other substances, so you may have to choose between zinc sulphate, zinc gluconate, zinc picolinate, and so on. Most testing has been done with zinc gluconate, and that's the variety most people choose. While zinc sulphate is also effective, it causes stomach upset in some users.

What's an effective dose? Since overdosing on zinc is a concern, calibrating effective dosage guidelines is important. A Danish study gave each volunteer a lozenge containing 4.5 milligrams of zinc every one-and-a-half waking hours and found this dose too low to be effective. Other studies have found that dosages of 13.3 to 23 milligrams of zinc every other waking hour relieved symptoms and shortened duration. These levels should only be taken for short periods of time, and maximum daily intake should not exceed 150 milligrams.

Tips for use. For best results, start taking zinc at the first onset of symptoms.

Are there side effects? Zinc tablets may cause mouth irritation and nausea in some people.

Caution! While zinc is an essential nutrient, too much can be harmful. Studies show that taking 200 milligrams a day can cause deficiencies of other important nutrients and may even contribute to anemia. Other studies have shown that dosages exceeding 300 milligrams daily actually *lower* immunity.

WHAT ELSE CAN YOU DO?

When you have a really nasty cold, cough, or upper respiratory infection, you definitely want to hit it with everything you've got. Don't overlook these tried and true helpers.

GO WITH GARLIC

Over the past decade, garlic has gotten so much publicity for its cancer-fighting, heart-helping capabilities that its older uses have been overshadowed. That's too bad, because garlic has a long and honorable reputation when it comes to colds, flu, and other infections. It turns out that quaint Old-World wisdom about the powers of garlic is absolutely true. The source of these powers? Test tube and other studies have shown that substances in garlic have a powerful antiviral effect. Moreover, many strains of bacteria and microbacteria are extremely vulnerable to garlic. For more about garlic, see chapter 7.

THE POWER OF GINGER

If you have clogged sinuses, the idea of ginger tea, with its sharp flavor and pungent scent, may sound especially appealing. Ginger is more than just a good idea—whether in tea or capsule form, ginger really *can* help when you have a cold. Here is yet another folk remedy that turns out to have solid grounding in science. The reason? When chemically analyzed, ginger has been found to contain several different substances that act specifically against cold viruses. For more about ginger, see chapter 11 on the Digestive System.

STOP A COUGH WITH LICORICE

Licorice (not the candy or the flavoring) is also known as glycyrrhiza, glycyrrhizin, or glycyrrhizic acid and is a long-standing favorite for suppressing coughs. Some reputable nutritionists claim there is ample scientific support for this, while others say the jury is still out. If you want to try licorice for a cough, remember that many commercial syrups and lozenges contain no real licorice at all. Buy from a reputable health food store or vitamin shop, and watch out for candylike remedies that may contain only flavoring and sugar.

Also, be aware that unless licorice is treated, it is glycyrrhized, and prolonged ingestion of glycyrrhized licorice can have serious side effects, including elevated blood pressure. Because of this you must limit use to a temporary basis—no longer than four to six weeks. Using deglycyrrhizinated licorice is one way to avoid problems, and many herbalists recommend products made from it even though it is less potent than glycyrrhized licorice. Finally, licorice is not recommended for use by people with cardiovascular disorders.

A detailed discussion of licorice can be found in chapter 11, on the Digestive System.

CHAPTER NINE

You Can Overcome
Depression

Prozac may be a depression sensation in the United States, but in Germany a safe, natural substance outsells it by a wide margin.

Without a doubt, depression is an exceptionally common disorder. The American Psychiatric Association estimates that anywhere from 7 to 18 percent of us will suffer a bout of clinical depression at some point in our lives. While prescription medications can help a good deal, most chemical antidepressants have very uncomfortable side effects. Moreover, they can be quite expensive. Today, an effective natural antidepressant is helping millions of people around the world, without the objectionable side effects and at about one-eighth the cost.

THE PROBLEM

Everyone has a down day now and then, and everyone goes through ordinary periods of sadness. Feeling gloomy, disappointed, or heartbroken in response to events such as loss, death, or divorce are normal and should not be considered cases of depression. However, if these feelings persist beyond a more or less normal period, or if they arise seemingly "out of nowhere," when life is going on much as it was before, one may well be suffering from depression.

WHO GETS DEPRESSION?

Some people are far more likely to get a case of the blues than others. Of course, life circumstances can affect one's outlook, but *what* happens doesn't seem to be as important as *who* it happens to. The two factors that most influence one's chances of suffering from depression are:

- **Family history.** Depression runs in families, and the nature–nurture controversy comes down in this case on the side of nature. In other words, it isn't a pattern of nurturing and child-rearing that contributes to the problem, but a biological predisposition that is passed along.

- **Being a woman.** Women are approximately twice as likely as men to report feelings of depression. Why this is so has been the subject of much speculation. Some insist that women find themselves in depression-promoting circumstances such as poverty and dependency more often than men do. These arguments haven't won acceptance among clinicians, who are more inclined to look at hormonal and other factors. Also, many suggest that depressed women manifest classic signs of the disorder, while depressed men are more likely to act out their feelings through aggression, alcoholism, and in extreme cases, acts of violence.

WHAT ARE THE SYMPTOMS?

Depression can make itself known in many ways, not all of them obvious. Few people have all the possible symptoms of depression, but most depressed people have several of the following:

- **Feelings of pervasive sadness.** You feel blue much of the day, almost every day.
- **Feeling bad about yourself.** Feelings of worthlessness and unwarranted guilt are common features of depression.
- **Loss of pleasure.** Activities that used to make you happy no longer do so. There is little in life that gives you true pleasure.
- **Apathy.** You are uninterested in work, hobbies, projects, friends, and family. You often feel you "just don't care" about anything anymore.
- **Difficulty concentrating.** Your mind tends to wander and even routine mental tasks challenge your ability to focus.
- **Lethargy and fatigue.** You don't have much energy, and even small chores seem to call for a major effort.
- **Restlessness.** You may feel on edge and agitated, or your friends may ask you why you've become uncharacteristically jumpy and fidgety.
- **Change in sleep patterns.** You may find it difficult to get enough sleep or may find yourself sleeping far, far too much.
- **Change in eating patterns.** You may overeat, over-

indulge in junk foods, or lose your appetite and find it difficult to eat anything at all.

WHAT'S THE OUTLOOK?

Left untreated, bouts of depression can last several months. After that, they may vanish completely or improve somewhat, leaving behind a welter of troubling symptoms. People can have a form of low-grade depression, known as dysthymia, that extends across years. Even when depression resolves itself, it is likely to come back, and many clinicians feel depression should be looked at as a chronic disorder.

All of this may sound glum, but fortunately, depression can be treated. Antidepressants, therapy, and counseling, or a combination, have helped millions of people bid a permanent farewell to the blues.

WHAT YOU NEED TO KNOW

Although we use the term depression to describe feelings of sadness that won't go away, there are several specific types of depression, as well as several degrees of severity. For example, you have undoubtedly heard of manic-depression, the old term for bipolar disorder where bouts of depression are interspersed with periods of unusual euphoria. There is also psychotic depression, in which the person literally loses touch with reality, and suicidal depression, in which the person has recurrent thoughts of escape through death.

All these depressions are quite serious and require prompt attention from a trained therapist. There is no evidence that any of the strategies described in this chapter will work for these most serious forms of depression.

PROVEN MIRACLES

ST. JOHN'S WORT

WHAT IS ST. JOHN'S WORT?

Don't be confused by the word wort—it has nothing whatever to do with the bumpy little skin condition, wart. "Wort" is the Old English word for "plant," and an indicator of just how long this remedy has been around. The flowering tops of the plant are the most potent parts and are generally used in preparation of the extracts that are sold throughout the world. Today, you might find products made from this plant referred to either as St. John's wort or by variations of its scientific name, hypericum perforatum. You might also hear references to "LI 160," the form of the extract used in many European studies.

THE MIRACLE EFFECT

Dozens of studies have shown that extract of St. John's wort, taken internally, is effective for mild to moderate depression. In particular, many specific, troubling symptoms of depression have proven extremely responsive to it. These include:
- Feelings of sadness
- Feelings of worthlessness
- Apathy
- Anxiety
- Lethargy

- Feeling tired and fatigued
- Sleep disturbances

One study has found that St. John's wort also works for people who have seasonal affective disorder (SAD), the form of depression that comes in the late fall and winter months and is related to the loss of daylight.

What makes St. John's wort so effective? Surprisingly, despite its long history of success, researchers haven't quite pinned down the answer. For some time, it was suggested that St. John's wort works like the group of synthetic antidepressants known as MAO inhibitors, or MAOIs. These drugs work by interfering with monoamine oxidase, a brain chemical that breaks down certain mood-regulating neurotransmitters. However, studies agree that the MAOI-like activity of St. John's wort is probably not strong enough to explain its effectiveness. Other researchers have suggested that St. John's wort works like Prozac, preventing the reabsorption of the mood-regulating neurotransmitter, serotonin. Other studies have investigated the effect of St. John's wort on other neurotransmitters, but no clear-cut answers have emerged. In fact, research is still under way to determine which substance, or combination of substances, in the plant make it so effective for dealing with depression.

In addition to effectively combating the symptoms of depression, St. John's wort has another feature that makes it popular with users: lack of troublesome side effects. Prescription antidepressants can produce several uncomfortable side effects, including dry mouth, weight gain, and loss of sex drive. None of these have been reported by users of St. John's wort.

HAS ST. JOHN'S WORT BEEN USED BEFORE?

St. John's wort has been used for a variety of medicinal purposes since the era of Hippocrates, more than 2,000 years ago. Its use as an antidepressant dates back at least to the Middle Ages. Like many natural remedies, it fell into disuse in the nineteenth and early twentieth centuries. In the early 1980s German researchers, prompted by favorable reports on St. John's wort tea, revived interest in the plant. Today, St. John's wort is listed in the official pharmacopoeias of several European countries and is especially popular in Germany where it accounts for more than half of all antidepressant medications sold. *New York Times* consumer health writer Jane Brody has noted that by 1994 Germans were using sixty-six million doses daily, and German doctors turned to prescription drugs only when St. John's wort proved ineffective.

RESEARCH FINDINGS

St. John's wort is one of the most-tested natural remedies in existence, and so many studies have produced such positive reports that even the most staunch disbelievers can find little to argue about. Here are results of just a few of the carefully conducted studies:

- In one of the earliest large trials of St. John's wort, conducted by Drs. Sommer and Harrer of Salzburg University, 105 people with mild depression were divided into two groups. Sixty-seven percent of the group who received St. John's wort reported significant improvement after four weeks of treatment, while those in the group receiving look-alike placebo pills did not.

- In a study published in 1994, Germany's Dr. W. D. Hubner and colleagues treated half of thirty-nine patients suffering from depression with St. John's wort. After four weeks of treatment, 70 percent of these patients were completely free of depression-related symptoms such as fatigue, lethargy, and disturbed sleep.

- St. John's wort measures up well against prescription medications. Results of several studies have shown St. John's wort to be as effective for relieving moderate depression as prescription medications. When Vorbach, Hubner, and Arnoldt compared St. John's wort to the popular chemical antidepressant imipramine, they concluded that there were "comparable results in both treatment groups," although St. John's wort produced "fewer and milder side effects."

- In 1997 Swedish researchers published a report in *Lakartidningen,* analyzing the findings of twenty-five independent clinical trials of St. John's wort. It was found that 61 percent of the patients improved on a very low dose of St. John's wort, while 75 percent improved on a higher dosage similar to the amount given in other trials.

OTHER WAYS ST. JOHN'S WORT CAN HELP

The remarkable and proven effectiveness of St. John's wort as an antidepressant has prompted researchers to investigate other potential healing properties—with some surprising results. A number of reports have found that St. John's wort has a significant effect against viruses and retroviruses in lab studies. Because of its activity against retroviruses, it is currently being evaluated as a potential agent in the battle against AIDS.

St. John's wort may turn out to be a helper on another major battlefield as well: cancer. Two reports, one published in 1994 and the other in 1996, suggest it may have a chemotherapeutic effect against gliomas, the most common group of cancers affecting the brain.

HOW TO TAKE ST. JOHN'S WORT

What form does it come in? Although St. John's wort can be bought in dried form and ingested as a tea, there are no studies indicating how effective this form of the herb might be. Most people take it as an extract in pills or capsules.

What's an effective dose? The majority of European studies tested people on a daily dosage ranging from 300 to 900 milligrams total of extract LI 160 per day, divided into three doses. Since the form you may purchase may be standardized to a different potency, be sure to follow the manufacturer's package instruction.

Tips for use. Like chemical antidepressants, St. John's wort isn't an instant cure. While some people may feel an improvement in the first two weeks, many people find that the full benefits of the herb are not felt until they have been taking it for three to five weeks. Since many people respond to St. John's wort at a low dosage, we suggest starting with the minimum recommended by the manufacturer and increasing the dosage only if you fail to see results in a reasonable time.

Are there side effects? People taking St. John's wort have reported fewer and milder side effects than people taking prescription antidepressants. In clinical trials, less than 1 percent of those on St. John's wort stopped taking it because they experienced uncomfortable side effects, while 3 percent stopped taking the prescription medications for this reason. Sexual dysfunction, dry mouth, and headache often associated with chemical antidepressants have not been reported with St. John's wort.

Side effects most commonly associated with use of this herb are gastrointestinal upsets, fatigue, and restlessness. One study estimated that 0.5 percent of those who tried the herb had an allergic reaction to it characterized by a skin rash. These discomforts are reversible and disappear when use is discontinued.

In addition to these minor side effects, a more serious problem has been reported. In extremely rare cases, a few users have developed photosensitivity—itching and sores on areas of the skin exposed to light. Again, the problem abated when the herb was withdrawn.

Caution! St. John's wort should never be taken in combination with any other type of antidepressant. If you have recently stopped taking antidepressants, allow a two-to-four-week "washout" period before beginning St. John's wort.

Since several drugs, including tetracyclines, can increase the risk of photosensitive reactions, consult your doctor before taking St. John's wort, if you are taking any form of medication.

Finally, St. John's wort has been proven to cause uterine contractions in lab animals and, to be on the safe side, should be avoided by pregnant women.

WHAT ABOUT THE MAOI FACTOR?

One thing that makes the class of prescription antidepressants known as MAO inhibitors (or MAOIs) difficult to take is the list of dietary restrictions that goes with them. Chemical substances in red wine, aged cheeses, salami, and other foods can interact with MAOIs to cause dangerous rises in blood pressure. Since St. John's wort has some MAOI-like action, people wonder whether the same dietary restrictions apply. There are no reports of this kind of adverse reaction, and researchers point out that in recommended doses the chances of such a reaction are negligible. However, some experts feel that caution should be taken. If you have any questions, or experience a flush or tingling when using this herb, consult your doctor at once.

WHAT ELSE CAN YOU DO?

Although St. John's wort is the most effective nutrient known for cases of mild to moderate depression, there are a few other factors you should consider if you can't seem to shake the blues.

THE GLUTAMINE CONNECTION

Back in 1976 a promising study appeared in a well-respected psychiatric journal published in Belgium. In the study, forty-three adults with depression improved on L-glutamine supplement. Although the study wasn't followed up, there is reason to believe the researchers were on the right track. Glutamine, a common amino acid in the human body, facilitates a brain chemical known as GABA, one of several mood-influencing neurotransmitters in the central nervous system.

LIGHT IT UP

If you suffer from seasonal affective disorder, which results from loss of light during the winter months, you might consider light therapy. Exposure to very bright light for a period of time each day can improve mood considerably. Although it was previously thought this light worked by entering the body through the retina, researchers at Cornell University found that shining a 13,000 lux light on the back of the knees was as good as shining it on the eyes. Authors of the study added that the backs of knees had been chosen as an arbitrary site, and asserted that shining the light anywhere on the skin would have produced similar results.

CHAPTER TEN

Protect Against
Diabetic Damage

*If you have diabetes, you already know of the
many health complications it can cause. But do
you know what complementary medicine can
do about them? You will after you read this
chapter.*

Diabetes bears the dubious distinction of being one of
the fastest-growing diseases in America today. Whether
it is the type that develops early in life or the type that
begins in middle age or later, diabetes is a disorder that
must be taken seriously. Medical management is a must.
But that doesn't mean there's nothing you yourself can
do to improve your overall health. With a few alterations
in your vitamin and nutrient program, you may be able to
do yourself more good than you know.

THE PROBLEM

If you have diabetes, you understand that this disorder
involves much more than watching what you eat.

Diabetes weakens veins, arteries and capillaries. Infections of the legs and feet and, in severe cases, even

gangrene can occur when blood fails to carry oxygen to the extremities. Hemorrhages in tiny capillaries can destroy vision. And kidney damage can be serious enough to require dialysis.

Although medical science has made great strides in managing this disease, it hasn't yet found a cure. That's why so many diabetics feel frustrated. It's dispiriting to follow doctor's advice to the letter and know your efforts won't yield perfect results.

Nevertheless, taking care of yourself will help make diabetes a disease you can live with and manage. And the recent findings on nutritional therapy described in this chapter make that task easier than ever before.

WHO SUFFERS FROM DIABETIC DAMAGE?

Diabetes is a complex disease. It is also a disease whose chemistry changes from day to day. This is why, if you have diabetes, it is important to be vigilant about diet and blood monitoring. The daily stress diabetes puts on the body becomes even greater when there is no control.

Unfortunately, many people may be walking around with untreated diabetes. According to one recent estimate, only about half of the sixteen million Americans who have diabetes are aware of their condition. With that in mind, it pays to review the leading risk factors for diabetes. They are:

- **Family history.** Diabetes has a strong genetic link. If you have a parent or sibling with diabetes, you are at risk.
- **Ethnic group.** Some groups are especially vulnerable to diabetes. In the United States, Native Ameri-

cans, African Americans, and Latinos have higher rates of this disorder than others.
- **Weight.** Being even moderately overweight adds to the risk of developing diabetes.
- **Age.** Juvenile diabetes usually becomes apparent before the person reaches adulthood. The most common form of diabetes, adult-onset (or Type II) diabetes, usually develops after the age of thirty.

WHAT ARE THE SYMPTOMS?

Your first line of defense against diabetes is to get it properly diagnosed. This is important, since many people develop the adult onset (Type II) form of the disease and live with it for some time without knowing they have it.

Consult a doctor if you frequently suffer from one or more of these symptoms:
- Excessive thirst
- Unexplained weight loss
- Periodic bouts of blurry vision
- Extreme and persistent fatigue, even when you get enough sleep

WHAT'S THE OUTLOOK?

Juvenile (Type I) diabetes is the most serious form of the disorder, and requires lifelong medication and management. The more common form, adult-onset (Type II) diabetes, is far more responsive to intervention. Many people can eliminate or greatly improve the condition by losing weight, monitoring their diet, and making other lifestyle changes.

WHAT YOU SHOULD KNOW

As we said above, the first and most important thing you should determine is whether or not you have diabetes. This is easy to find out and doesn't involve expensive or exotic testing. If you've had a physical lately, a routine check for diabetes was certainly one of the tests performed. If you haven't had a checkup lately and are at risk for this disease, make an appointment today.

PROVEN MIRACLES

OPC
(FOUND IN PYCNOGENOLS, GRAPE SEED EXTRACT, AND OTHER SOURCES)

WHAT IS OPC?

OPCs, pycnogenols, pine bark extract, grape seed extract—what *are* these substances anyway? Let's set the record straight right now. OPCs (short for oligomeric proanthocyanidin) are antioxidant flavonoids. Like other flavonoids, OPCs are found in a variety of plants. Two plant sources are especially rich in OPCs: pine bark extracts (marketed as pycnogenols) and grape seed extract.

In other words, if you take pine bark extract (pycnogenols) or grape seed extract, you will be taking OPCs in each case, but in a different mix because they are derived from different sources. In Europe, OPCs have been found so effective that they are available as patented medication.

THE MIRACLE EFFECT

In recent years, researchers have begun to look at diabetes in a whole new way. Instead of focusing only on insulin problems, they are looking at the damage it does to the body. Much of this damage, it is now suggested, is the result of free radicals, harmful chemical molecules that can damage cells and tissues.

This certainly would explain why OPCs, powerful antioxidants capable of mopping up many harmful free radicals, are one of the most effective nutrients available for minimizing diabetic damage.

Numerous trials indicate that OPC preparations are effective for a wide-ranging set of problems related to diabetes, including:

- **Retinal damage** due to tiny, ruptured capillaries. This condition is also known as diabetic retinopathy.
- **Poor circulation,** especially to the feet and lower limbs.
- **Kidney damage,** also known as nephropathy.

Scientists believe OPCs protect against this damage by vastly improving the strength of the blood vessels. In particular, OPCs seem to prevent tiny capillaries from rupturing.

HAVE THESE SUBSTANCES BEEN USED BEFORE?

We know from records of European explorers that Native Americans chewed pine bark to prevent scurvy during the winter months. The miracle bark was rich in OPCs.

The newcomers from Europe didn't pick up the habit. OPCs had to be discovered all over again, this time in

Europe. The strengthening effect of OPCs on capillaries was documented in the 1950s. French researchers, especially, took the lead, and OPC-rich products are officially approved for the treatment of diabetic retinopathy in France.

OPC-based products are now used by millions of people in Europe, South America, Australia, New Zealand, and Asia. In the United States, pycnogenols and grape seed extract, leading sources of OPCs, are rapidly gaining popularity.

RESEARCH FINDINGS

Numerous reports support the use of OPCs for problems that arise with diabetes. Some of these findings include:

- French doctors found that diabetics who took an OPC supplement daily significantly decreased the risk of damage to their vision. Rupturing of the tiny capillaries in the retina was reduced by as much as 90 percent.
- One diabetic patient with extremely poor circulation complained of numbness, pain, and coldness in a lower limb. When given OPC supplements on a regular basis, these symptoms dramatically improved. Doctors noted that blood flow in the main artery to the foot increased—so much so that the skin temperature of this previously cold limb actually rose.
- Excessive excretion of albumin, a protein, predicts kidney damage in diabetics. Bringing down this rate has been shown to be an effective strategy for postponing this damage. Numerous studies have shown that OPC supplements keep the body from excreting excessive amounts of this important substance.

OTHER WAYS OPC CAN HELP

You needn't be diabetic to profit from the benefits of products rich in OPCs. As study after study has shown, nutrients such as grape seed extract and pycnogenols are great all-around helpers for capillaries, veins, and arteries. Because of this, OPCs are especially beneficial to people suffering from:

- **Varicose veins.** As the name implies, this disorder afflicts only the veins, not the whole blood vessel system. While horse chestnut has been found specifically effective for varicosities, OPCs also help. In one study, nearly 80 percent of varicose vein sufferers treated with OPCs experienced some degree of improvement. (For more on horse chestnut and varicose veins, see chapter 24.)
- **Cardiovascular problems.** OPCs' ability to strengthen blood vessels, the pathways on which the heart depends, makes them essential for anyone with heart disease (see chapter 5 on Blood Vessels).

HOW TO TAKE OPC

What form does it come in? OPC products come in tablets and capsules. Depending on the source of the OPCs they contain, you may find them under a variety of different names, such as grape seed extract, pycnogenols, and so on.

What's an effective dose? Studies have found that a daily dose of 50 to 100 milligrams of OPCs (standardized to 85 percent active substance) is sufficient to strengthen blood vessels. Since the product you buy may be standardized to a different level, be sure to follow the manufacturer's package instructions.

Tips for use. When purchasing a product, be sure to check the standardization to see the percent of active OPCs it contains. The level should be quite high—80 percent or above. Another thing to remember is that continued use is necessary to get the full benefits of these nutrients.

Are there side effects? In human trials, OPC products have been extremely well tolerated. However, there is always the possibility that an individual will have an adverse reaction. If you experience discomfort or rash, discontinue at once.

ALPHA LIPOIC ACID

WHAT IS ALPHA LIPOIC ACID?

Alpha lipoic acid (also known as ALA and thioctic acid), is not a vitamin but a coenzyme. In addition to working as a powerful antioxidant on its own, it forms part of what one researcher has called an antioxidant network, and its presence strengthens the effect of other antioxidants, including vitamins C and E.

THE MIRACLE EFFECT

Alpha lipoic acid is especially helpful in preventing and reversing nerve damage (neuropathy) due to diabetes. Studies have shown that it can:

- Decrease pain
- Decrease burning sensation
- Decrease tingling "pins and needles" feeling
- Decrease numbness
- Improve blood flow to nerves

How does alpha lipoic acid accomplish these miracles? To date, researchers have focused on its antioxidant powers. In the body, alpha lipoic acid works on its own to mop up harmful free radicals. The body also converts some alpha lipoic acid to an even more powerful antioxidant called dihydrolipoic acid. Both of these helpful acids go after a free radical known to play a role in the development of atherosclerosis (hardening of the arteries) and certain neurological disorders.

Alpha lipoic acid also helps clear sugar from the blood, helping out the body's faulty insulin mechanism. The complete workings of alpha lipoic acid are still being studied. In time, researchers may discover that it has yet other beneficial actions.

HAS ALPHA LIPOIC ACID BEEN USED BEFORE?

Alpha lipoic acid wasn't discovered until 1951, and its value as an antioxidant wasn't appreciated until much later. One of the first studies on its help in treating diabetic neuropathy appeared in a German medical journal in 1975. Although the study showed that it helped nearly 90 percent of the patients who tried it, little follow-up research was done.

In the late 1980s, alpha lipoic acid at last began to receive the attention it deserved. A series of studies in the mid-1990s confirmed its helpfulness in dealing with nerve damage. In Germany it's been officially approved by Commission E as safe and effective for diabetic neuropathy, and many people take it on a daily basis.

RESEARCH FINDINGS

Alpha lipoic acid's effectiveness for diabetic nerve damage came to light as early as 1975. A German study of eighty-nine patients with diabetes and symptoms of neuropathy were given oral supplements of alpha lipoic acid. One-third of the group received 100 milligrams of the nutrient daily, while the other two-thirds received 200 milligrams daily.

Even in the lower dosage group, alpha lipoic acid was remarkably successful. Twenty-three of the twenty-nine patients improved significantly. In the group that received a higher dosage, the results were even better, with fifty-one of sixty patients improving.

Since this initial report, many studies have evaluated the effectiveness of alpha lipoic acid. All of the trials we reviewed had favorable results, including a large study involving 328 patients at several different clinics.

Another study, by Low and colleagues, tried the nutrient on patients whose blood flow to nerves was only half as much as in healthy people. Patients were randomly assigned low, medium, or high doses of lipoic acid.

Although the group receiving the highest doses showed greater gains in the beginning, the other two groups caught up over a period of weeks. At the end of three months, all three groups had improved dramatically. In fact, their measured blood flow to nerves was not significantly different from that of healthy people without nerve damage.

OTHER WAYS ALPHA LIPOIC ACID CAN HELP

Alpha lipoic acid's ability to neutralize free radicals makes it an ally in protecting against cancer (see chapter 6, page 126). Its ability to increase the effect of other cancer-preventing antioxidants (such as vitamins C and E and coenzyme Q-10) also makes it an important anti-cancer nutrient.

HOW TO TAKE ALPHA LIPOIC ACID

What form does it come in? Alpha lipoic acid comes in capsules.

What's an effective dose? There are no established government guidelines for this nutrient. Although some studies we reviewed used doses of 600 milligrams a day, doses of 200 milligrams a day were also found to be effective.

Tips for use. Alpha lipoic acid should be used on an ongoing basis to be effective. For best results, take in divided doses with meals.

Are there side effects? Alpha lipoic acid has been found safe when taken in the doses recommended above.

WHY *NOT* CHROMIUM?

A good deal has been written about the effectiveness of chromium for preventing and even reversing diabetes. Some ads and articles are so enthusiastic one wonders why anyone bothers to take insulin anymore. If you think these promises sound too good to be true, you're wise to be skeptical. Despite the claims, there are some problems with chromium.

While individual success stories have been reported, large-scale placebo-controlled studies have not yet been done. No one knows what the effects of large doses of chromium would be over the period of years most people would need to take it.

And, unfortunately, most people would need larger rather than smaller doses. A study reported by Anderson and colleagues in 1997 highlighted this fact. To achieve results, individuals with diabetes needed to take chromium in amounts larger than those considered to be safe and effective.

While the patients in the study were under constant medical supervision, there is a real danger that others might be tempted to try chromium on their own, without appropriate monitoring. Because diabetes is a complex disorder that changes from day to day, this is a very risky strategy.

For these reasons, most responsible researchers feel the benefits of taking chromium for control of diabetes are unproven, while its long-term risks remain unknown. "Is chromium toxic or essential?" Senft and Kohout asked in a 1996 report. Their answer: "It is both."

Until researchers find a safe, reliable strategy for enlisting it as an aid in treating diabetes, we recommend that you leave it alone.

WHAT ELSE CAN YOU DO?

Diabetes is a complex disorder, one that requires team-work between doctor and patient. If you have diabetes, you already know the facts, and you know that diet and exercise are also a part of the health equation. Here is something else to consider as well.

THE ANTIOXIDANT NETWORK

If one antioxidant, alpha lipoic acid, is good, are more antioxidants better? Very possibly. Antioxidant therapy to help buffer the damage done by diabetes is a fresh—and promising—area of research.

One recent study divided eighty patients with diabetes into four groups. One group took nothing, one group took alpha lipoic acid, another group took selenium, and the final group took vitamin E. At the end of three months, symptoms of nerve damage in all three groups that received supplements were significantly less than symptoms in the group that took nothing.

The authors of the study concluded that adding anti-oxidant nutrients to appropriate traditional care could well help reverse complications of diabetes.

CHAPTER ELEVEN

Nutrients to Heal the
Digestive System

*Stress, illness, even antibiotics. All can take a
toll on your digestive system. Is there help?
Yes—and from some surprising sources.*

Few systems in the body are exposed to the unique set of
stressors the digestive system is subjected to.

Challenge #1: Break down food without also breaking
down the tissues of the esophagus, stomach, and intestines.

Challenge #2: Make nutrients readily available to the
body without making them available to harmful bacteria and molds hiding out in the digestive system, waiting to gain a toehold.

Challenge #3: Adhere to this agenda while digesting an
ever-widening menu of strange foods and processing
chemicals, odd beverages, and other items evolution
never foresaw.

Challenge #4: Do all this in an organism (the modern
human) that often eats irregularly, exercises too little,

sleeps too little, works too much, and is frequently under stress.

It's no wonder the process often goes astray. Fortunately, there are things you can start doing today to get back on track.

THE PROBLEM

The vast majority of digestive ills are caused by poor eating habits, microorganisms run amok, lifestyle habits, or a combination of these. Some common digestive system problems include:

- **Heartburn.** Medically known as esophageal reflux, heartburn has nothing to do with your heart. Instead, it is a burning sensation caused when stomach acids wash back up into the esophagus. Two common causes of heartburn are being overweight and eating large meals too close to bedtime. Certain foods (such as spicy dishes, peppers, and so on) can also trigger reflux, and some people are more prone to it than others. Persistent heartburn is serious because stomach acids are antagonistic to the cells that line the esophagus. Some researchers believe there is an association between escalating rates of heartburn and similarly escalating rates of esophageal cancer in the United States.

- **Indigestion.** All of us have had the feeling of a meal that didn't sit quite right. It may have been what we ate, the fact that we ate too quickly, or that we had an argument with someone sitting across from us. For whatever reason, the digestive process was subverted, either by an outpouring of stomach acids or by a nervous system that interfered with the usual measured contraction of the stomach and intestines.

- **Ulcers.** For decades people thought ulcers were solely stress related. Today we know that a bacterium, *Helicobacter pylori* (*H. pylori*, for short), causes chronic infection of the stomach that sets the stage for ulcers, stomach cancer, and possibly even heart disease. Ulcers are caused by the formation of raw, open lesions on the lining of the stomach or duodenum. Stomach acid further irritates these open sores, causing pain and, in some cases, uncontrolled bleeding. Although diet and stress and other factors play a role, the underlying cause is often the bacterium, which, fortunately, can be medically treated.

- **Yeast and other infections.** From the mouth to the large intestines and beyond, the digestive system is host to innumerable microorganisms, some necessary and helpful and some detrimental. When the harmful ones get out of hand, chronic discomfort follows.

- **Inflammatory bowel diseases.** This is a general term that includes two chronic intestinal problems, ulcerative colitis (often referred to simply as colitis) and Crohn's disease. Although these are different disorders, they have similar symptoms. Colitis is an inflammation of the inner intestinal wall. In Crohn's disease, a much rarer condition, the inflammation penetrates several layers of tissue and, in severe cases, can cause internal bleeding.

- **Irritable bowel syndrome.** This somewhat vague term refers to a condition rather than a specific disease. It can be caused by microorganisms, drugs, diet, psychological factors such as anxiety, or an interplay of these. The patient with irritable bowel syndrome suffers bouts of indigestion, diarrhea, gas, and other upsets.

- **Diverticulitis.** It isn't uncommon for small sacs of intestinal lining to poke through the intestinal wall. In fact, about half of people over age sixty are thought to have this condition, although they never realize it. In a small number of cases, these protruding sacs become inflamed, a painful condition known as diverticulitis.

WHO SUFFERS FROM DIGESTIVE PROBLEMS?

There are a few obvious factors that can lead to problems, such as bacterial infection, a diet that includes too much sugar, and not eating enough roughage. However, some conditions, such as inflammatory bowel diseases and diverticulitis, remain something of a medical puzzle. Individual factors, such as body chemistry and nervous system sensitivity, seem to play an interactive role in many digestive system problems. In addition, many medications (including aspirin, ibuprofen, and acetaminophen) can irritate the stomach.

WHAT ARE THE SYMPTOMS?

The symptoms of digestive problems are often so uncomfortable that people think of them as disorders unto themselves. Warning signals to pay attention to include:

- **Nausea.** Nausea is a symptom with numerous causes. Emotional upset, viral infection, pregnancy, inner ear disturbances, motion sickness, medication, and chemotherapy are the most common causes of nausea.

- **Weight loss.** Stomach and intestinal disorders can result in a loss of appetite as well as the poor or partial digestion of food. When this happens, the body is unable to absorb the nutrients it needs.
- **Tenderness and pain.** Stomachaches, tender spots, and sharp pains all should be evaluated.
- **Constipation.** One of the most common complaints of our era, constipation, can be an outcome of a disorder such as diverticulitis or merely an indicator of a diet that doesn't contain enough bulk.
- **Cramps and diarrhea.** Like constipation, cramps and diarrhea can signal a more serious problem or may be the temporary result of diet. Microorganisms are also a frequent cause of diarrhea.
- **Flatulence.** Although gas can be a symptom of a disorder, most instances are merely the by-product of the food you eat—including such healthy, high-fiber foods as broccoli, beans, and cabbage.

WHAT'S THE OUTLOOK?

Most digestive problems are temporary. But some can become worse if they're ignored. It's important to stop infections and inflammation before they gain a toehold. You may need to be a bit vigilant, but your efforts will be well worthwhile.

WHAT YOU SHOULD KNOW

The disorders described above are serious and require medical attention. But they are generally not immediately life threatening, except in the case of bleeding ulcers. Sometimes things go wrong that *do* require immediate help, such as appendicitis or bowel obstruction. If you have any of the following symptoms, check with a doctor as soon as possible.

- Severe, unremitting abdominal pain
- Abdominal pain accompanied by fever
- Vomiting of blood
- Bloody diarrhea or feces

PROVEN MIRACLES

PROBIOTICS
THE DIGESTIVE SYSTEM SUPERSTAR

WHAT ARE PROBIOTICS?

In addition to the harmful microorganisms that get into the digestive system, there are numerous helpful ones as well. These probiotics, also referred to as friendly bacteria, play an essential role in holding harmful microorganisms in check. Unfortunately, factors in modern life have upset the natural balance. Antibiotics, for example, attack both helpful and harmful bacteria, as does the fluoride frequently added to drinking water.

There are literally thousands of probiotic microorganisms, and researchers are just beginning to identify which strains work best against specific problems.

THE MIRACLE EFFECT

When you take probiotics, the helpful bacteria go to work against the harmful bacteria you didn't even know you had. Suddenly the bouts of indigestion, diarrhea, and gas you've been suffering from disappear. This may sound too good to be true, but it isn't. The overgrowth of harmful bacteria play at least a contributing role in *most* digestive system disorders. Even people with serious disorders can benefit from probiotics. The disorders and symptoms that probiotics can improve include:

- Yeast infections
- *E. coli* infections
- *H. pylori* infections
- Indigestion
- Constipation
- Diarrhea

HAVE PROBIOTICS BEEN USED BEFORE?

The idea of using probiotics has been around for a while. In fact, you've probably already come across one form of probiotic therapy. If you've seen ads for yogurt with "active cultures" or noticed acidophilus milk on your grocer's shelves, you've seen food items making use of one of the best known probiotics, *lactobacillus acidophilus*, which aids people with difficulty digesting dairy products (lactose intolerance).

At one time, the "big three" probiotics were *lactobacillus acidophilus, bifidobacterium*, and *lactobacillus bulgaricus*. Beginning in the mid-1990s, a flurry of new reports began to appear, finding ever more effective strains of bacteria to use against specific problems. According to many researchers, probiotics offer more than a way to restore "lost" bacteria. In the future, specially engineered probiotics may serve as easy-to-take, easy-to-distribute, extremely inexpensive medicines, leaving humans as well as the animals we use as food free from numerous viral, bacterial, and other infections.

RESEARCH FINDINGS

Since few humans would willingly expose themselves to bacteria for the sake of research, some of the best studies come from lab animals. For example, when mice with various strains of harmful microorganisms ate food treated with probiotics, their diarrhea stopped within three days. The same friendly bacteria stopped several other notorious microorganisms, including *E. coli, Shigella dysenteriae,* and *Salmonella typhosa.*

In another study, untreated mice and mice given a probiotic were both fed large amounts of the bacterium that can cause ulcers, *H. pylori.* Mice that didn't get probiotics became ill, but the mice treated with probiotics remained healthy.

Since warm-blooded animals host many of the same microorganisms, these animal studies are accurate predictors of how humans will react. And human studies done to date bear this out. For example:

- Infants with lactose intolerance improved when fed a specific strain of *lactobacillus.*
- Thirty patients with indigestion caused by loss of helpful bacteria were given a probiotic capsule every morning with breakfast. After one week abdominal pain, pressure, bloating, and gas were milder, and within two weeks a further and significant improvement was seen. Patients in this group who described themselves as lactose intolerant saw an improvement in that condition as well.

• One of the largest studies of probiotics to date, by Smyrnov and colleagues, monitored some eight hundred patients with a variety of digestive problems at clinics in Kiev, Dnepropetrovsk, and Moscow. When given the probiotic *bisporin*, acute intestinal infections cleared up and bacterial balance in the stomach was returned to normal.

OTHER WAYS PROBIOTICS CAN HELP

Bacteria can colonize in any warm, moist body tract. In women, vaginal yeast infections are especially common. The same probiotics that help the digestive system have been found effective for inhibiting yeast overgrowth in the vagina. An even more exciting potential use of probiotics involves the treatment of cancer. A specific strain of *acidophilus bulgaricus* has been shown to slow tumor growth and inhibit metastases in humans. Whether or not probiotic treatment can become an effective and side-effect-free form of chemotherapy remains to be seen, as does the possibility of taking probiotics as a cancer preventative.

HOW TO TAKE PROBIOTICS

What form does it come in? The most convenient and effective way to take probiotics, and the best way to guarantee adequate dosage, is in capsule form.

What's an effective dose? Since probiotics are microorganisms, they can be packaged easily. A single daily capsule can contain billions of live bacteria. A dosage study has found two billion effective for eliminating digestive problems in humans.

Tips for use. When you buy probiotics, you are buying a fragile product. If not handled correctly, the friendly microorganisms will die and become ineffective. In addition, be sure to read and follow the manufacturer's package directions regarding proper storage methods. Many products must be refrigerated to remain effective.

Are there side effects? No side effects have been reported in any of the studies we reviewed. Probiotics seem to be extremely well tolerated, even when given in large amounts.

GINGER
FOR INDIGESTION AND NAUSEA

WHAT IS GINGER?

The same part of the ginger plant that's used for cooking, the underground stem or rhizome, is used in herbal preparations.

THE MIRACLE EFFECT

At one time, researchers thought that ginger was effective for motion sickness because it influenced the workings of the inner ear. This has now been ruled out. In fact, one of the truly amazing things about ginger is its ability to stop all sorts of nausea, not just nausea related to motion. How it accomplishes this remains something of a mystery. Researchers agree that ginger's effectiveness is due to its volatile oils and oleoresins, but the chemical mechanism at work has yet to be identified.

HAS GINGER BEEN USED BEFORE?

The use of ginger for upset stomach dates so far back it's hard to determine exactly where it began. The Chinese, for example, have used ginger both as a medicine and in cooking for at least 2,500 years.

The first controlled investigations of ginger's effectiveness were done in the mid-1980s. Scientific proof of folk-wisdom fact revived interest in ginger, even in the usually skeptical medical community. Germany's Commission E has approved ginger not only to combat nausea and indigestion once they have developed, but also to prevent nausea due to motion sickness.

RESEARCH FINDINGS

In the mid-1980s, an herbal researcher discovered that ginger prevented vomiting attacks during a bout of the flu. Intrigued, he and a colleague enlisted volunteers to participate in a formal study. Mowrey and Clayson asked thirty-six people with motion sickness to take either ginger or dimenhydrinate (the active ingredient in nonprescription remedies), then sit in a rotating chair. The results? Not only was ginger effective, it was *more* effective than the popular medicine proved to be.

Two years later, a Swedish research team (Grontved and colleagues) gave naval cadets unaccustomed to high seas one gram of ginger before sailing. The ginger effectively reduced nausea, vomiting, sweating, and feelings of dizziness.

Some of the most interesting uses of ginger may be where you'd least expect them—in hospital settings. At least one study has shown it to be effective in reducing nausea in patients given a particular chemotherapy drug. Other studies have tried giving ginger to postoperative patients who often experience nausea as a result of anesthesia.

One of these studies found ginger was as effective for nausea and vomiting as the prescription medication the hospital usually dispensed, and more than twice as effective as a placebo. Other studies have borne out this finding, both for major surgery and minor day-surgery.

Not all studies have found ginger to be effective. However, the negative studies that we reviewed used small amounts of ginger (500 to 1,000 milligrams), while studies finding ginger effective used twice that amount. Moreover, as researchers themselves point out, there are many kinds of ginger, of varying chemical composition. It's possible that using a weaker form of ginger also contributes to negative findings.

OTHER WAYS GINGER CAN HELP

Ginger has long been valued as an aid for the common cold. Until recently, people supposed it was the sharp, pungent taste and smell that were responsible for opening clogged sinuses. Perhaps. But recent investigations have discovered that the substances in ginger act specifically against cold-causing rhinoviruses (see chapter 8).

Another new use for this age-old product is in the promise it holds for rheumatoid arthritis sufferers. Although few studies have been done on this, some encouraging findings have been produced, suggesting that ginger may help reduce joint pain as well as improve mobility (see chapter 2).

HOW TO TAKE GINGER

What form does it come in?   Although large amounts of raw ginger can be effective, the most convenient way to take ginger is in concentrated capsule or tablet form.

What's an effective dose?   Doses below one gram (1,000 milligrams) have generally been found ineffective for quelling nausea, while doses of one to two grams have been found effective.

Tips for use.   If you are taking ginger to prevent motion sickness, swallow capsules twenty to thirty minutes ahead of time. You can also take ginger after nausea has set in, but it will take approximately half an hour to work.

Are there side effects?   Ginger is nontoxic and side effects have not been reported in studies. Some users, however, may experience stomach upset.

Caution!   Pregnant women are warned against taking ginger in large amounts because it may cause uterine contractions. People taking medications for diabetes or heart disease and people on blood-thinning drugs should also avoid ginger.

LICORICE
FOR HEARTBURN AND ULCERS

WHAT IS LICORICE?

You might find the candy delicious, but it has very little to do with herbal uses. In fact, "licorice" candy is often a sugary sweet flavored with anise. The root of the licorice plant, also known by its botanical name, *glycyrrhiza glabra*, has long played a role in herbal medicine.

We include licorice here because, when properly used, it has been proven highly effective for digestive problems; however, certain precautions in its use must be taken (see Caution, page 206).

THE MIRACLE EFFECT

Stomach acids and unfriendly bacteria, such as *H. pylori*, irritate the lining of the esophagus and stomach. If the irritation is severe enough, ulcerations form. Ulcers do not appear overnight, but are the end result of a process often perceived as heartburn and indigestion by those who suffer from it. The good news is that licorice can interrupt this process. In fact, for many people, licorice can heal ulcers that have already formed.

The reason for licorice's effectiveness is chemically complex. By influencing certain digestive enzymes, it raises the concentration of prostaglandins. These prostaglandins, in turn, promote the secretion of mucus that soothes and, ultimately heals, ulcers. In the case of duodenal ulcers, licorice stimulates Brunner's glands, which produce the mucus secretions that protect the duodenum.

HAS LICORICE BEEN USED BEFORE?

The use of licorice as an ulcer remedy was pioneered more than fifty years ago by a Dutch physician, who noted that ulcer patients improved on a concoction containing 40 percent licorice extract. The physician, F. E.

Revers, publicized his findings and numerous trial studies were done.

While the studies confirmed the effectiveness of licorice, they also confirmed a serious drawback Revers had noticed. Depending on the amount ingested, licorice could cause fluid buildup and swelling of the limbs and the face. Although the condition reversed itself when licorice use stopped, Revers was concerned.

Later researchers recorded cases of death due to heart failure associated with large amounts of licorice consumption. Researchers have also found that a safe, deglycyrrhizinated form is not as effective as the more dangerous original.

Much of the work done on licorice has been geared toward finding safe levels and preparations. Outside the United States licorice-derived medicines such as carbenoxolene have been successfully used by ulcer sufferers and have been looked on for years as one of the best available treatments.

Germany's Commission E has approved licorice for the treatment of ulcers, with specific guidelines limiting the length of time patients may take this medication to four to six weeks.

RESEARCH FINDINGS

Many anecdotes and individual case studies attest to licorice's beneficial effect on the digestive system. In animals, licorice-coated aspirin has been found to prevent the stomach irritation and bleeding usually caused by aspirin.

The most decisive human test is one outlined in the *British Medical Journal* report by Morgan, McAdam, and Pacsoo. In this study, licorice-based carbenoxolene was tested against the nonlicorice medicine, cimetidine. The results? The licorice-based medicine was every bit as effective for healing ulcers as the non-licorice one.

OTHER WAYS LICORICE CAN HELP

Licorice has long been valued for soothing coughs and sore throats, though many insist that most popular preparations contain so little licorice the effect is largely placebo.

A more exciting potential use for licorice may be its ability to protect against viruses. Mice injected with glycyrrhizin once before and twice after being given a lethal dose of flu virus had a 100 percent survival rate, while untreated mice in a control group died. Preliminary research suggests that licorice may inhibit far more serious viruses that afflict humans, including HIV, hepatitis B, and Epstein-Barr. However, whether licorice can be given in doses that are both safe and effective remains to be seen.

HOW TO TAKE LICORICE

What form does it come in? Licorice comes in capsules, tablets, and chewable tablets.

What's an effective dose? To avoid possible toxic effects, Germany's Commission E recommends taking no more than 200 to 600 milligrams of glycyrrhizin daily and continuing this regimen for no more than four to six weeks.

Tips for use. For safety's sake, you may wish to use a deglycyrrhizinated form of licorice. If not, be sure to purchase a standardized product so you can calculate exactly how much you're taking.

Are there side effects? Prolonged use of licorice has life-threatening side effects. See Caution below.

Caution! We can't repeat it too often. Unless it has been deglycyrrhizinated, licorice can be dangerous. Excessive or prolonged use causes serious side effects, including high blood pressure and heart failure. Do not, under any circumstances, take licorice for—at the very most— more than four to six weeks at a time.

Licorice should not be taken at all by pregnant women or by people with cardiovascular problems, liver or kidney disease, or potassium deficiency. It should also not be used by people on hormone therapy or people receiving treatment for hypoglycemia.

PEPPERMINT OIL
FOR INDIGESTION AND IRRITABLE BOWEL SYNDROME

WHAT IS PEPPERMINT OIL?

Derived from the leaves and flowers of the peppermint plant, peppermint oil has a very high menthol content (more than 50 percent) and a long, time-honored tradition as a natural healer. It is this concentrated oil that is of interest to modern herbalists, not the flavoring or the candy.

THE MIRACLE EFFECT

Peppermint oil has complex chemical activity, and lab studies have shown that it acts directly on the intestinal tract. To be specific, the menthol component of peppermint oil appears to inhibit the smooth muscle spasms that cause pain, cramping, indigestion, and diarrhea.

HAS PEPPERMINT OIL BEEN USED BEFORE?

Peppermint oil is one of the oldest medicines on earth. The most ancient of all known medical texts, the Ebers papyrus (which dates back to Egypt, c. 1550 B.C.) recommends peppermint oil for stomach ailments. Mankind has heeded this advice for nearly four thousand years.

Although peppermint is used mostly as a flavoring in the United States, peppermint oil is widely used in Europe, and Germany's Commission E has officially approved its use for digestive problems.

RESEARCH FINDINGS

Most of the research on peppermint oil comes from Europe, where it figures as an ingredient in several commercial preparations. A study of one such product, which combines peppermint and caraway oils in a 9:5 ratio, tested the product against a placebo in a double-blind study involving thirty-nine patients with pain and indigestion. The peppermint oil product significantly outperformed the placebo, and after four weeks of treatment 89.5 percent of patients receiving the active preparation reported a significant lessening of pain.

Another product encapsulates peppermint oil in a coating designed to delay digestion until the capsule reaches the intestine. This product was tested against a placebo in 110 men and women with irritable bowel syndrome. Peppermint oil was superior to the placebo in every measure, as these findings show:

	TREATED GROUP	PLACEBO GROUP
Reduced abdominal pain	79%	43%
Reduced bloating	83%	29%
Reduced diarrhea	83%	32%
Reduced stomach rumbling	73%	31%
Reduced gas	79%	22%

OTHER WAYS PEPPERMINT CAN HELP

The same menthol component that makes peppermint oil an effective antispasmodic when taken internally also appears to work externally. When applied to the temples and forehead, peppermint oil has been found helpful in relieving the pain of tension headaches (see chapter 12, page 211).

HOW TO TAKE PEPPERMINT OIL

What form does it come in? Peppermint oil comes in gelatin capsules and coated capsules. If you are taking peppermint for a stomach problem, look for a gelatin capsule that will break down quickly. If you are seeking help for a bowel problem, look for a coated product (sometimes labeled entero-coated) that will remain intact until reaching the intestine.

What's an effective dose? Since the size of capsules varies from manufacturer to manufacturer, follow the package directions for the product you have purchased.

Tips for use. Swallow the capsules whole. Undiluted peppermint oil will cause heartburn.

Are there side effects? Peppermint oil is safe and easy to tolerate. However, some people may have an allergic reaction. If you experience rash or itching, rapid heartbeat, muscle spasms, or increased indigestion, discontinue use at once.

WHAT ELSE CAN YOU DO?

PSYLLIUM:
NATURE'S GREAT REGULATOR

Also known as plantago and ispaghula, psyllium seed husks can be helpful to anyone with irregularity problems. Both constipation and diarrhea can arise on their own, with no seeming cause, or they can be symptoms of other digestive system problems, such as irritable bowel syndrome. Psyllium's main use is as a laxative.

In double-blind studies, 3.25 grams of psyllium taken three times daily was deemed more effective than 7 grams of wheat bran taken three times daily.

Psyllium has also been found effective for diarrhea. In a study of patients with irritable bowel syndrome, twenty of twenty-six patients reported a significant improvement after eight weeks of treatment.

In another report children with chronic, nonspecific

diarrhea were divided into two groups. One group was treated with psyllium while the other group made dietary changes. While dietary changes helped some children, almost twice as many children in the psyllium group improved.

Psyllium may have another benefit. Like much-touted bran fiber, psyllium seed husks appear to have a cholesterol-lowering effect, especially when coupled with changes in diet. Some people are allergic to psyllium but for most people it is both safe and effective.

If you decide to try psyllium, follow the package directions and be sure to drink plenty of fluids with it.

THE GOOD OF GARLIC

Garlic has a well-established reputation for defending the body from numerous bacteria, microbacteria, and yeasts. Many of the harmful microorganisms that garlic attacks are those that wreak havoc in the digestive system. For more about garlic, see chapter 7 on cholesterol and triglycerides.

VITAMIN SUPPLEMENTATION

If you have an inflammatory bowel condition, there may be a chance that you're malnourished. Study after study has shown that these disorders interrupt the digestive process and interfere with the natural absorption of nutrients. To minimize the damage, make sure you take a good multivitamin supplement daily.

CHAPTER TWELVE

Effective Prevention for
Headaches

*Aspirin might help a headache once it starts.
But these nutrients may keep you from getting
the headache at all.*

There are few things more miserable than a headache.
And, like ants at a picnic, where there is one there are
likely to be more. People who have headaches tend to
have *lots* of headaches—and as most sufferers know,
over-the-counter pain remedies don't always provide the
relief they promise.

Now many sufferers are finding a better way to prevent pain—avoid getting the headache in the first place.

THE PROBLEM

Not all headaches are alike. They have different causes
and even different symptoms. Among the basic types of
headaches are:

- **Migraine headache.** The pain and discomfort of a
  migraine are due to changes in the blood vessels of

the temples. A migraine headache can last for days. Often it involves such additional symptoms as dizziness, nausea, and visual disturbances.

- **Cluster headache.** Like migraines, cluster headaches are caused by vascular changes. Said to be the most intense of all headaches, the pain often centers around one eye. Typically the pain lasts for a few hours, fades, then returns again a few hours later. Bouts of these headaches can last for days or months at a time. Medical science has not yet discovered the cause.

- **Tension headache.** Tension headaches can occur occasionally or, for some people, on a daily or near-daily basis. As the name implies, they are related to mental stress, physical stress, or both. This type of headache can also be caused by a wide variety of physical conditions, such as spinal problems or exposure to environmental toxins.

- **Headache due to disease.** In very rare cases, headaches are a symptom of disease. This can be anything from an infectious illness, such as meningitis, to vision or hearing disorders or even a tumor. While the vast majority of headaches are not due to such problems, persistent or recurrent headaches should be checked out by a physician to eliminate the possibility.

WHO SUFFERS FROM HEADACHES?

Anyone can get a headache, but some people seem to suffer far more from them than others do. Unfortunately, many of the risk factors for headaches are ones that can't be easily controlled.

Risk factors associated with chronic headache include:

- **Genetic inheritance.** Headaches often run in families. This is especially true of migraine headaches.
- **Female hormones.** Fluctuating hormone levels, which occur just before or during menstruation, are a frequent cause of migraines. This is why the majority of people who suffer from migraines—70 percent—are women.
- **Being a male.** Just as women are the primary sufferers when it comes to migraines, nearly all cluster headache sufferers—90 percent—are men.
- **Personality.** According to the National Headache Foundation, headache sufferers tend to share certain personality traits. As a group, headache-prone people are ambitious, energetic people who often strive for order and perfection.
- **Stress.** Work and worry can both contribute to the development of headaches.
- **Diet and nutrition.** For some people, certain foods can trigger headaches. Smoking and withdrawal from caffeine can also cause headaches.
- **Dental and/or jaw problems.** Teeth that form a less than perfect bite or a jaw that is misaligned can cause headaches.
- **Sinus problems.** Chronic infections that leave sinuses clogged and inflamed are a prime cause of headaches.

WHAT ARE THE SYMPTOMS?

We call them headaches but the symptoms can include more than a simple ache. Headache hallmarks include:

- Pain and throbbing in the head
- Muscle ache, especially in the neck
- Nausea and/or vomiting
- Dizziness
- Visual disturbances
- Sensitivity to light, sound, or certain smells and tastes
- Fatigue

WHAT'S THE OUTLOOK?

If you're a chronic headache sufferer, you probably already know that headaches are somewhat cyclical. You may go through a period where headaches are frequent and severe, then a period, sometimes years long, where they are relatively rare. For women who get hormonal migraines, pregnancy and menopause often bring relief. Sufferers of other types of headaches may also "age out" of the problem, or be able to make changes that diminish the frequency or intensity of their headaches.

WHAT YOU NEED TO KNOW

As we said before, most headaches have nothing to do with more serious conditions. In a very few cases, however, they might be important signs that shouldn't be overlooked. For instance, frequently awakening with a headache that fades as the day progresses may be a symptom of high blood pressure.

Just to make sure you're not ignoring a problem that should be medically evaluated, we recommend discussing your headaches with your doctor.

PROVEN MIRACLES

FEVERFEW

WHAT IS FEVERFEW?

Feverfew is a plant whose leaves and other above-ground parts have been used by herbal practitioners for at least two thousand years.

THE MIRACLE EFFECT

If you have a headache right now, feverfew won't help. But if you want to avoid future headaches, you should consider this herbal helper.

To date, studies have shown that feverfew is especially helpful for migraine sufferers. However, the substances that make feverfew work have a special effect on the walls of the cerebral vessels. This action may make feverfew effective for other types of headaches as well, especially cluster headaches.

When tested on human migraine sufferers, feverfew was found to:

- Reduce the number of headaches
- Reduce the severity of attacks
- Reduce secondary symptoms such as nausea and vomiting

HAS FEVERFEW BEEN USED BEFORE?

The use of feverfew for headache dates back at least two thousand years, to the Greek physician Dioscorides, who also recommended it for menstrual discomfort. In 1597 the English herbalist John Gerard said it was especially helpful for common headaches, migraines, and dizziness.

Modern interest in feverfew dates from the 1970s. The herb is especially popular in Canada and the United States, where it has been used to prevent painful, disabling headaches.

RESEARCH FINDINGS

Several human studies have found that feverfew, taken on an ongoing basis, can reduce the number and severity of attacks in migraine headache sufferers.

The first controlled trial of feverfew, by Johnson and colleagues, was published in the *British Medical Journal* in 1985. The study involved seventeen migraine sufferers who had been chewing feverfew leaves to control their headaches. In place of the leaves, patients were given either a capsule containing feverfew or a placebo.

The group that received active feverfew did not notice any change. But the group that had given up their feverfew leaves for a placebo reported more frequent headaches, more severe headaches, and a worsening of secondary effects such as nausea.

This study provided the first scientific proof of feverfew's headache-stopping capabilities. It also demonstrated that feverfew taken in capsule form was at least as effective as chewing fresh leaves. This was important since, for many people, the leaves are an irritant that can cause ulcerations in the mouth.

The unusual nature of the study—beginning with patients already taking the substance in question—caused controversy as well. Because patients who took the placebo experienced a worsening of symptoms after giving up their feverfew leaves, critics suggested they were suffering from "post-feverfew syndrome." However, other studies have not borne this out.

A second, more ambitious study was undertaken by Murphy and colleagues. In the new study, seventy-two headache sufferers were divided into two groups. One group received feverfew while the other group received placebos. After four months of testing and a one-month washout period, the two groups traded regimens. As with the initial study, feverfew was found remarkably effective for reducing the number and severity of headaches.

OTHER WAYS FEVERFEW CAN HELP

At present, feverfew is recommended only as an aid in headache prevention. Although it has frequently been touted as an aid in dealing with rheumatoid arthritis, convincing studies are unavailable, and the jury is still out.

One intriguing report suggests that feverfew may have another use altogether. In an animal study, feverfew kept clots from sticking to the interior walls of rabbit aortas. This opens up the possibility that feverfew, working as an anti-clotting agent, may ultimately prove useful in the prevention of cardiovascular disease.

HOW TO TAKE FEVERFEW

What form does it come in? Feverfew comes in tablets and capsules. You can also buy fresh or dried leaves, intended to be chewed. Aside from not being standardized, leaves can irritate the mouth and tongue, and chewing them isn't recommended.

What's an effective dose? If you decide to buy feverfew, look for a product that is standardized to contain at least 0.2 percent of parthenolide, the active ingredient. Since experts consider 250 micrograms of parthenolide an effective daily dose, you would need to take 125 milligrams daily of a product standardized to the 0.2 percent guidelines. Since standardization may vary, be sure to follow the manufacturer's package instructions.

Tips for use. Feverfew must be taken daily to prevent headaches. It may take several weeks for you to notice a difference.

Side effects. Although most people tolerate feverfew well, some people may be allergic to it. Discontinue if you develop a rash, itching, or other discomfort.

Caution! Since feverfew can cause uterine contractions, it should not be taken by pregnant women.

MAGNESIUM

WHAT IS MAGNESIUM?

Magnesium is a trace mineral, important to the body for a variety of functions. Research has shown that low levels of magnesium are associated with migraine, cluster, and tension headaches.

THE MIRACLE EFFECT

Magnesium has an impressive ability to fight most types of headaches. As we noted above, low levels of magnesium are common in many headache sufferers. Magnesium supplementation works by compensating for this deficiency. In fact, it seems to work both as a preventative and a cure. For many people, magnesium may be able to:

- Prevent headache attacks
- Shorten duration of headache
- Reduce or eliminate headache pain
- Reduce or eliminate symptoms such as nausea and sensitivity to light and sound
- Prevent immediate recurrence of headache

HAS MAGNESIUM BEEN USED BEFORE?

Magnesium is essential to health and is included in multivitamin and mineral preparations. The idea of taking magnesium to prevent and cure headaches is relatively new, dating mostly from the mid-1990s.

RESEARCH FINDINGS

Numerous studies have concluded that magnesium has a dual benefit for headache sufferers. Taken on an ongoing basis, it can reduce the number of headache attacks. In one study, by Piekert and colleagues, oral magnesium supplements reduced headache attacks by 41 percent in chronic migraine suffers.

Magnesium can also bring relief when taken during an attack.

One of the most impressive studies done to date, by

Mauskop and colleagues, gave patients a single intravenous dose of 1,000 milligrams of magnesium during a headache attack. The group of forty patients, volunteers at a headache treatment clinic, included both men and women, ranging in age from fourteen to fifty-five. Patients suffered from a variety of headaches, including migraine, cluster, tension, and chronic headaches with migrainelike features.

For 80 percent of these patients, magnesium completely eliminated pain within fifteen minutes. More than half of the patients (56 percent) remained pain-free for twenty-four hours. Magnesium also eliminated symptoms such as nausea and sensitivity to light and sound.

Those who had the lowest levels of magnesium at the outset, researchers noted, were those who benefited most from magnesium supplementation. Researchers also noted that, as a group, sufferers with cluster headaches tended to have lower magnesium levels than people who suffered from tension or migraine headaches.

The same research team also performed studies that tested magnesium on, in one case, cluster headache sufferers only and, in another case, migraine sufferers only. In both of these studies, intravenous magnesium was found effective for eliminating pain in a significant number of patients, and for preventing recurrence of pain for at least twenty-four hours.

OTHER WAYS MAGNESIUM CAN HELP

Maintaining adequate magnesium intake is important for general health. In addition to its ability to help headache sufferers, studies indicate that magnesium supplements can also help women who suffer from premenstrual syndrome (see chapter 20, page 341).

HOW TO TAKE MAGNESIUM

What form does it come in? Magnesium comes in tablets. It is sometimes combined with other nutrients, such as calcium, or is part of a multivitamin.

What's an effective dose? Studies we reviewed used oral supplements of magnesium ranging from 360 to 600 milligrams a day.

Tips for use. For best absorption and to avoid side effects (see below), take with meals. To effectively prevent headaches, magnesium must be taken on an ongoing basis, and benefits may not be seen for several weeks.

Are there side effects? Magnesium may cause diarrhea and/or stomach irritation in some users.

Caution! Magnesium is extremely safe for most people when taken at recommended doses. However, it should be avoided by people with kidney problems, irregular or weak heartbeat, and ileostomy.

WHAT ELSE CAN YOU DO?

If you suffer from headaches, one of the best things you can do for yourself is to become an expert on what may trigger your headaches. You may find that eating certain foods results in a headache, or that bad lighting conditions need to be corrected. Developing some stress-reducing strategies can also help. In addition, there's one other pain-relief strategy you should know about.

PEPPERMINT AND EUCALYPTUS OILS

Want that throbbing in your forehead or temples to stop right now? There may be a way. According to researchers, rubbing a little essential oil on the affected area may help. Depending on the type of headache you have, you'll want to try either peppermint oil on its own or a combination of peppermint and eucalyptus. According to a study done at a neurology clinic in Germany, peppermint oil alone is more effective for pain related to migraine and cluster headaches, while a combination of peppermint and eucalyptus is more effective for headaches that involve muscle tension.

Oil can be applied several times throughout the day. Be a little cautious, however, as applying too frequently can cause skin irritation. Also, be sure to avoid getting oil in or around your eyes.

CHAPTER THIRTEEN

Protect Against

Heart Disease and Coronary Artery Disease

You feed the rest of your body, now it's time to feed your heart. Our menu of miracle nutrients not only nourishes—it actually helps reverse the disease process.

Despite massive publicity about the risk factors, heart disease (which includes coronary artery disease) is still America's number one killer. Why? Human nature. Most of us know that we should stop smoking, lose weight, eat less fat and more fruits and vegetables, get more exercise, and avoid stress. But knowing isn't the same as getting it done, and many of us wonder what else we can do to ward off disease.

We recommend making *all* the lifestyle changes mentioned above—and we also recommend learning about the terrific heart-helpers described in this chapter.

THE PROBLEM

"Heart disease" is a loosely applied, all-purpose term for a whole cluster of conditions affecting the heart.

Some heart diseases are congenital (conditions people are born with), while others involve specific viruses, infections, and cancers that attack the heart. None of these conditions are addressed in this chapter. The kind of "heart disease" we're concerned with here is the far more common set of symptoms, impairments, and life-threatening conditions that come about largely as a result of the lifestyle we live. These include:

- **Angina** (full name: angina pectoris). Angina isn't a disease in itself but a symptom of disease. It is the pain or squeezing sensation that radiates from the center of the chest and, in some cases, extends down into the left arm or up into the shoulders or jaw. Angina, the heart's signal that it is not receiving enough oxygen, is often linked to coronary artery disease.

- **Arrhythmia.** This refers to any change in the normal beating of the heart, including uneven pulse and rapid, fluttery pulse. One of the key causes of arrhythmia is the inability of the heart tissue to conduct the electrical impulse that regulates beating.

- **Ischemic heart disease.** This disease is the direct result of the heart receiving an inadequate supply of blood. The key causes of ischemic heart disease are clogged arteries, atherosclerosis (hardening of the arteries), and coronary artery disease.

- **Heart failure and congestive heart failure.** This condition occurs when the heart is unable to pump well enough to meet the body's demands. As a result, tissues do not receive adequate oxygen and other nutrients carried by the blood. The leading causes of heart failure in people over forty are atherosclerosis with blood clotting in the heart, uncontrolled high blood pressure, and disease of the heart valves. Congestive heart failure refers to the accumulation of fluids in body tissues (especially the lungs) as a result of the heart's impaired functioning.

- **Cardiomyopathy.** Any disease that damages the heart's muscle tissue.
- **Heart attack.** Often referred to by its medical name, myocardial infarction (MI for short), a heart attack occurs when one of the heart's arteries becomes blocked, shutting off the heart's blood supply. This blockage is usually the result of blood clots or coronary artery disease.
- **Coronary artery disease.** This is the diagnosis when either of the two arteries that lead from the heart becomes constricted. The most common cause of this disease is atherosclerosis, in which plaque adheres to the walls of the arteries, causing them to thicken and become rigid. As a result the arteries are unable to accommodate bits of plaque that loosen and enter the blood stream.

WHO GETS THESE DISEASES?

At one time, heart disease was looked on as a predominantly male disorder. No longer. Women seem to be catching up with men in this area, perhaps because they're catching up with them in other areas of life as well. Whether you're a man or a woman, here are the risk factors you need to be aware of:

- **Age.** If you're a man, age-related risk increases after forty-five. If you're a woman, risk increases if

you're over fifty-five or have gone through menopause or had your ovaries removed.

- **Family history.** Unfortunately, a predilection to developing heart diseases does seem to run in families. If you have a father or brother who suffered a
heart attack before age fifty-five or a mother or sister who had one before sixty-five, your own risk is
greater.
- **Weight.** Studies have found that being even mildly
overweight is a risk factor for heart disease, and the
risk is even greater for those who are massively
obese. Extra flesh also means extra capillaries and
greater blood volume than your heart was meant to
pump. To compensate, the heart tries to push more
blood with each beat, and this wear and tear can
cause abnormalities in the left ventricle. The good
news? When the extra weight is shed, the abnormalities seem to reverse.
- **Smoking.** Smokers are two to four times as likely
to develop coronary artery disease. Worse, smokers
are more likely to die from their problems than non-
smokers who develop coronary artery disease.
- **Cholesterol.** Having high cholesterol is a risk factor.
- **Homocysteine.** Researchers are finding out that
having high levels of this amino acid may be a significant risk factor for heart disease. How significant? According to the experts, homocysteine may
be more important than cholesterol and almost as
important as smoking (see also chapter 14 on
Homocysteine).
- **Blood pressure.** Having high blood pressure forces
the heart to pump harder to circulate blood. Left

untreated, high blood pressure can cause the heart to become enlarged, weakened, and less able to perform its work. The American Heart Association recommends maintaining a pressure reading of no higher than 140/90.

- **Lack of exercise.** The heart is a muscle and, like any muscle, requires exercise to stay healthy. For your heart's sake, get at least thirty minutes of aerobic activity three times a week.

- **Diet and nutrition.** Most people know that eating too much fat, sugar, and certain other foods can be harmful, but too few people know that what they *don't* take in can be just as important. Lack of certain nutrients—including vitamin E and coenzyme Q-10—has been linked to the development of heart disease and coronary artery disease.

- **Stress.** It isn't just a cliché. Tension, anxiety, frustration, and anger all have been linked to heart problems. For example, a British team studied more than ten thousand civil servants and found that those who had little control over their jobs were almost twice as likely to develop heart problems over the next five years. This was true regardless of salary, job status, or personal health factors.

- **Diabetes.** People with diabetes have higher rates of heart disease and coronary artery disease than nondiabetics. Since diabetes is sometimes a result of obesity, this may be a risk factor more within your control than you think.

- **Alcohol abuse.** Much publicity has been given lately to the beneficial effects of a glass of wine or so a day. Drinking in excess, however, is still considered a significant risk factor.

WHAT ARE THE SYMPTOMS?

Unfortunately, you can have heart disease and coronary artery disease without knowing it. The long process of deterioration may not be apparent until a good deal of damage has been done. For some people, the first "symptom" is a disastrous heart attack or heart failure. All this is a powerful argument for taking preventive measures, having regular checkups, and being alert to symptoms.

Not all symptoms of heart disease and coronary artery disease are obvious ones that involve chest pain. In addition, one person may have quite a different set of symptoms than another person, even though the underlying disease is the same.

Signs to be on the lookout for include:

- **Angina.** A feeling of pain or tightness in the chest. In some cases, the pain is also felt in the left arm and the jaw.
- **Rapid heartbeat.** Pulse is faster than normal or may feel fluttery.
- **Recurrent chest pain.** A sharp or squeezing sensation in the center of the chest that lasts a few minutes, goes away, and then recurs later should be evaluated by a doctor.
- **Radiant pain.** The pain that begins in the center of the chest may extend to the arms, neck, or shoulders.
- **Shortness of breath.** Chronic difficulty catching one's breath—not due to other causes, such as asthma.
- **Extreme fatigue.** Constant, overwhelming exhaus-

tion may indicate that the heart is not pumping enough blood and oxygen to the tissues of the body.

- **Bouts of dizziness.** Feeling light-headed or blacking out can be a sign of problems.
- **Swelling of the ankles or lower extremities.** Also known as edema, this condition may indicate that the heart is not pumping well.
- **Gastric discomfort.** Nausea or upset stomach can be symptoms of a wide range of ills, including heart disease.

Consult a Doctor Immediately if . . .
Chest pain or constriction is accompanied by dizziness, faintness, sweating, nausea, or shortness of breath.

WHAT'S THE OUTLOOK?

Heart disease and coronary artery disease are serious conditions. Left untreated, they only get worse. The end result is impaired quality of life and premature death. Sound grim? The good news is that these very serious disorders are amazingly responsive to management and intervention. Although it's better to start addressing the condition sooner rather than later, even people with advanced disease have seen remarkable reversals in their condition.

WHAT YOU SHOULD KNOW

The key to overcoming heart disease and coronary artery disease is to know whether or not you have them. Don't guess or assume things are fine because you have no symptoms. Risk factors may tell you more about your health than obvious symptoms. But don't guess—find out for sure. If you haven't had a checkup for a while, now is a good time to make an appointment. If you're under treatment for these conditions, work with your doctor to manage the disorders, and don't stop taking any medications your doctor has prescribed.

PROVEN MIRACLES

COENZYME Q-10

WHAT IS COENZYME Q-10?

You've probably heard the words or seen the product. Suddenly, everyone is talking about coenzyme Q-10, also referred to as coQ-10, ubiquinol-10, and ubiquinone. But chances are good that, like thousands of others, you don't know exactly what it is. Neither do the experts. At present, there's a serious debate about whether this powerful antioxidant is a vitamin or simply operates like one. But even those who don't agree on this point agree on something far more important: coenzyme Q-10's benefits. This amazing substance, found in small amounts in some foods and produced within the body, has a dramatic effect on heart health.

THE MIRACLE EFFECT

Coenzyme Q-10 plays two important roles. As an antioxidant, it scavenges free radicals, the molecules that wreak havoc on healthy cells. It also kindles the chain reaction that allows cells to produce energy. This second, energizing role is especially important for the heart, an organ that must find the energy to beat over 100,000 times a day, day in and day out.

It's not surprising that the heart muscle has high concentrations of coenzyme Q-10—in healthy people, that is. Studies have established a clear and direct link between lack of coQ-10 and heart disease, and people with advanced heart failure have significantly less coenzyme Q-10 in their heart tissue than people with milder forms of the disease.

Fortunately, oral supplements of synthesized coenzyme Q-10 are well absorbed by the body. In fact, a researcher who compared absorption from food to absorption from supplement found no significant difference between the two.

For people with heart disease, congestive heart failure, angina, or arrhythmia, coQ-10 can cut symptoms dramatically, improve quality of life, and even forestall premature death. One researcher observed that two out of three patients had a positive response to this easy to take supplement. The news may be even better than that. Studies that tracked patients during a longer period of use (six months to one year) reported positive response rates, hitting or topping the 80 percent mark.

CoQ-10 works to improve a range of symptoms that arise from heart disease and coronary artery disease. Taking the supplement for as little as two months can:

- Reduce shortness of breath, when at rest as well as during exertion.
- Reduce cyanosis, the bluish discoloration that signals skin and tissues aren't receiving enough oxygen.

- Improve lung function and reduce fluid accumulation in the lungs.
- Reduce fluid buildup (edema) in the ankles.
- Normalize heart rate.
- Improve blood pressure, both systolic (upper reading) and diastolic (lower reading).

HAS COENZYME Q-10 BEEN USED BEFORE?

Is coenzyme Q-10 really amazing? Yes—enough to win the world's most prestigious scientific accolade. In 1978 Peter D. Mitchell was awarded the Nobel prize for chemistry when he discovered how coQ-10 works to produce cell energy.

At the time he won the prize, Mitchell was working on a little-known nutrient. Coenzyme Q-10 was discovered in 1957 by a Purdue University researcher, Frederick Crane. In the late 1960s, pioneer Japanese researchers discovered that coenzyme Q-10 was found in especially high concentrations in the muscle of the heart. They also demonstrated that this hitherto unknown enzyme played a crucial role in energizing cells.

Other researchers now became interested in coenzyme Q-10 as a possible aid for people with heart disease. In the early 1980s, Folkers and colleagues studied its use on patients with heart failure. Since then, the effectiveness and safety of coQ-10 have made it an international favorite, used successfully by people throughout the world.

RESEARCH FINDINGS

Numerous case reports and over a dozen clinical trials have proven that CoQ-10 is one of the most powerful heart nutrients available anywhere. These studies have included large numbers of people suffering from various types and stages of heart disease and, in some cases, have tracked them over long periods of time. For example:

- In the early 1990s, Italian researchers Morisco, Trimarco, and Condorelli assessed coenzyme Q-10's benefit to elderly men with congestive heart failure. The double-blind, placebo-controlled investigation involved 641 men, all of whom continued to take their regular medication. During the year-long study period, 118 men from the placebo-taking half of the group were hospitalized for complications of their disorder—but only 73 men taking coenzyme Q-10 required hospitalization. Moreover, disease-related incidences of edema or asthma were each slashed by more than half.

- One of the most ambitious trials of coenzyme Q-10 was an Italian investigation headed by Biaggi and colleagues. The study included 2,664 patients with heart disease under treatment at 173 locations. Over a three-month period, these results were seen:
  - **79.8%** of patients had less sweating.
  - **78.6%** of patients had less fluid retention.
  - **78%** of patients had less pallor, a sign of better circulation.
  - **78%** of patients had less fluid in their lungs.
  - **75%** of patients experienced fewer heart palpitations.
  - **73%** of patients had less dizziness.
  - **72%** of patients had improved jugular vein circulation.

- **63%** of patients had less irregular heartbeat (arrhythmia).
- **53%** of patients had less shortness of breath.
- **49%** of patients had improvement of enlarged liver.

Most patients in the study enjoyed more than one improvement, and 54 percent saw improvement of at least three disease symptoms.

OTHER WAYS COENZYME Q-10 CAN HELP

Coenzyme Q-10 is such a recent discovery that researchers have not yet discovered its complete healing potential. Some areas that bear watching are listed below.

- **Antihypertensive.** Coenzyme Q-10 helps combat high blood pressure.
- **Nerve and muscle rejuvenation.** A report by Folkers and Simonsen has shown that patients with nerve and muscle damage from a variety of diseases benefited significantly from coenzyme Q-10. In a double-blind, placebo-controlled study, those receiving 100 milligrams of coenzyme Q-10 daily showed ''definitely improved physical performance'' compared to patients who received only a placebo.
- **Cancer therapy.** Clinical trials have included coenzyme Q-10 as one of several nutrients given to women whose breast cancer was considered high risk because of metastasis. The results were exceptionally promising, with both tumor spread and mortality rate being dramatically lowered. (See chapter 6 on Cancer). CoQ-10 may help cancer pa-

tients in another way as well, by preventing toxicity from the chemotherapy drug, Adriamycin.

HOW TO TAKE COENZYME Q-10

What form does it come in? The most commonly available form of coQ-10 is capsules.

What's an effective dose? Clear guidelines on how much coQ-10 to take have yet to emerge. In studies, patients improved on dosages ranging from 50 milligrams to 150 milligrams per day. One study used a dosage of 2 milligrams per kilo (2.2 pounds) of body weight.

Tips for use. Coenzyme Q-10 isn't a one-time cure. To get the full benefit, you need to take it on a daily, ongoing basis. Be aware that it may take a few weeks to begin to feel an improvement. The amino acid carnitine seems to enhance the effectiveness of coQ-10 (see What Else Can You Do? below).

Are there side effects? Coenzyme Q-10 is considered safe and nontoxic. A very small number of people (0.8 to 1.5 percent) have reported side effects, usually in the form of nausea, upset stomach, and/or diarrhea.

Caution! There have been some reports that coenzyme Q-10 blocks the beneficial effects of warfarin, a common heart medication. If you're already taking this or any other drug, be sure to consult your doctor before trying coenzyme Q-10.

HAWTHORN

WHAT IS HAWTHORN?

Hawthorn (known as weissdorn in Germany) is a thorny, tree-sized shrub native to Europe. Its leaves, white flowers, and scarlet berries have been used in herbal preparations. But current research shows that preparations made with the leaf and flowers only are the most effective.

THE MIRACLE EFFECT

Hawthorn's reputation as the eminent heart herb is well earned. According to herbal authority Christopher Hobbs, who has researched hawthorn extensively and whose own father is a living success story, "It is the first herb, besides garlic, that should be added to one's daily dietary regimen when there is any suspicion of problems of cardiovascular disease."

Chemically analyzed, hawthorn has been shown to have strong antioxidant activities, probably because it is rich in flavonoids and OPCs, the active substance in pycnogenols and grape seed extract. (For more on OPCs, see chapter 5 on Blood Vessels.)

However, researchers point out that hawthorn's beneficial effects are so significant that other chemical activities, yet to be identified, may also be at work. Documented effects of hawthorn show that it can:

- Reduce symptoms of congestive heart failure.
- Reduce angina.
- Reduce arrhythmia and help to regulate the heartbeat.

- Improve overall cardiac function and efficiency.
- Help keep coronary arteries relaxed and properly dilated, allowing more blood to fuel the heart with oxygen.
- Protect against future coronary disease.
- Improve stamina.
- Halt or retard further deterioration.

HAS HAWTHORN BEEN USED BEFORE?

Hawthorn has been known for at least two millennia and has a long tradition in Chinese medicine. In the Western world, early herbalists focused on the plant's bark and found it mildly useful for sore throat. Later practitioners discovered that the healing bite of this plant is in its flowers, berries, and leaves. Its use as a heart medicine was first noted in France in the 1600s.

In nineteenth-century Ireland, a doctor named Green gained fame by giving patients with heart ailments a concoction of his own making. After his death, his daughter revealed the secret ingredient in his life-saving mix: hawthorn berries. Another nineteenth-century doctor, the German homeopath Assman, preferred it to digitalis (foxglove) because it was effective and safer to use.

As is the case with many other herbal preparations, hawthorn's use as a modern-day heart aid was pioneered in continental Europe. Thousands of European doctors prescribe it for their patients, in Germany especially, where the government's Commission E has approved it for use as a supportive medicine in cases of mild coronary problems.

Now that hawthorn can be easily purchased in America, it's becoming increasingly popular throughout the United States.

HARD EVIDENCE

Hawthorn has been the subject of numerous lab, animal, and human studies. When tried on humans, hawthorn has been proven especially helpful for problems associated with insufficient blood supply to the heart, a key result of vascular disease. People with this condition are often unable to perform even mild activities without suffering angina and disturbed heart rhythms.

But studies done in Germany show that hawthorn can change this picture. To test hawthorn's effect, two evaluations are made. At the beginning of a study, patients are monitored during exercise on stationary bicycles. This test is repeated after taking hawthorn for a period of several weeks. These patients have shown significant improvement on a number of points, including greater stamina, less fatigue, and the ability to exercise for longer periods of time. Their hearts were able to pump a greater volume of blood, and both blood pressure and heart rate during exercise declined. To guard against a placebo effect, an inactive product was given to half of the people in each study group. Hawthorn outperformed placebo every time.

A 1996 report by Weikl and colleagues underscores a sometimes overlooked reason to try hawthorn—the progressive nature of heart disease. The eight-week trial involved giving half of 137 patients a placebo and half a standardized hawthorn preparation. Each patient was evaluated at the beginning of the study, and records of individual symptoms were kept. At the end of the study, patients were evaluated again to see if their individual symptoms had improved. Patients who received hawthorn experienced an improvement in their symptoms. However, those who received only a placebo saw their symptoms worsen over this short period of time. The difference between these two groups was reflected in one more evaluation—those who took hawthorn reported a greater sense of mental well-being.

Animal studies have examined the internal physiological effects of hawthorn. In one study, researchers concluded that hawthorn can actually protect heart tissues from the damage caused by clogged arteries and an insufficient supply of oxygen.

OTHER WAYS HAWTHORN CAN HELP

Hawthorn's chief usefulness is as a supportive therapy in treating heart disease and factors associated with heart disease. In addition to the benefits described in this chapter, hawthorn may play a role in lowering high blood pressure. It also has been shown to lower the level of lipids in the blood, the insoluble fats that contribute to cholesterol (see chapter 7).

HOW TO TAKE HAWTHORN

What form does it come in? Hawthorn comes in capsules and drops. Make sure you buy a formulation made from the leaves and flowers (not the berries), as that is what has been proven most effective according to Commission E's most recent evaluation.

What's an effective dosage? There is little consensus on ideal dosage for this herb, and recommendations can be confusing due to manufacturers' different formulations. If you are healthy and want to take hawthorn as a preventative measure, follow the manufacturer's package instructions. If you are under treatment for heart problems, ask your doctor's advice.

Tips for use. Although studies have noted improvements after as little as eight weeks of use, herbal authority Christopher Hobbs stresses that hawthorn is really a long-term preventative. According to him, benefits become established at the three-month mark and, with regular use, continue to strengthen and nourish the heart over a period of years.

Are there side effects? Though not common, some people have reported some cases of nausea, sweating, and rash on the hands.

Caution! Although hawthorn is considered generally safe, adverse reactions are possible. Discontinue use at once if you experience breathing difficulty, rash, or sweating.

Because hawthorn has a significant cardiovascular effect, it may interact with other heart medicines. Hawthorn is not intended for self-medication, so be sure to consult your doctor before trying it.

VITAMIN C AND FLAVONOIDS

WHAT ARE VITAMIN C AND FLAVONOIDS?

Vitamin C is a powerful antioxidant, meaning that it scavenges free radicals, the harmful, cell-transforming chemicals that are largely the by-products of body metabolism. The changes free radicals bring about in healthy cells underlie many of our most dreaded diseases, including heart disease and cancer.

Flavonoids (also referred to as bioflavonoids) are a huge group of vitaminlike substances found in plants. Studies indicate that flavonoids facilitate the body's use of vitamin C, and some have been proven to boost its effectiveness in combating heart disease. You may not realize it, but you've already done a good deal of reading about the effects of flavonoids on the heart. Remember all those articles about the heart-healthy benefits of a glass of wine with dinner? One of the best known of all flavonoids, quercetin, is found in abundance in the skin of grapes. This would explain how a single glass of wine daily, with its dense concentration of nutrients, could benefit the heart.

THE MIRACLE EFFECT

In the early 1980s, writing in the *Journal of Human Nutrition,* medical researchers Horsey, Lively, and Dickerson asserted that, "ascorbic acid deficiency may be one of several preventable 'risk' factors contributing to the present epidemic of IHD (ischemic heart disease) in the Western world."

That's a bold statement, but subsequent research does suggest that vitamin C plays an amazing role in heart health. In particular, it seems to cut the risk of coronary artery disease.

When a diseased artery becomes completely blocked, triggering a heart attack, two things are actually at work. First, the artery has become narrowed through the accumulation of plaque or because it is blocked with clotted blood. But something else is happening as well. Healthy arteries are flexible, and the cells lining their interior walls expand and contract as they move the blood along. Diseased arteries lose their flexibility and become hard and rigid—which explains why the popular term for atherosclerosis is hardening of the arteries. Unable to dilate properly, the artery cannot accommodate the flow of blood and the heart becomes starved for nourishment and oxygen. Tissues in the heart become weakened, further impairing the heart's ability to function.

Vitamin C works on both problems. It helps control cholesterol and keeps blood platelets from clumping together into artery-clogging clots. In fact, it can even help break up clots that have already formed. Vitamin C also strengthens and nourishes the tissues of the coronary arteries and the heart itself.

Researchers have linked low tissue levels of vitamin C with high rates of heart disease. One reason for this is the fact that vitamin C helps keep coronary arteries relaxed and able to dilate; they can accommodate a greater blood flow and are less likely to be blocked by bits of arterial plaque. Inside the arteries, vitamin C may also have a Teflon-like effect that makes it more difficult for plaque to stick to artery walls.

When arteries do become narrowed and blood flow is restricted, vitamin C goes right on protecting—an animal study that duplicated the effects of coronary artery blockage found that heart tissues nourished on vitamin C sustained less damage.

Flavonoids are useful not only because they enhance vitamin C's effectiveness, they work independently to halt coronary artery disease. Grape skin products rich in quercetin, for example, have been shown to promote relaxation and dilation of aortic tissues in lab animals.

The flavonoid rutin also strengthens blood vessels. Combining rutin with vitamin C and another flavonoid, hesperidin, has been shown to significantly increase blood flow in people with heart disease.

HAS VITAMIN C BEEN USED BEFORE?

Vitamin C has long been used for general health, but its role in helping people with heart disease is relatively new. Interest began in the 1970s, when physicians and researchers noted that rates of heart disease in Western industrialized countries were on the increase while dietary intake of vitamin C was decreasing.

RESEARCH FINDINGS

Many studies have shown a link between high intake of vitamin C and lower rates of heart disease. Results of one of the largest such survey, which included 6,624 American men and women, were released to the public in 1998. In this study, those who had the highest blood levels of ascorbic acid (chemical equal to vitamin C) had 27 percent less prevalence of coronary artery disease than groups whose levels were the lowest. Researchers also found that an increase of just half a milligram of ascorbic acid per one-tenth of a liter of blood could drop disease rates by 11 percent.

Findings like this always invite questions from skeptics. Isn't it likely that people who take in more vitamin C are more conscious about other aspects of health as well? Is vitamin C getting all the credit when, in fact, these people may also weigh less, smoke less, and exercise more? Yes, it is possible, but most studies take care to adjust for or eliminate such variables.

A study done by Levine and Frei at the Boston University Medical Center offers proof that's hard to contest. In this test, forty-six patients with coronary artery disease were divided into two groups. Everyone in both groups underwent an ultrasound exam to determine how well the main artery in the upper arm was able to dilate.

Patients in one group received a single 2,000-milligram dose of vitamin C, while patients in the other group took a placebo. The ultrasound exams were repeated two hours later. While arteries in the placebo-taking group showed no change, the arteries of those who received vitamin C showed far greater ability to dilate.

What's more, those whose arteries had been the most rigid showed the greatest measure of improvement. Almost all patients in this group had 50 percent more dilation than previously.

OTHER WAYS VITAMIN C CAN HELP

Vitamin C is truly a multi-talented vitamin, and it plays a role in dealing with everything from short-term illnesses like the common cold to major, life-threatening diseases like cancer. In cardiovascular health alone, it not only protects the heart and arteries, it helps control cholesterol and may help control high blood pressure in some people. The same factors that make vitamin C effective for protecting the arteries of the heart work to protect the arteries that feed other organs, including the brain. A report published in the *British Medical Journal* in 1995 noted that people who had the highest intake of dietary vitamin C had the lowest risk of stroke.

HOW TO TAKE VITAMIN C AND FLAVONOIDS

What forms do they come in? Both vitamin C and flavonoids come in tablets. Vitamin C is also available in chewable tablets and powder.

What's an effective dose? Studies suggest that higher than average doses of vitamin C are needed to combat heart disease. For example, the Levine and Frei study that successfully dilated arteries of people with coronary artery disease used a daily oral dose of 2,000 milligrams.

Similar doses have also been used in studies showing vitamin C's ability to break up clots in the blood. While this dosage is considerably higher than the government recommendations, many practitioners and researchers are convinced that "standard" guidelines for C fall far short of what is really needed.

There are no established government guidelines for flavonoids, and advice from the experts varies a great deal. Your best option is to follow the package directions for the specific product you buy.

Tips for use. If you want to take large doses of vitamin C, don't shock your system—start at a low dose and build up. To avoid possible side effects (see below) divide your daily intake into several smaller doses and take throughout the day.

Are there side effects? While vitamin C is considered safe and nontoxic, it can cause stomach irritation and/or diarrhea. (See Tips for use, above.)

Caution! Some doctors warn against taking high doses of vitamin C during pregnancy, so be sure to consult your obstetrician before taking more than the recommended daily minimum of this vitamin.

WHAT ELSE CAN YOU DO?

The heart is an elegant example of how deeply interdependent the body's systems are. It's impossible to take care of your heart and ignore other factors. If you really care about heart health, you'll also want to find out what you can do about cholesterol (chapter 7) and homocysteine (chapter 14).

There are a few other things you should know about as well.

CONTROL BLOOD PRESSURE

The nutrients you've just read about all have been shown to play some role in controlling blood pressure under certain circumstances. However, high blood pressure is a serious and complex condition. Over time, untreated high blood pressure can cause the heart to become enlarged and severely weakened. And, unfortunately, there is no miracle nutrient or drug that will work reliably on its own.

If you have high blood pressure, you must work with your doctor to develop an overall strategy to bring your blood pressure down. This may include changes in diet, nutrition, exercise, and lifestyle habits. In some cases medication may also be needed.

These adjustments require commitment and effort on your part, but the results are measured in extra years of life and health.

CARNITINE:
AMINO ACID FOR THE HEART

The amino acid carnitine plays a large role in heart health. Carnitine deficiency can damage the heart's muscle tissue, while an adequate supply of carnitine can help protect the heart from damage caused by decreased oxygen supply. Congestive heart failure interferes with the production of carnitine, making an already bad situation even worse. However, a study done on people with congestive heart failure showed that carnitine supplementation can help. Taking 900 milligrams a day increased energy and ability to exercise. Another interesting finding suggests that carnitine may be more effective when taken with coenzyme Q-10.

DON'T OVERLOOK TAURINE

Taurine is another amino acid that should interest anyone concerned with cardiovascular health. In particular, it strengthens the heart muscle and improves its ability to contract. A placebo-controlled study of people with heart disease found that almost 80 percent of the group receiving this amino acid reported some benefit from the supplement.

CHAPTER FOURTEEN

Cut Heart Attack and Stroke Risk with
Lower Homocysteine

There may be a potential killer loose in your body, one you don't even know about. Luckily, there's a remedy that's simple, safe, and sure.

In one generation, the word *cholesterol* went from unknown to notorious. Now the word is *homocysteine*. Doctors are discovering that this little-known substance is a risk factor for life-threatening heart attack and stroke. Fortunately, there's a way to foil homocysteine, and it's readily available.

THE PROBLEM

Homocysteine is a by-product of protein metabolism. When all goes well, homocysteine is converted to a harmless substance and quickly cleared from the blood. However, several factors can interfere with this process, causing homocysteine levels to rise. As early as 1969, Dr. Kilmer McCully began to suspect that this condition played a role in cardiovascular disease.

We now know that Dr. McCully was right. A high level of homocysteine can have a lethal effect on the body. It dramatically raises the chances of heart attack and stroke because it hardens and clogs arteries (including the arteries that feed the heart and brain) and promotes the formation of blood clots in both veins and arteries. One study found that elderly men with high levels of homocysteine were twice as likely to have clogged arteries as men whose levels were low. Men with high levels of homocysteine are nearly three and a half times more likely to have a heart attack as men with low homocysteine, and the risk factor for women is only slightly less.

Unlike high cholesterol, which can take years to cause problems, homocysteine is a relatively fast worker. People born with a genetic inability to clear it from their blood will, if not treated, usually develop severe atherosclerosis and die before the age of 15. In animal studies, damage could be noted after just one week of exposure to high homocysteine levels.

WHO SUFFERS FROM HIGH HOMOCYSTEINE?

Abnormally high levels of homocysteine should be a rare occurrence, but they aren't. It's been estimated that 33 percent of people middle-aged and older have this problem. Some of the known factors that contribute to this are:

- **Deficiencies of folic acid and other B complex vitamins.** Studies show a remarkable correlation between high levels of homocysteine and low intake of folic acid (a B vitamin) and vitamins B6, and

B12. Unfortunately, this is quite a common deficiency. A 1993 report, published in the *American Journal of Clinical Nutrition*, found that 59 percent of middle-aged men were deficient in folic acid, 56 percent lacked enough B12, and 25 percent did not get enough B6. Studies of women have found similar—and often greater—deficiencies of these important B vitamins.

- **Genetic inheritance.** A common genetic mutation puts people at risk for high homocysteine.
- **Age.** The older one gets the higher the level of homocysteine is likely to be. Whether this is due to declining nutrition, greater demands for certain vitamins, or some other factor has not yet been established.
- **Alcoholism.** In a hospital study, active alcoholics were compared to both nondrinkers and recovered alcoholics. The active alcoholics had significantly higher levels of homocysteine than the other two groups, and recovered alcoholics had no higher levels of homocysteine than nondrinkers. When the active alcoholics stopped drinking, homocysteine levels fell within one to two weeks.
- **Coffee and cigarettes.** A Norwegian study determined that men age forty to forty-two who drank nine or more cups of coffee a day had 18 percent higher blood levels of homocysteine than men who drank no coffee. For women, levels were nearly 30 percent higher. Those who combined cigarette smoking (twenty or more a day) with coffee drinking had the highest levels of homocysteine.

WHAT ARE THE SYMPTOMS?

High homocysteine doesn't give you a headache, stomachache, rash, or any other mild warning signal. Unless you have your blood analyzed, there is no way to tell whether you have high levels of homocysteine.

WHAT'S THE OUTLOOK?

High homocysteine levels take an equally high toll on the body's circulatory system and can lead to stroke, heart attack, coronary artery disease, blood clots in veins and arteries, and other extremely serious health problems. Homocysteine levels do not fall by themselves. In fact, they tend to increase as we age. Fortunately, however, this is one degenerative process that can be halted and turned around—not with drugs from your doctor but with supplements of B vitamins.

WHAT YOU SHOULD KNOW

Are you getting enough B vitamins in your diet? Probably not. Many people fail to take in the amounts of folic acid, B6, and B12 recommended by the government. To complicate matters even more, there is a raging controversy about how much is "enough." At one time, the United States government recommended a daily allowance of 400 micrograms of folic acid. In the 1990s, this was lowered to 200 micrograms for men and only 180 for women. Studies like those referred to in this chapter persuaded the government to raise the recommended allowance back to 400 micrograms, but many researchers feel an even higher dose of folic acid is necessary to reverse homocysteine levels once they have begun to rise.

PROVEN MIRACLES

FOLIC ACID, B6, AND B12

WHAT ARE FOLIC ACID, B6, AND B12?

Folic acid, B6, and B12 are all members of the B-vitamin family. Folic acid appears to be the key player in terms of homocysteine, but B6 and B12 are also important. Although all of these are available in food sources, most of us probably don't ingest enough of these nutrients.

THE MIRACLE EFFECT

Since a great many Americans and others who eat a contemporary Western diet probably don't get enough B vitamins, researchers have wondered whether compensating for these deficiencies with B-complex supplements could help lower homocysteine. The answer so far is a resounding *Yes!*

Tufts University researcher Jacob Selhub, who has conducted several studies on the effects of high homocysteine, has concluded that, "regimens of vitamin supplementation (including folic acid, vitamin B12, and vitamin B6) effectively lower moderately elevated plasma homocysteine concentrations to the normal range."

Even readings at the high end of normal may be

enough to put your health at risk. While the normal range for homocysteine is 4 to 17 micromoles per deciliter of blood, readings above 12 have been linked to increased rates of cardiovascular disease.

As far as researchers have been able to determine, the body utilizes supplemental B-complex vitamins in the same way it utilizes dietary forms of these vitamins or at least effectively enough to keep homocysteine from climbing to abnormal levels.

Researchers are confident that lowering homocysteine levels with supplements of folic acid and vitamins B6 and B12 will keep many people from developing the problems that lead to stroke, heart attack, and premature death. Sarah Beresford, a University of Washington researcher whose 1995 article in *The New England Journal of Medicine* helped draw attention to the problem, has estimated that upward of fifty thousand lives could be saved annually if people would take the time to get enough of these essential vitamins.

HAVE THESE VITAMINS BEEN USED BEFORE?

Folic acid, vitamin B6, and vitamin B12 are considered essential for health, and the U.S. government has established recommended daily allowances for all three. Unfortunately, these allowance were established before research on homocysteine came to light and there is a consensus among researchers that the guidelines are far too low. For example, Dr. Joel Mason of Tufts University School of Medicine has noted that homocysteine levels began to rise when folic acid intake fell.

RESEARCH FINDINGS

Research studies leave little doubt that higher intake of folic acid and other B vitamins dramatically decreases disease. One of the largest studies ever undertaken has tracked eighty thousand female nurses since 1980 to evaluate the long-term impact of nutrition and lifestyle habits on health. After all other health factors were adjusted for, B vitamins were seen to have an enormous impact on the health of these women. For example:

- Women whose intake of folic acid exceeded 545 micrograms per day were 31 percent less likely to suffer a heart attack or fatal case of coronary artery disease than women whose intake was less than 150 micrograms per day.
- A daily intake of 5.9 milligrams or more of vitamin B6 was associated with a 33 percent lower risk of heart attack and coronary artery disease.
- Women with the highest intake of both folic acid and vitamin B6 had a 45 percent lower risk of heart attack and coronary artery disease than women with the lowest combined intake of these vitamins.
- Up to certain maximum levels, more folic acid may mean less disease. Between ranges of 150 micrograms and 700 micrograms of folic acid intake per day, each increase of 100 micrograms was associated with approximately 6 percent less risk of disease.

Sarah Beresford's research supports the idea that doses above the government's recommended allowances are needed to lower elevated homocysteine levels. In her study, when men with high homocysteine took 650 micrograms of folic acid each day, levels fell by 42 percent.

A large-scale British study also revealed a dramatic reduction in homocysteine levels. The study involved 1,114 individuals, ages twenty-three to seventy-five, in twelve different trials. Daily doses above 500 micrograms of folic acid dramatically lowered homocysteine. The authors of the study concluded that among people who eat a typical Western diet, adding these B vitamins could "reduce blood homocysteine concentrations by about a quarter to a third."

How much will reducing high homocysteine levels help? Research has shown that just as risk escalates with high levels, it de-escalates with even partial reduction. Experts believe even a slight reduction will decidedly reduce the risk of disease.

OTHER WAYS THESE VITAMINS CAN HELP

Any woman who's had a baby is probably familiar with folic acid. Taken as a supplement, this vitamin protects against several major birth defects, including the crippling spina bifida. In adequate amounts, these B-complex vitamins help normalize blood pressure, regulate mood, keep female hormones in balance, and stimulate the immune system.

HOW TO TAKE FOLIC ACID, B6, AND B12

What form does it come in? B vitamins come in a dizzying array of tablets and capsules, and are sold alone as well as in combination (B complex) preparations.

What's an effective dose? Experts agree that we need more of these vitamins than government guidelines endorse, and a good B vitamin complex will exceed government recommendations. Most studies have achieved good results with just 500 to 750 micrograms of folic acid daily—good news, since too much of this B vitamin can be harmful (see Caution, below).

Tips for use. Since these vitamins work together and influence each other, it's important to take all three. The most convenient way to do this is in a B-complex capsule, but be sure to check the label before you buy, since some formulations we checked lacked adequate levels of folic acid.

Are there side effects? High doses of these vitamins may cause gastric upset, gas, bloating, and diarrhea.

Caution! Many physicians feel that long-term use of high doses of folic acid poses a risk of kidney damage, so don't take more than 800 micrograms a day without consulting your doctor.

Don't take high doses of folic acid if you have anemia, since it could mask your condition and prevent you from receiving proper treatment.

CHAPTER FIFTEEN

Sleep Away Your
Insomnia

If you're reluctant to take prescription remedies that can be habit forming and over-the-counter products that leave you groggy, help is on the way. Tossing and turning can become a thing of the past with natural sleep-inducers!

Without a doubt, insomnia is one of mankind's oldest and most pervasive problems. It's been estimated that nearly 40 million Americans suffer from some form of insomnia. And, to make matters worse, we're getting less sleep all the time—about 20 percent less than just a century ago. While there's an abundant supply of both prescription and over-the-counter remedies available, many people find the side effects (ranging from addiction to next-day "hangover") intolerable. Research has gone full circle, and now finds that some of the best hangover-free solutions don't come from the pharmacy shelf but straight from Mother Nature's cupboard.

THE PROBLEM

Everyone has different rest requirements. If you don't sleep much and have plenty of pep and energy, that's fine. But if you don't meet your body's own sleep requirements, you'll end up dragging through life and feeling sleepy during the day. One or two nights of troubled sleep probably won't make a big difference in your life, but if the problem becomes chronic, the effects can be significant, ranging from flatness and irritability to physical aches and pains to reduced ability to concentrate or perform tasks.

WHO GETS INSOMNIA?

All sorts of conditions can lead to insomnia, including physical problems, psychological problems, and lifestyle variables. If you're having trouble sleeping, ask yourself whether any of the following risk factors may be contributing to your problem.

- **Anxiety and worry.** For some perverse reason, nighttime is often the right time for our fears to run rampant. Symptoms can range from mild sleeplessness to all-out anxiety attacks, complete with pounding heart and racing pulse.
- **Depression.** Many people associate depression with sleeping too much, but insomnia is almost as common, especially if the depression is mixed with symptoms of anxiety.
- **Stress.** Overwork, studying hard, the end of a relationship, or a rocky patch in a marriage—all these forms of stress rob you of tranquillity and make it hard for you to sleep.

- **Changes in day-to-day schedule.** Changes in work hours, mealtimes, and other routines can send your body all the wrong signals.
- **Positive changes.** Good things can also affect sleeping patterns adversely. Typical in this category are receiving a job promotion, moving to a new home, starting a new relationship, having a baby, and planning for a major celebration, event, or vacation.
- **Bad bedroom habits.** Do you watch TV, work, or eat in bed? Is your bedroom too light, too noisy, or too quiet? If so, you may be sabotaging your own chances for a good night's sleep.
- **Lack of exercise.** Your mind may be tired, but if you're a chronic couch potato, your sedentary lifestyle may be preventing you from falling asleep. The body needs to be tired, too! (Just don't exercise too close to bedtime.)
- **Drinking alcohol or smoking too close to bedtime.** Alcohol can make you drowsy, but it can also make you wake up after only a short period of sleep. Cigarettes, on the other hand, can act as a mild stimulant.
- **Drinking caffeine.** Coffee and cola drinks are obvious no-no's, but also avoid those teas that contain caffeine.
- **Eating too much too close to bedtime.** Like drinking, eating can make you drowsy—but undigested food can also lead to heartburn that wakes you up.
- **Medication.** Some prescription medications can cause insomnia, so if your troubles began about the same time your prescription did, check with your doctor.

- **Pain.** If you have a condition that causes chronic discomfort (such as arthritis), you may find that pain keeps you from getting the rest you need.
- **Allergies and other breathing problems.** Any condition that causes you to cough, wheeze, or struggle for breath will interfere with your ability to get a good night's sleep.
- **Menopause.** Night sweats and hot flashes are common causes of wakefulness in women.
- **Age.** Sleep patterns shift markedly with age, and about half of all those over sixty-five suffer chronic sleep disturbance.
- **Restless leg syndrome.** Older people are often kept awake by this harmless but mysterious condition, which causes the legs to twitch and move restlessly during the night.
- **Thyroid imbalance.** Overactive thyroid can interfere with natural sleep patterns.
- **Hypoglycemia.** Falling blood sugar levels can trigger a chain reaction that results in the brain getting an internal "wake up" call long before the alarm goes off.

WHAT ARE THE SYMPTOMS?

There are several patterns of insomnia. The one most often associated with the word is difficulty in falling asleep. However, many people with insomnia fall asleep easily but are unable to stay asleep long enough to get adequate rest. They either wake too early in the morning or awaken frequently and for prolonged periods throughout the night. Finally, you may be someone whose sleep is abnormally restless or troubled by nightmares. All of these patterns prevent you from getting the rest your mind and body need, and are considered forms of insomnia.

WHAT'S THE OUTLOOK?

Most cases of insomnia take care of themselves. It's very common to go through bouts of sleeplessness that last a few days or even a few weeks, then reestablish a normal sleep pattern. However, some people have chronic sleep problems. Bouts of sleeplessness may last a month or more and recur so frequently that normal sleep is the exception rather than the rule. Although sedatives and other prescription medications may help, they also have side effects (such as morning grogginess and addictive potential) that make them unsuitable for long-term use. If you're a chronic problem-sleeper, you'll want to try natural solutions that don't have these potentially harmful side effects.

WHAT YOU NEED TO KNOW

Not everyone who's short of sleep suffers from insomnia. With the helter-skelter pace of modern life, many of us work too many hours, have too many obligations, and find our days so crammed with things to do, we literally don't have *time* to sleep. Before you decide you have insomnia, check your schedule. If you only allow six hours for sleeping when you really need seven or eight, free up some extra sack time.

Assuming that time in bed isn't your problem, remember that insomnia can be a secondary symptom of a whole host of problems. Try pinpointing what's causing your sleepless nights. If the underlying cause is one of those listed on pages 258–260, find out what measures you can take to treat or minimize that specific cause.

PROVEN MIRACLES

VALERIAN

WHAT IS VALERIAN?

Valerian is a plant with no nutritive value and a rather unpleasant taste. Its root, however, is another matter. Valerian root (and products made from it) has great value as a natural aid for sleep and relaxation. Despite the fact that valerian is often called natural Valium, it's important to understand that Valium is not derived from valerian and is not chemically related to it.

THE MIRACLE EFFECT

What is the secret of valerian? Actually, there are two secrets. Scientists have identified two substances, contained within the root, that have distinct pharmacological effects. Valepotriates and sesquiterpenes both work on the central nervous system. They are mildly sedating and promote sleep by slowing central nervous system activity and relaxing the mind and body.

One of valerian's big benefits lies in what it does not do—namely, leave users with a "hangover" or interfere with normal sleep cycles. While valerian users enthusiastically report more and better sleep, they do not report episodes of morning grogginess as a result of use, nor do they say they have trouble recalling their dreams—a common complaint with prescription medications.

HAS VALERIAN BEEN USED BEFORE?

Valerian has been used for well over two thousand years. Ancient Greek physicians prescribed it for a wide variety of problems. Galen, the most famous physician of the early Christian era, prescribed it specifically for insomnia. Its use has persisted throughout the centuries, and it was especially popular in nineteenth-century Europe, where it was used either on its own or as an ingredient in calmatives and nerve tonics.

RESEARCH FINDINGS

Although valerian's reputation as an all-purpose sedative stretches back for centuries, it wasn't until the 1980s that scientific studies tracked its effects on large numbers of human subjects. Numerous studies have now confirmed what proponents of this miracle root knew all along: Valerian works!

Double-blind studies, in which one group receives a realistic-looking placebo while a second group receives an authentic substance, show that valerian helps people fall asleep more quickly, stay asleep longer, and get a more restful night's sleep. In one Portuguese study, conducted in the late 1980s, 89 percent of those who received valerian in a double-blind study described their sleep as "much improved," and a full 44 percent said their sleep was "perfect." Studies done on the elderly have shown valerian to be equally effective on older people.

Germany's Commission E, a massive, state-sponsored inquiry into the medical effectiveness of all sorts of herbs and nutrients, found this herb so effective it recommends drinking valerian tea throughout the day to calm nerves and soothe tensions.

OTHER WAYS VALERIAN CAN HELP

Because valerian is a mild sedative, it has been recommended for all sorts of problems related to tension, including stomach upset, backache, headache, and general anxiety. In 1992 a Japanese research team published a report concerning valerian's effect on mice. The team concluded that valerian may be useful as an antidepressant, though much further study is needed.

HOW TO TAKE VALERIAN

What form does it come in? Valerian comes in a variety of forms, including capsules, extracts, and tinctures. Valerian tea is also popular and can be found in most health food stores.

One of the plant's strong points, from an herbalist's point of view, is that it combines well with other substances. For this reason, many sleep-promoting and anxiety-reducing products use valerian as an ingredient with substances such as hops and lemon balm.

What's an effective dose? Studies vary when it comes to establishing an effective dose of valerian, possibly because different potencies were used in testing. However, several studies suggest that lower doses are as effective as higher ones, and that one form is likely to be as effective as another.

Tips for use. Since valerian works well with other sleep-inducing herbs, you might want to try one of the many products that deliver this miracle in combination form. If you find a bedtime cup of tea soothing, you might want to replace your usual brew with an infusion made of valerian root dried and sold for this purpose.

Are there side effects? Unlike synthetic sleep aids, valerian is virtually free of side effects. When taken in recommended doses, it is also safe, and adverse reactions have not been reported. It has been noted that valerian in excessive amounts can make some people feel nauseated.

Caution! Valerian should not be taken with alcohol, as the two can interact to cause excessive drowsiness. Terry Willard, president of the Canadian Association of Herbal Practitioners, points out that while valerian is not addictive, it can be habit-forming, and stronger doses are needed over time. For this reason, he suggests taking valerian only on a short-term basis of no more than one month. He also cautions that pregnant women should not take valerian until further human studies have been done.

PASSIONFLOWER

WHAT IS PASSIONFLOWER?

If you have a garden, you may be growing a blue-flowering plant you know as passionflower. Alert: This isn't the plant we're talking about, so don't race to the garden to make your own preparations. The garden plant—*Pas-*

siflora caerulea—contains toxic substances, and this has led to much confusion over the safety of passionflower preparations. The plant used in sleep aids is *Passiflora incarnata,* and it does not contain toxic substances.

THE MIRACLE EFFECT

The full riddle of passionflower's effectiveness has yet to be unraveled. In studying preparations made from this plant, scientists have focused on two groups of substances, alkaloids and flavonoids. Passionflower contains several specific types of each, some of which produce a sedative effect. However, most researchers are not quite satisfied with this answer, and note that the observed effect of passionflower is stronger than the chemical amounts present in the plant would indicate. This means that either the substances have a synergistic effect or other substances within the plant are responsible for the plant's soothing properties.

HAS PASSIONFLOWER BEEN USED BEFORE?

Passionflower has been used to calm nerves and promote sleep for centuries. It was popular in America in the early 1900s and was a common ingredient in numerous over-the-counter preparations. In 1978 the FDA found that not enough human studies had been done to confirm passionflower's status. They ruled that passionflower could not be recognized as "safe and effective," thus prohibiting its use as an ingredient in nonprescription medications. Despite the U.S. ruling, passionflower remains a popular and highly regarded ingredient throughout Europe and is a leading ingredient in numerous calmatives and sleep aids.

RESEARCH FINDINGS

One of the problems proponents of this miracle herb face in establishing its scientific credentials is the fact that human studies have yet to be conducted. However, lab studies on both mice and rats have proven that passionflower extract has a definite and positive effect on sleep and relaxation. Studies on mice have shown that even in low doses it significantly reduces motor activity. Other studies, done on rats, confirmed that passionflower extract not only calmed motor activity but significantly lengthened sleep. After a review of the studies, Germany's Commission E judged passionflower as safe and effective for use.

OTHER WAYS PASSIONFLOWER CAN HELP

An interesting study, published in 1973, suggested that passionflower may have a use very different from its traditional one. This study found that passionflower extract worked as an antimicrobial agent for fighting yeast, molds, and bacteria. Unfortunately, this interesting research thread has not been followed up and begs for further exploration.

HOW TO TAKE PASSIONFLOWER

What form does it come in? Passionflower comes in extract and tincture form, in capsules, and in a loose, dried form meant to be steeped and drunk as an infusion. Like valerian, it is also a good ''combiner'' and is an ingredient in several good, safe, and natural over-the-counter products.

What's an effective dose?   Since human studies have not yet been done, guidelines for an effective dose have not yet been established. Because of this and because various products will differ in strength, be sure to follow the manufacturer's package directions.

Tips for use.   While there is no evidence that one form of passionflower is more effective than another, many people find a steaming cup of tea, brewed as an infusion, especially relaxing.

Are there side effects?   When taken according to manufacturers' directions, passionflower is considered safe and free of side effects. However, taking passionflower in excessive doses may have side effects, and should be avoided.

Caution!   Excessive amounts of passionflower may be harmful for pregnant or breast-feeding women and must be avoided. Also, excessive use of passionflower should be avoided by people taking MAOI medications for depression, as excessive sedation may result.

WHY *NOT* MELATONIN?

Without a doubt, melatonin is one of the best-selling sleep aids on the market today, with Americans buying an estimated $250 million worth of the pills each year. But that doesn't mean that melatonin is effective—or safe. The fact is, the jury is still out on both of these questions. So far, melatonin is more an unknown than a miracle.

Despite all the hype, respondents to a survey conducted by *Consumer Reports* magazine gave melatonin relatively low ratings as a sleep aid. While 25 percent of four hundred people questioned said melatonin was helpful, almost 50 percent said it had no benefit at all.

More worrisome to physicians is the safety question. Melatonin is a naturally occurring hormone, produced in small amounts by the body's pineal gland. Melatonin levels rise naturally before sleep, and research leaves little doubt that this hormone plays a role in regulating sleep rhythms and the body's natural clock. However, hormones are powerful agents, and artificially raising or lowering them can have profound effects on the body. Dr. Gary Richardson, assistant professor of medicine at Brown University, has pointed out that some studies suggest that melatonin may make insomnia worse and even, for some users, cause blood vessels to narrow. Dr. Richard I. Wurtman, a Massachusetts Institute of Technology researcher, believes that small levels of melatonin can be helpful but points out that this unregulated substance is commonly sold in dosages that raise blood levels of melatonin to ten times or more above normal—a situation that could have long-term consequences for users.

With melatonin's efficacy still unproven and its long-term safety still unknown, we can't recommend it for use as of yet.

WHAT ELSE CAN YOU DO?

Instead of counting sheep when you can't sleep, try some of the strategies below for this age-old problem!

KAVA

Kava is a wonder-worker when it comes to calming the nerves. But, for a certain percentage of people, it has also been found to be an effective sleep aid. To find out more about this amazing gift from the South Pacific, read about it in chapter 1 on Anxiety.

HOPS CAN HELP

Have you ever noticed that drinking beer makes you drowsy? The reason isn't the alcohol, but the hops. We don't recommend drinking beer before bed, as the alcohol is counterproductive to a good night's sleep, but hops may do the trick. Take hops in a product that combines them with other herbs, brew hops tea, or take as a tincture.

Hops should be taken only in moderate amounts—no more than half a gram of dried hops daily, according to Germany's Commission E. People with depression *should not* take hops, as this natural sedative may make the condition worse.

REISHI MUSHROOMS

Although reishi mushrooms aren't yet well known in the West as insomnia-fighters, president of the Canadian Association of Herbal Practitioners Terry Willard says they are his personal treatment of choice for tension-related sleep problems. This is one mushroom you probably won't want to eat, as the taste is not at all pleasant. Try taking it in tablet form, according to the manufacturer's package directions.

CALCIUM AND MAGNESIUM

Calcium's importance for maintaining strong bones and teeth has overshadowed its other health benefits, which include regulating heartbeat and blood pressure and transmitting nerve messages in the central nervous system. Calcium also works with magnesium to relax muscles.

Magnesium has a strong role to play in nervous disorders of all sorts, and people with abnormally low levels of magnesium have been found to have higher levels of mental disorders and sleep disturbances. Make sure you get your recommended daily requirements of these miracle minerals, which can be purchased separately or in combined form. For best results, take calcium and magnesium in a 2:1 ratio (twice as much calcium as magnesium).

ST. JOHN'S WORT

If your insomnia is associated with mild depression, you might want to give St. John's wort a try. Not only does it help lift mild cases of the blues, at least one study has found it specifically helpful for cases of mood-related insomnia. St. John's wort is discussed in detail in chapter 9.

TAKE TEA

While many teas contain caffeine and should be avoided before bedtime, several herbs are ideal for sleep-promoting teas. We've already mentioned that valerian, passionflower, and hops can be brewed as tea. You might also want to consider teas containing:

- Lemon
- Catnip
- Chamomile
- Kava

Be sure to explore the shelves of your local health food store, as there are also many good sleep-promoting teas made of various combinations of herbs.

CHAPTER SIXTEEN

Stop the Formation of
Kidney Stones

Even in people predisposed to form kidney stones, simple, natural strategies are proving effective in warding off stones permanently.

As chronic health problems go, kidney stones carry a low risk of death. That's the up side. If you've ever had kidney stones, you know what the down side is: excruciating pain as the stone works its way through the urethra for elimination. Once you're at this point, you need medical help, and kidney stones can be promptly and safely treated by a doctor. However, the simple and effective strategies in this chapter may prevent stones from forming in the first place.

THE PROBLEM

Kidney stones form when minerals and other insoluble waste substances become so dense in the urine that they can no longer be broken down and passed painlessly out of the body. Instead, they form crystals and the crystals form stones. Inside the kidney, the stones may cause relatively little pain. When pieces break off and enter the urethra, the pain can be intense. The agony of passing a kidney stone has been described in any number of creative ways. Even the smallest stones are larger than the urethral passage, and the crystals found on the surface of each stone are sharp and jagged, scraping tender tissue as they are forced along.

WHO GETS KIDNEY STONES?

Risk factors associated with kidney stone formation include:

- **Being a man.** Although women can and do develop stones, men are far more likely than women to suffer with this problem.
- **Having had kidney stones before.** People who've had stones once are at high risk for developing them again.
- **Family history.** Stones run in families, probably because both fixed factors (such as individual biology) and flexible factors (such as dietary habits) are passed from generation to generation.
- **Having a bladder infection.** Bladder infections can start a chain reaction in urinary chemistry, ultimately causing urine to become highly alkaline, a condition that can lead to stone formation. (To find out more about what you can do, see chapter 4 on Bladder Infections.)
- **Underlying medical condition.** Hyperthyroidism, hyperparathyroidism, and a few other medical conditions can cause kidney stones to form. Once these

conditions are treated, stone formation is usually no longer a problem.

WHAT ARE THE SYMPTOMS?

The most memorable symptom of a kidney stone is pain—strong, sharp, and continual. Although this pain usually radiates from the urethra, lower back pain can also be part of this disorder. In addition, there can be blood in the urine, usually caused by the scraping of the stone's sharp edges against the delicate tissue lining the urethra. Complete blockage is a rare but serious and even life-threatening possibility. When it occurs, the sufferer can develop fever and other signs of kidney failure.

WHAT'S THE OUTLOOK?

What did people do before medical treatment was available for kidney stones? The lucky suffered pain and incapacity until the stones were passed, while a few unlucky ones died of kidney blockage and failure.

The lesson: Kidney stones are nothing to fool with. Stones that have formed require prompt medical attention. Fortunately, there are now several effective treatments available, most of them nonsurgical. Unfortunately, certain people seem prone to stone formation, and having stones once increases the likelihood that you will have them again.

If you don't want to spend a lifetime suffering recurrent bouts of kidney stones, there *are* things you can do. While there is no drug to prevent recurrence of stones, there is a growing consensus in the medical community that recurrence can be effectively prevented with a few simple, inexpensive strategies.

WHAT YOU SHOULD KNOW

If you pass a kidney stone, try to retrieve it and take it to your doctor for analysis. Knowing what kind of stones your body is forming will help you choose a strategy to prevent future recurrence.

The vast majority of stones are made of calcium, magnesium, phosphate, and oxalic acid or uric acid, but there are several other types as well. While some prevention strategies are effective for all stones, some are more effective for a particular type of stone. Stones related to urinary tract infections, for example, are not calcium stones and are best prevented by eliminating the infections that cause them.

PROVEN MIRACLES

THREE SIMPLE STRATEGIES

Dr. Gary Curhan, a leading practitioner and researcher, has written that "Clearly, efforts to prevent or at least reduce the likelihood of developing a kidney stone would be an important component of the care of patients at risk. In particular, modifiable dietary factors appear to play an important role in the formation of calcium oxalate stones."

Although a leader in the field, Dr. Curhan is not alone in this opinion. Over the past decade, several studies have focused on the cause-and-prevention aspect of kidney stone formation. The results are now in, and several studies suggest that stone prevention may be easier and far more effective than previously believed.

STRATEGY #1: INCREASE URINARY OUTPUT

Producing more urine is one way of preventing new stones from forming. The more urine the body passes, the greater the volume of insoluble wastes it can excrete. According to Dr. Curhan, a good goal to aim for is an output of 2 liters (a little less than 2 quarts) a day. You can meet this goal without taking prescription diuretics if you:

- **Drink more water—and we do mean water.** People who think they're drinking plenty of water are often mistaken. What they're drinking plenty of is coffee, sodas, and other liquids. These don't necessarily increase urine output, and some—such as salty soups or broths—may even contribute to fluid retention and decreased urine flow.

- **Consider goldenrod** (also written as *golden rod*). While goldenrod's amazing uses are not well known in North America, its reputation in Europe dates back more than two hundred years. A text dating from 1788 notes that after drinking goldenrod infusion for several weeks, a young boy was able to pass numerous large stones and a quantity of gravellike smaller ones. Although the exact chemical reasons for its effectiveness are not known, several studies have concluded that it does reliably increase urine production.

    Commission E, Germany's massive task force on the safety and usefulness of plant medicines, endorses goldenrod as a bona-fide diuretic and has found no harmful side effects associated with its use.

    In America, Varo Tyler, an authority on herbal

medicine, is one of the first to have noted the benefits of goldenrod, calling it the safest and most effective of the diuretic herbs recommended for prevention of kidney stones. Although the herb is not yet as familiar to Americans as to Europeans, goldenrod is available in the U.S. without prescription and usually comes in liquid extract form. If you decide to try goldenrod, be sure to follow the specific manufacturer's instructions for use.

STRATEGY #2: SOLVE THE CALCIUM PARADOX

Since most kidney stones contain calcium, cutting down on calcium should help cut down on stone recurrence, right? Well, the problem is a bit more complex than that, and the correct answer is both *yes* and *no*.

For many years, physicians routinely told kidney-stone patients to restrict the number of calcium-rich foods in their diet. Beginning in 1980, Dr. Gary Curhan and colleagues began a long-term study of calcium intake and kidney-stone formation in women. The study, conducted over a period of ten years, asked more than 90,000 women to fill out questionnaires about dietary habits, use of nutritional supplements, and incidence of kidney stones. Not surprisingly, results showed that women who took calcium supplements were about 20 percent more likely to suffer from kidney stones than women who did not take supplements.

But this finding was overshadowed by the big surprise. After the data had been analyzed, Curhan and his colleagues discovered that women who had more calcium in their diets (by choosing calcium-rich foods) cut their risk of developing stones dramatically. To be specific, women eating 1,000 milligrams of calcium in food sources daily had only half as many incidences of stones as women who ingested only 500 milligrams of the supplement per day!

The researchers theorized that calcium can help prevent stone formation by keeping oxalate from being absorbed from food. They noted that 67 percent of the women taking calcium supplements took them without food, and speculated that taking supplements with meals could equalize the imbalance.

Another large study by the same research team, begun in 1986 and lasting through 1990, followed over 45,000 men ranging from forty to seventy-five years of age. Although the men did not take calcium supplements in significant amounts, the findings for dietary calcium intake was the same. For both men and women, high intake of *dietary* calcium decreases the risk of stone formation.

Caution! If you're taking calcium to ward off osteoporosis, don't stop or cut back for fear of developing kidney stones. Try getting more calcium from foods like low-fat dairy products and tofu.

STRATEGY #3: PAY ATTENTION TO DAILY VALUES

While taking more than the recommended daily dosage of vitamins and nutrients won't prevent stones from forming, correcting deficiencies might help. Make sure you have enough of the following nutrients:

- **Magnesium.** Stanley Gershoff, dean emeritus at Tufts University School of Nutrition, believes that magnesium helps prevent calcium oxalate from forming into crystals. Although the exact chemical interaction remains unknown, Gershoff has conducted studies that back up his claim. In one study, 149 people with a history of recurrent calcium kidney stones took 300 milligrams of magnesium per day. Ninety percent of the people in the study had no stones over a four-year period, and those who did had few incidences of recurrence. If you think low magnesium may be your problem, Dr. Gershoff recommends taking it under a doctor's supervision and working to find the lowest dose that works for you.

- **Vitamin B6.** Taking supplements of vitamin B6 has also been associated with a decrease in kidney-stone formation. In addition to magnesium, participants in the study cited above took 10 milligrams of the vitamin per day. Another study, conducted in India, found that people cut their risk of recurrence when they took 40 milligrams of B6 as a daily supplement. Dr. Fred Coe, of the University of Chicago Pritzger School of Medicine, explains that B6 deficiency can promote stone formation but adds that, in his opinion, "most stone-formers aren't B6 deficient." He cautions that people taking the vitamin as a supplement should not exceed 50 milligrams a day and should stop if there is any numbness in the hands or feet.

- **Potassium.** Low levels of potassium can increase the risk of kidney-stone formation. If your diet includes plenty of fruits, vegetables, and grains, you probably don't need to worry about potassium deficiency.

WHAT ELSE CAN YOU DO?

There are a few more simple steps that can pay off in permanent relief from kidney stones.

PAY ATTENTION TO DIET

For some people, there's a close link between diet and kidney-stone formation. If you're serious about preventing recurrence of kidney stones, cut down on your use of:

- **Oxalates.** Oxalates, chemical substances that contribute to the formation of kidney stones, are found in many of the foods we eat every day. To decrease your chance of developing stones, cut back on oxalate-rich foods, which include beans, cocoa, parsley, rhubarb, and spinach.
- **Salt.** Lowering dietary sodium can reduce the amount of calcium in the urine, cutting your risk of stone formation. Try flavoring foods with herbs or lemon juice, and avoid fast and processed foods that have a high salt content.
- **Sugar.** Too much sugar packs a double whammy. First, it decreases urine output. Second, it increases calcium in the urine. This two-step process leads to a higher concentration of urinary calcium, a factor in stone formation.
- **Protein.** If you eat more than 10 ounces of meat a day, you may be setting yourself up for problems. Animal protein increases your body's levels of both

calcium, a common stone component, and uric acid, a less common component of kidney stones.

DON'T GO OVERBOARD ON VITAMINS

If taken in very high doses, both vitamins C and D may cause recurrence of kidney stones. If you are prone to kidney stones, consult your doctor before taking more than the standard recommended daily amount of either of these.

BE SELECTIVE ABOUT BEVERAGES

Both alcohol and caffeine are somewhat dehydrating and should be avoided or limited, because they tend to decrease urinary output. Caffeine is found not only in coffee but in certain teas and carbonated beverages. If you enjoy these drinks, switch to decaffeinated varieties. If you're a soda drinker, be sure to check the label for sodium, which can add a lot of salt to your diet.

For overall kidney and bladder health, the best choice is water. Two to three quarts a day will help your body get rid of calcium and other insoluble wastes—*before* they form crystals that can cause you pain and problems farther down the road.

CHAPTER SEVENTEEN

The Secret of a Healthy
Liver

Did you know that an innocuous weed is the most powerful agent there is for protecting your liver from cancer-causing agents and disease? Dramatic new evidence shows that milk thistle is even effective against damage done by hepatitis and cirrhosis!

Quick—name three things your liver does. Can't come up with an answer? That's the problem. Most people know all about the heart and its importance, but the liver—just as necessary for life and every bit as vulnerable—is often overlooked. That's too bad, because this football-shaped organ performs more than a dozen important functions. According to the American Liver Foundation, the liver:

- Neutralizes and destroys toxins
- Cleanses blood of bacteria and waste products
- Stores certain vitamins, minerals, and sugars
- Manufactures proteins
- Produces bile, essential for proper digestion
- Regulates production and excretion of cholesterol
- Produces quick energy on demand
- Metabolizes alcohol

- Regulates fat transport
- Monitors and regulates the blood levels of many chemicals and drugs
- Maintains hormone balance
- Helps regulate blood clotting
- Boosts the immune system to help resist disease
- Stores iron
- Replaces its own damaged tissue

Enough said? If you've taken the health of your liver for granted, now's the time to start paying attention!

THE PROBLEM

Is your liver healthy? Are you sure? Fortunately, most people don't have liver disease—but that doesn't mean their "healthy" livers aren't being damaged slowly and significantly, day by day over a period of years. The fact is that just by going about your daily business, you're subjecting your liver to all sorts of stress.

The liver is one of the body's major waste-filtering organs, targeting and removing bacteria and other organic toxins from the blood. The modern liver has a new and even bigger job to do. In addition to dealing with organic wastes, it must deal with a whole host of *inorganic wastes*—the chemicals from air pollution, aerosols, synthetic fibers, cosmetics, cleaning fluids, dyes, and thousands of other products that find their way into our bodies. Even beneficial products, including some prescription and over-the-counter medications may sometimes harm the liver.

In addition to the ordinary assaults of modern life, the liver can be threatened by a number of diseases. The most common are:

Fatty Liver. Though not a disease in itself, fatty liver is a symptom of other health problems. As the name suggests, this condition results when fat accumulates in the liver. Prime causes of fatty liver are heavy alcohol consumption, extreme overweight, and diabetes. If these problems are treated, the condition usually improves on its own.

Though fatty liver does not itself impair the liver's ability to function, it can be a warning signal of more serious troubles to come and should not be ignored.

Hepatitis. Lumped together under the word "hepatitis" are several distinctly different forms of inflammatory liver disease. The various types of viral hepatitis are distinguished by letters of the alphabet, as in hepatitis A, hepatitis B, and so on. Each of these types is caused by a different virus, and each has a different transmission route and different outcome. In America, the most common forms of viral hepatitis are:

- *Hepatitis A.* Hepatitis A is spread through fecal matter, through contaminated shellfish, through anal sex, and through kissing. Although there is no specific treatment other than rest, most people make a full recovery in six months or less, with no permanent damage.

- *Hepatitis B.* More serious than hepatitis A, hepatitis B is spread through bodily fluids (including saliva, blood, semen, vaginal secretions, tears, and breast milk). Although most people recover from hepatitis B, 5 to 10 percent will become permanent carriers of the virus. A small percentage do not make a full recovery. An estimated 5 to 10 percent eventually develop serious liver problems, including chronic liver disease, cirrhosis, and cancer.

- *Hepatitis C.* Hepatitis C is transmitted through blood. Since rigorous testing of donated blood has all but eliminated risk associated with transfusions in the United States, the people most at risk for contracting this form of the disease are drug users who share needles. The Centers for Disease Control associates the risk of sexual transmission with multiple partners and recommends the use of condoms. Hepatitis C is a serious disease. Up to 85 percent of people who get it will develop chronic hepatitis and are at increased risk for cirrhosis and cancer of the liver.

Other forms of hepatitis: In addition to viral hepatitis, people can also suffer from chronic hepatitis—caused by viral infections, medications, metabolic disorders, or immune system disorders—and alcoholic hepatitis, caused by heavy drinking.

Cirrhosis. In cirrhosis, normal liver cells become damaged and are replaced by scar tissue. The decreased amount of healthy tissue makes it impossible for the liver to perform all its functions, and advanced cirrhosis can be fatal.

Excessive drinking of alcoholic beverages is the primary cause of cirrhosis, but it certainly isn't the only cause. People can also develop cirrhosis as a result of chronic hepatitis, diabetes, inherited diseases and conditions, bile-duct diseases, long-term exposure to environmental toxins, severe adverse drug reaction, and parasitic infection.

Cancer. Cancer that originates in the liver is *not* common. However, having another form of liver disease, such as hepatitis B or C, increases the risk of developing cancer of the liver.

WHO GETS LIVER DISEASE?

Factors linked to developing a liver disease are:

- Heavy alcohol consumption
- Contact with virus-contaminated blood
- Intravenous drug use
- Unprotected sex
- Exposure to contaminated water, food, etc.
- Long-term exposure to environmental toxins
- Travel to countries with high rates of hepatitis
- Certain inherited disorders, such as having too much iron or copper in the liver
- Prolonged obstruction of bile ducts
- Unidentified factors. Although the above conditions increase the chances of liver disease, a significant number of people who get liver disease have *no* identifiable risk factor.

WHAT ARE THE SYMPTOMS?

Although symptoms vary depending on what type of liver disease is present, general warning signals include:

- Jaundice, marked by yellowing of the skin or whites of the eyes
- Dark-colored urine
- Loss of appetite, nausea, and/or vomiting
- Passing or vomiting blood

- Changes in stool color. Grayish or yellow stools are cause for concern, as are black stools, which can indicate intestinal bleeding
- Abdominal swelling or pain
- Fatigue, loss of stamina, or loss of sex drive
- Generalized itching that does not go away
- Unexpected weight loss or gain

WHAT'S THE OUTLOOK?

Outcome varies depending on what type of liver disease is present. As we mentioned above, some liver problems, such as hepatitis A, are relatively mild, and most people can look forward to a full recovery. Other problems can be thwarted by identifying and treating the underlying cause before too much damage is done. However, liver diseases can be quite serious. Some people end up with permanently damaged livers, while others—an estimated 25,000 Americans each year—will die of liver disease.

WHAT YOU NEED TO KNOW

Even people who are well informed about cardiac fitness sometimes take liver health for granted. Just like the heart, the liver has a staggering job to do and is constantly under stress. Learning to protect your liver is a health basic. With a little attention from you, your liver will reward you with years of healthy living.

PROVEN MIRACLES

MILK THISTLE

WHAT IS MILK THISTLE

Considered a weed in most places, milk thistle grows throughout much of Europe, the United States, and the United Kingdom. Although the young leaves of the plant are tender and edible, they do not contain high concentrations of the plant's helpful substances. Therefore, most people take milk thistle in capsule form, as an extract prepared from the fruits of the plant.

THE MIRACLE EFFECT

Milk thistle contains silymarin, a flavonoid group that has a natural affinity for the liver. Perhaps the most amazing thing about milk thistle is that the chemically active substances in silymarin don't just work one way. Instead, silymarin acts in multiple ways to protect and heal. Here's what milk thistle can do for you:

- **Protects against toxins and pollutants.** Milk thistle helps protect liver cells from being damaged by certain toxins and harmful substances, including those in certain prescription medications. Though this mechanism isn't completely understood, it seems that milk thistle's active substances make liver cell walls especially impervious to toxins. In one study, milk thistle even had an antidotal effect. Given shortly after powerful toxins were given to lab animals, it reduced liver damage and lowered the death rate.

- **Stimulates regeneration of liver tissue.** One of the problems with liver disease is that liver tissue, once damaged, is slow to replace itself. Active substances in milk thistle increase the rate of regeneration, improving the liver's ability to function.
- **Offers a better outlook for people with hepatitis.** Milk thistle extract has been effective for people with hepatitis B as well as chronic hepatitis, and researchers suspect it may help those with hepatitis C as well. In studies, people had decreased levels of the enzymes that indicate liver damage, and improved liver functioning was also noted.
- **Improves the outlook for people with cirrhosis.** Milk thistle is a remarkable helper for people battling cirrhosis. There is dramatic evidence that milk thistle is effective for all types of cirrhosis, including alcohol-related cirrhosis, which makes up the majority of cases of this disease. In one study, cirrhosis sufferers who took milk thistle had substantially lower mortality rates than cirrhosis sufferers who were not given this miracle of nature. In addition, milk thistle's amazing ability to improve functioning in a damaged liver has allowed people with diabetes-related cirrhosis to actually *lower* their intake of insulin.
- **Protects against cancer.** Among other substances, silymarin contains silybin, a potent antioxidant that consumes cancer-promoting free radicals. Recently researchers have discovered that milk thistle's cancer-protective abilities may be even more potent than previously thought. When researchers exposed

mouse skin to tumor-causing agents, skin treated with milk thistle extract proved highly resistant to tumor development.

- **Increases glutathione levels.** Glutathione, an anti-oxidant, is a powerful natural cancer fighter. The silymarin in milk thistle increases glutathione levels in the liver.

HAS MILK THISTLE BEEN USED BEFORE?

The use of milk thistle in human medicine dates back at least two thousand years. Romans employed it as a liver tonic, and its white-veined leaves led some to believe it could stimulate milk production in new mothers. Milk thistle's popularity outlasted the Roman empire. It was used throughout Europe well into the nineteenth century, when the rise of chemically refined and synthetic medications overtook the use of natural medicines.

In the last twenty years, milk thistle has become popular once again. In the late 1970s, German researchers began releasing results of scientific studies done on milk thistle. Since then, an overwhelming amount of evidence has accumulated, and even the toughest-minded researchers agree that milk thistle is a *highly effective medicine* for promoting health and reversing the disease process in the liver.

RESEARCH FINDINGS

Numerous studies on both animals and humans have confirmed milk thistle's effectiveness. Germany's Commission E has reviewed the evidence and given milk thistle its official seal of approval. For more than a decade, they have endorsed the use of milk thistle as beneficial in treating liver diseases such as hepatitis and cirrhosis. Here are just a few of the remarkable findings:

- In one of the largest studies ever done on milk thistle, German researchers tracked over 2,600 patients with a variety of liver problems, including hepatitis, cirrhosis, and fatty liver. After taking milk thistle extract for eight weeks, a majority of people in the study reported a dramatic decline in symptoms. The study, published in 1992, also showed that actual signs of disease (such as enlarged liver, elevated enzymes, and so on) diminished dramatically.

- Researchers at the University of Vienna divided 170 men, women, and children with cirrhosis into two groups, each group containing cases of both alcoholic and nonalcoholic cirrhosis. One group received milk thistle extract while the other group received a look-alike placebo. Other than this, all patients received the same medical treatment for their condition, and each patient was tracked for an average of three years and five months. After adjusting for dropouts, who were not counted, each group contained seventy-three members at the end of the study. The final results, published in the *Journal of Hepatology* in 1989, were startling: While thirty-one people in the placebo group died of liver disease during the course of the study, the mortality rate in the milk thistle group was much lower, with a mortality count of just eighteen. For more than a dozen people in the group, milk thistle had literally proved to be the difference between life and death!

- In a study published in *Biochemical and Biophysical Research Communication* in 1997, researchers at Case Western Reserve University found that milk thistle extract shows high cancer-fighting potential. In the study, researchers first applied silymarin, the active substance in milk thistle, to mouse skin. They then applied two chemical substances known to cause tumors to the skin. In the case of the first chemical, silymarin was 100 percent effective in blocking cancer—no tumors formed in the skin tissue. In the case of the second chemical, silymarin blocked tumors in 85 percent of the samples. Moreover, it discouraged proliferation when cancer did occur—only 6 percent of the samples showed the kind of multiple tumors one would ordinarily expect to see.

  These dramatic results caused the authors to conclude that silymarin has enormous potential as a tumor suppressor.

OTHER WAYS MILK THISTLE CAN HELP

At present, other benefits of milk thistle have not been documented. However, at least one group of researchers has suggested that it may have broad-based tumor-protective potential that should be fully explored.

HOW TO TAKE MILK THISTLE

What form does it come in? Most people take milk thistle in concentrated form in capsules. Concentrated liquid extract is also available.

What's an effective dose? Milk thistle often comes in 200-milligram capsules, standardized to contain 70 to 80 percent (140 to 160 milligrams) silymarin. Several studies on humans support the finding that three of these capsules a day is an effective average dose.

Tips for use. Even if you're a purist who prefers to drink your medicine as a tea, that isn't a good option when it comes to milk thistle. The reason: You simply can't get enough concentrated silymarin to do any good.

Are there side effects? Side effects are mild, uncommon, and temporary. They are limited to gastrointestinal upsets, such as nausea and upset stomach. We have not been able to find reports of any more serious side effects or of adverse reactions to milk thistle.

WHAT ELSE CAN YOU DO?

The bad news is that diseases of the liver are often serious and sometimes life threatening. The good news is that *most liver disease can be prevented.* Here are some important steps to take if you want to safeguard your liver.

BE SMART ABOUT ALCOHOL

Milk thistle is *not* an open invitation to drink heavily. If you're serious about taking charge of your health, you must make changes in your lifestyle. Alcohol may taste good to you, but to your liver it's a toxin. If you have cirrhosis or any other type of liver disease, don't drink *any* alcoholic beverages. If you don't have liver disease, limit your alcohol consumption to no more than two drinks a day.

DON'T OVERMEDICATE

When you really need medication, the benefits outweigh the risks. Unfortunately, some people adopt a "why not?" attitude when it comes to medicine. Because even helpful medications tax the liver, avoid taking medication unless you really need it. This warning applies to prescription as well as nonprescription preparations. Remember that even relatively mild over-the-counter medications combined with liquor can deliver a punishing wallop to the liver. The same goes for prescription medications. To be safe, don't mix any drugs or medications—prescription, over-the-counter, or other—with alcohol.

MINIMIZE YOUR RISK OF GETTING HEPATITIS B

You might want to talk to your doctor about being vaccinated for this form of hepatitis, especially if you're in a high-risk job (such as health-care work) or are traveling to a country where rates of the disorder are especially high. Also, avoid high-risk activities such as having unprotected sex or sharing toothbrushes, razors, etc. If you're exposed to this form of hepatitis, consult your doctor immediately. Prompt vaccination and treatment are usually effective in preventing the disease.

AVOID TOXINS AND POLLUTANTS

None of us can completely avoid the contaminants that come with modern life, but we should try to eliminate as much risk as possible. This means common sense measures such as making sure rooms are well ventilated whenever you are working with paints, solvents, and other chemicals; avoiding workplace environments that don't meet government safety standards; and so on.

BE VIGILANT ABOUT HEALTH PROBLEMS

The best way to keep your liver for life is to stop disease before it damages your liver. Make sure you get regular checkups in order to get treatment for any of the symptoms described above (see pages 287–288) as well as any other health conditions you may have. Even problems that aren't directly related to the liver can have an impact on this organ if they're ignored. Untreated diabetes and gall bladder problems, for example, can both compromise the health of your liver.

CHAPTER EIGHTEEN

Unlock the Secrets of

Male Sexuality and Fertility

What man wouldn't want to energize his sex life? The nutrients in this chapter are just the ticket for greater potency.

Impotence. Infertility. Both can undermine a relationship and destroy a man's self-confidence. Sometimes these problems are closely related and sometimes couples face one but not the other. Fortunately, there's help for both.

THE PROBLEM

Let's be clear right from the start: Impotence and infertility *are not* the same problem. A man can be infertile without being impotent and vice versa.

Impotence is the inability to achieve and maintain an erection. Infertility just refers to the difficulty a man has impregnating a viable partner. Obviously, a man who isn't able to maintain an erection will have trouble impregnating his partner. But very often infertility is an independent problem. Few men are completely sterile.

More often, the problem is low fertility. This may be because there are too few sperm or because the sperm aren't mobile enough.

WHO SUFFERS FROM THESE PROBLEMS?

Neither impotence nor infertility is a sign that a man isn't "really" a man.

Unfortunately, many men don't see it that way. They feel there is something profoundly wrong with them, or that they have insurmountable psychological problems. Would it surprise you to know that, for both impotence and infertility, the cause is usually physical rather than psychological?

Until the 1990s, impotence was thought to be largely psychological. Some still think it is, but they're wrong. According to Ajay Nehra, a Mayo Clinic specialist, "The causes are physical in 85 percent to 90 percent of cases."

Leading causes of impotence include:
- **Age.** Declining levels of the hormone testosterone and other age-related problems are probably the leading reasons men lose sexual desire and ability.
- **Chronic disease.** Diabetes, heart disease, kidney disease, and circulatory problems are all common causes.
- **Prescription medication.** A common side effect of many medications, including many high blood pressure drugs, is difficulty achieving and maintaining an erection.

- **Low testosterone levels.** This can be due to medication, disease, or other factors.
- **Psychological factors.** Although most causes are physical, state of mind can definitely influence a man's sexual health. It will come as no surprise that the key culprits are stress, anxiety, and depression.
- **Drug or alcohol use.**
- **Removal of prostate gland.**

Leading causes of infertility include:

- **Physical conditions.** A number of treatable physical conditions can result in lowered fertility. These include varicose veins in the testicles, undescended testicles, and pituitary disorder.
- **Heat.** Wearing tight-fitting briefs and trousers that hug the testicles close to the body raise the temperature and lower fertility. Spending too much time in hot tubs can have the same result.
- **Environmental factors.** Exposure to environmental toxins can decrease fertility.
- **Sexually transmitted diseases.** STDs, such as gonorrhea, can scar the sperm ducts and block passage.
- **Prescription and nonprescription drugs.** Some drugs used in chemotherapy, as well as marijuana and alcohol, can lower fertility.
- **Genes.** Some men may have a genetic defect that affects sperm production.
- **Testicular damage.** Injuries and infections, such as mumps, can lead to infertility.

WHAT ARE THE SYMPTOMS?

Impotence can involve a range of symptoms, including lack of desire, inability to get an erection, and inability to maintain an erection.

Infertility has only one symptom: the inability to impregnate a viable partner. A man can have an active sex life and still be infertile, and the only way to know for sure is to visit a doctor.

WHAT'S THE OUTLOOK?

Sometimes, impotence and infertility are the result of temporary factors, such as illness, that quickly correct themselves. In other cases, the underlying causes are chronic and call for long-term changes or treatment.

WHAT YOU SHOULD KNOW

In recent years, treatment options for both of these conditions have improved dramatically. In the field of sexuality and impotence especially, traditional medicine has made great leaps in understanding the complex matter of male potency. New and better treatments are also available for infertile couples. In addition to the highly beneficial nutrients described in this chapter, you may want to make an appointment with your family physician or a urologist to discuss the problem.

PROVEN MIRACLES

GINSENG FOR SEXUAL ENERGY
AND INFERTILITY

WHAT IS GINSENG?

You've probably heard of ginseng, the plant whose root has been used for centuries in Asian medicine. Actually, there are several types of ginseng, and not all types are equally effective. Throughout this chapter, we are discussing one specific type of ginseng: red panax ginseng. Often referred to as Chinese or Korean ginseng, this is the variety most widely used throughout most of the world, including the United States. It is also the only variety proven to be an effective stimulant for male sexuality and infertility.

THE MIRACLE EFFECT

Ginseng boosts male sexuality. A large percentage of men who use it report increased satisfaction with their sex lives. Measurable test results show that it can:

- Help maintain erection longer
- Increase size and firmness of erection
- Increase sexual desire
- Raise testosterone levels
- Increase sperm count
- Increase sperm mobility

Although researchers do not completely agree on the exact reason for ginseng's potent effect, many have suggested that the ginsenocides it contains stimulate hormone production.

HAS GINSENG BEEN USED BEFORE?

Ginseng is a traditional herb used widely in Chinese medicine. Native Americans also used a variety of ginseng, but European settlers dismissed its potential usefulness and it did not become popular here until this century. Today, millions of people around the world use ginseng as an overall tonic and aphrodisiac.

RESEARCH FINDINGS

Sexual research is a difficult undertaking. Most people don't want observers in their bedrooms, monitoring the effect of this or that nutrient. On the other hand, asking for a subjective opinion may lead to findings that are more wish fulfillment than reality. But research on ginseng includes positive findings from both humans and animals, making the big picture much clearer.

When male rats were fed ginseng supplement for sixty days, their testosterone levels rose. In another study, male rats fed ginseng supplement mated more often than healthy males who did not receive supplements.

While animal studies have been undertaken for some time, scientific studies of ginseng's effect on humans didn't begin until the 1990s. In one study, published in the *International Journal of Impotence Research* in 1995, a group of ninety men complaining of impotence were divided into three groups. One group received ginseng, another received a placebo, and a third received a popular antidepressant medication.

Not only did ginseng outperform the placebo, it also outperformed the antidepressant drug. Though no man was completely "cured" of his problems, 60 percent of men taking ginseng reported a dramatic improvement in their sex lives, and increased satisfaction.

To make sure the effect was more than just wishful thinking, researchers used a machine to monitor penile response. Men taking ginseng achieved erections easily and more often, had larger and firmer erections, and maintained them with less difficulty.

In another important study, men with low fertility volunteered to take ginseng supplement. Blood analysis showed an increase in testosterone. More important, other tests showed that taking ginseng increased both the number and quality of sperm. More sperm were present in each milliliter of fluid, and the mobility of individual sperm was also much improved.

OTHER WAYS GINSENG CAN HELP

In recent years, ginseng has been widely touted as an energy booster. According to our research, this is definitely true if you are a rat or a mouse. Unfortunately, tests done on humans haven't supported this claim.

A more promising use for ginseng is as an aid to mental alertness. It has been shown to improve mental capabilities under stress. It also works as a memory aid and helps buffer the effects of aging on the brain (see chapter 19).

HOW TO TAKE GINSENG

What form does it come in? Ginseng comes in capsules and in dried form to make into tea. Capsules are a better choice because they ensure a standardized dose. As we mentioned above, make sure you buy only red panax ginseng. Other varieties haven't been proven effective when it comes to enhancing sexuality and fertility.

What's an effective dose? The key to getting an effective dose starts with a reliable product. Since ginseng is expensive, some manufacturers might cut corners by adulterating their products. Make sure you buy a standardized product from a reputable manufacturer. Since strength varies from product to product, follow the manufacturer's package direction for your product.

Tips for use. Don't look for instant results—ginseng is not Viagra. It may take a few weeks to see results, especially if you are using it for fertility problems. For best results, take it with food or water, and avoid taking it with stimulants such as caffeinated coffee, tea, or cola beverages.

Are there side effects? A few years ago, there was a ginseng scare when one report linked its use to elevated blood pressure. However, there were several problems with the way the study was done. Most researchers agree that the alarm was blown out of proportion, and no such dangers have been found in more carefully controlled studies. The bottom line: Ginseng is considered safe and generally nontoxic in moderate doses.

Some individuals may be allergic to ginseng. If you

develop heart palpitations or chest pain, nausea, head-ache, agitation, or insomnia, discontinue at once.

Caution! Although ginseng is safe at recommended doses, some people have been tempted to have better sex sooner by overdosing. This is dangerous since ginseng can be toxic in very large amounts. Moreover, overdosing will cause a decrease in potency rather than an increase.

Ginseng should not be taken by people taking one class of antidepressant medications, MAO inhibitors, also referred to as MAOIs. If you are taking a drug of this type for depression or anxiety, your doctor will already have told you that you cannot eat certain foods, including aged meats and cheese and red wine. Ginseng should also be avoided by people who are taking antipsychotic medications and people who are receiving hormone treatment.

VITAMIN E FOR INFERTILITY

WHAT IS VITAMIN E?

Vitamin E is a powerful antioxidant vitamin. Low levels of this key nutrient have been linked to a number of problems, including cancer and, research is now finding, low fertility in men.

THE MIRACLE EFFECT

If low levels of vitamin E are linked to low male fertility, will bolstering those levels help? Apparently, yes. And the added vitamin E needn't come from food sources, it can come from a simple vitamin supplement.

When researchers raised levels of vitamin E in men with low fertility, they also raised the number and quality of sperm. Microscopic analysis of sperm showed they had improved mobility and were better able to attach to the unfertilized egg. But the best results haven't come from microscopic analysis. They've came from test subjects who've reported "real life" results: pregnancies and healthy babies in place of disappointment and frustration.

Researchers believe the reason for the E miracle is its antioxidant activity. The manufacture of healthy sperm is a delicate process and vulnerable to all sorts of disruptions. Free radicals, chemical molecules that damage cells, may interfere with the process. Decline in the number of sperm, as well as deformities that make sperm unable to do their job, may be the direct result of our increased exposure to a wide variety of free radicals. Vitamin E knocks out these harmful molecules and prevents the damage.

HAS VITAMIN E BEEN USED BEFORE?

Vitamin E has always been included in the human diet. However, as that diet has changed and as industrialization has exposed us to a wider range of the chemicals that produce free radicals, our need for extra vitamin E may have grown. Millions of people around the world now take vitamin E in supplement form every day.

RESEARCH FINDINGS

It sounds too good to be true, but for a significant percentage of infertile couples, vitamin E may be the answer they've been looking for. In fact, studies suggest it's at least as effective—and possibly *more* effective—than expensive high-tech procedures.

A report by Kessopoulou and colleagues, which appeared in 1995, offered the first solid, convincing proof of the vitamin's effectiveness. In this study, thirty men with low fertility were divided into two groups. For three months, one group took 600 IUs of vitamin E daily while the other took a placebo. Sperm counts were measured and analyzed.

After a one-month rest period, the two groups changed routines. This time the group that had taken placebo pills took vitamin E, and vice versa. This kind of test is considered the most accurate available, because it gives researchers a chance to measure the effects of both placebo and active substance in the same individual.

For both stages of the test, sperm potency dramatically improved under the influence of vitamin E. According to measuring standards used by the researchers, taking vitamin E supplement made sperm two and a half times as potent as they had been before supplementation began.

Another study, conducted at the Asir Infertility Center in Saudi Arabia, used a larger study group. Over one hundred couples unable to conceive due to low male fertility volunteered. In half of the group, males took daily vitamin E supplement, while the other half received a look-alike placebo. During the test period, none of the females in the placebo group became pregnant. By contrast, more than 20 percent of those in the vitamin E group conceived—a much higher success rate than *in vitro* fertilization can boast!

OTHER WAYS VITAMIN E CAN HELP

Vitamin E's ability to clean up free radicals makes it potent on two other health fronts. It is one of the very best natural cancer-fighters available (see chapter 6), and countless studies have linked high levels of vitamin E to low rates of a wide variety of cancers.

Anyone interested in cutting the risk of heart attack and stroke will also be interested in vitamin E. Studies attest to its effectiveness in lowering artery-clogging cholesterol and preventing blood from clumping and forming dangerous clots (see chapter 7).

HOW TO TAKE VITAMIN E

What form does it come in? Vitamin E comes in capsules, tablets, and drops.

What's an effective dose? In studies, a daily dose of 600 IUs of vitamin E was used. Although no problems were noted, this is more than the amount recommended in government guidelines. Because very large doses can have adverse effects, don't take more than 800 IUs a day.

Tips for use. Studies have shown that vitamin E is more effective when taken with another key antioxidant, vitamin C. The reason may be that when a vitamin E molecule is damaged by interacting with a free radical, C converts it back to its original form, giving it, in effect, a second life. To minimize stomach upset, take vitamin E at mealtimes or with a snack.

Are there side effects? Vitamin E can cause diarrhea and stomach upset (see Tips for use, above).

Caution! People with anemia, poorly clotting blood, liver disease, or overactive thyroid should not take vitamin E supplements without consulting a doctor.

WHY *NOT* YOHIMBE?

In recent years, yohimbe has been widely advertised as a sexual tonic for men. There's just one catch: Yohimbe has a number of dangerous side effects. It can cause insomnia, anxiety, rapid pulse, high blood pressure, nausea, and vomiting, even in otherwise healthy men. For these reasons we join Germany's Commission E and other reputable sources in *not* recommending this herb.

WHAT ELSE CAN YOU DO?

If you really want to improve your sexual potency, don't neglect the importance of diet, exercise, and other lifestyle factors. In addition to these, there's one other fertility-building nutrient that shouldn't be overlooked.

SELENIUM:
THE MALE MICRONUTRIENT

Since the late 1980s, researchers have noted that selenium deficiency lowers reproduction rates in man as well as animals. Selenium is needed for production of testosterone. It's also been noted that when selenium levels are low, sperm are immobile because the tail is weakened or deformed.

Many nutritionists and researchers feel that selenium deficiency is common, even among well-nourished people. In one double-blind trial, low-fertility men who took selenium supplements increased the mobility of their sperm by 100 percent!

CHAPTER NINETEEN

Boost Your
Memory and Mental Alertness

Must you lose your mental edge as you get older? According to researchers, not necessarily. And these nutrients may help.

Have you ever had difficulty summoning a name or fact from memory? Or felt confused and unable to think straight? We've all had these mental glitches from time to time. Unfortunately, as we grow older, the likelihood is that we will have more of these incidents. For some, there may be a real difficulty in carrying on life as usual.

The good news is that research is finding ways to help us forestall and even reverse the problem. And some of the best miracle workers aren't expensive, prescription-only drugs—they're nutrients you can go out and buy today.

THE PROBLEM

We often think of the mind as a thing apart, a unique thinking entity that is somehow separate from the body. But, of course, this isn't exactly true.

The brain is very much a part of the body. It is subject to the same rules of biology as the rest of the body. Like the rest of the body, the brain must be fed and nourished. In fact, the brain is one of the biggest energy users in the body. It must have oxygen, glucose, and other nutrients. When it doesn't get them, it suffers. It cannot process information efficiently and may be unable to access or assemble bits of stored data. Most people experience some decline in memory and mental alertness as they age. Usually the decline is not great and does not affect the person's ability to function or enjoy life.

In addition to common memory problems, there are also diseases that involve wide-scale memory loss. Instead of being unable to recall a few insignificant dates or facts, the person is unable to remember family members, friends, and major facts about his or her own life. This is the case with Alzheimer's disease as well as dementia (sometimes called senile dementia), disorders which may well impair a person's ability to live independently.

WHO SUFFERS FROM THESE PROBLEMS?

A number of factors influence our mental functioning. Some, such as illness or extreme fatigue, are temporary. Our mental abilities come back with a good night's sleep or the return of physical health.

Other factors cause chronic problems with memory and mental alertness. These factors include:

- **Age.** Getting older is the biggest single risk factor for declining memory and alertness.
- **Insufficient blood supply.** Oxygen, carried by the blood, reaches the brain through a system of arteries and capillaries. When arteries are clogged or diseased, as with atherosclerosis, the brain is constantly deprived. The medical word for this condition is cerebral insufficiency, and it plays an enormous role in loss of memory and alertness.
- **Alzheimer's disease.** This age-related disease causes progressive memory loss.
- **Dementia.** Also known as senile dementia, this condition involves severe and large-scale memory loss. It can come about as a result of Alzheimer's disease, cerebral insufficiency, a stroke, or other conditions.
- **Stress.** Under stressful conditions the brain produces excess cortisol, which interferes with memory.
- **History of stroke, cardiac arrest, or head injury.** During a stroke or cardiac arrest, blood supply to the brain is interrupted. A head injury can also cause problems with memory and mental functioning.
- **Other diseases.** In addition to Alzheimer's disease and dementia, other chronic disorders—including Parkinson's and Huntington's chorea—can also cause memory disturbances. Nonchronic disorders, such as infections, can also cause these problems.
- **Nutrition.** Especially among the elderly, maintaining a standard level of nutrition is extremely important.
- **Certain medications.** Some prescription drugs can

cause problems. Foggy memory, difficulty in concentrating, and other symptoms are side effects, not signs, of permanent damage.

WHAT ARE THE SYMPTOMS?

As the following list shows, not all signs associated with these problems are obvious. Symptoms can include:

- Inability to recall
- Difficulty recognizing people and/or places
- Distraction and absent-mindedness
- Confusion
- Lethargy
- Dizziness
- Ringing in ears (tinnitus)
- Headaches
- Uncharacteristic behavior
- Emotional disturbances such as depression, paranoia, or anxiety

WHAT'S THE OUTLOOK?

Since most of these problems are the result of chronic conditions, such as aging or stress, the problems are also chronic. In the case of aging, they may also be progressive. However, this doesn't mean there is nothing you can do. As this chapter will show, even very serious disorders, such as Alzheimer's disease, can be significantly slowed.

WHAT YOU SHOULD KNOW

As we've noted, mild memory or alertness problems are often the result of normal conditions such as aging, stress, and other factors. If you or a relative has problems that seem severe, or seem to be getting worse, you should by all means consult a doctor. Before using the nutrients in this chapter, make sure you have an accurate diagnosis and are not suffering from an underlying disease that requires different treatment.

PROVEN MIRACLES

GINKGO

WHAT IS GINKGO?

Ginkgo is the oldest living tree species on the earth today. Its familiar, notched, fan-shaped leaves are the source of its healing power.

THE MIRACLE EFFECT

Ginkgo has a proven effect on a wide range of problems related to memory loss and impaired mental functioning. Studies have shown that it improves overall mental functioning and slows progression of such serious disorders as:

- Alzheimer's disease
- Cerebral insufficiency
- Dementia
- Impaired cerebral functioning

In particular, ginkgo has been shown to help specific symptoms of these disorders, including:

- Decision-making abilities
- Attentiveness

- Reaction time
- Memory
- Mental functions such as reasoning, perception, learning, and understanding
- Dizziness
- Ringing in ears (tinnitus)
- Vision disturbances
- Concentration and memory difficulties related to depression and anxiety

How can ginkgo improve such a wide set of symptoms? Although we do not yet know all there is to know about this age-old healer, researchers believe that it has several chemical actions rather than just one.

Like other age-related diseases, loss of memory and declining mental function are thought to be at least partially related to damage done by free radicals. Ginkgo contains numerous antioxidants—flavonoids such as quercetin and rutin—which act to neutralize many free radicals. Flavonoids also play a role in strengthening capillaries, which can improve blood flow to the brain. Ginkgo also contains substances that work to prevent the accumulation of fluids in the brain. According to still other researchers, gingko may help by influencing chemical messengers in the brain.

HAS GINKGO BEEN USED BEFORE?

Ginkgo is among the oldest medicines in the world, and has been used by the Chinese for almost five thousand years.

Today ginkgo is one of the world's best-selling herbal remedies. It's number one in Germany, where the government has officially approved its use as a remedy for cerebral circulatory problems. Ginkgo is also extremely popular in France and other European countries, where millions of doses are sold each year.

In the past few years, ginkgo has become popular in America, where recent research and publicity have given it a boost in the public's mind.

RESEARCH FINDINGS

There have been dozens and dozens of lab, animal, and human studies done with ginkgo. With few exceptions, the results have been extremely positive. While we don't have room to include all of the findings, here's a summary of ginkgo's effects on humans:

- Perhaps the most famous study of ginkgo, which grabbed headlines in 1997, was conducted by LeBars and colleagues at the New York Institute for Medical Research. Previous studies had tested people with mild or moderate memory loss, but the LeBars study worked with 309 patients who had severe problems due either to Alzheimer's or stroke-related dementia. Half of those in the study received ginkgo, while the other half received a placebo. Their progress was monitored over the course of one year.

  At the end of fifty-two weeks, a significant number of patients in the ginkgo group showed improvement in areas such as reasoning, memory, and learning. They also showed better social functioning. Even for patients who didn't experience significant gains, many benefited by not getting worse. Ginkgo effectively slowed the progress of the disease for many people.

People in the placebo group did not achieve significant gains, and many got worse as their disease progressed.

- One of the earliest proofs of ginkgo's effectiveness was a reported by Taillandier and colleagues in 1986. In the study, 166 patients with age-related brain disorders were given either a placebo or ginkgo supplement. Three months into the study, researchers concluded that ginkgo use resulted in significant improvement. Even better, mental functioning was still improving at the six-month mark when the study ended.

- Seventy-two volunteers with cerebral insufficiency were given a battery of memory and learning tests; they were then given either daily ginkgo supplements or placebos. At the end of just six weeks, tests showed that individuals taking ginkgo had significant gains in short-term memory. At the end of twenty-four weeks, when the test ended, the ginkgo group also showed substantial improvement in learning ability. No such gains were seen in those who took placebos.

- Ginkgo can have an immediate effect, according to a study by Allain and colleagues. In this test, eighteen elderly men and women with slight age-related memory problems were given either a placebo or a single dose of ginkgo extract. One hour later, they were asked to perform various mental tests. The test was repeated at a later date, this time with the placebo-takers receiving ginkgo and ginkgo-takers receiving the placebo. In both phases of the test, individuals who took ginkgo were able to process information more rapidly.

OTHER WAYS GINKGO CAN HELP

Ginkgo's ability to improve circulation in the brain may make it useful for other circulatory problems. One promising line of research suggests it may help stop leg cramps due to poor circulation (see chapter 5).

Another line of research suggests that it may also be useful for people with cardiovascular problems, both by helping to correct irregular heartbeat and by acting as a natural blood-thinner.

HOW TO USE GINKGO

What form does it come in? Ginkgo comes in many forms, including tea. Tea, however, will not provide enough of ginkgo's active ingredients to be effective. The best way to take ginkgo is in capsule form.

What's an effective dose? Most of the studies we reviewed recommended a dosage of 120 milligrams per day.

Tips for use. Ginkgo is most effective when divided into three doses and taken throughout the day. Although some studies show that ginkgo has an immediate effect, most studies show that long-term continuous use is necessary to get ginkgo's real benefits.

Are there side effects? Studies we reviewed did not report side effects. Ginkgo is considered safe and nontoxic; however, some experts have cautioned that stomach upset can occur.

Caution! Ginkgo acts as a natural blood-thinner. If you take blood-thinning medications (including aspirin) on a regular basis, avoid ginkgo.

ACETYL-L-CARNITINE

WHAT IS ACETYL-L-CARNITINE?

Acetyl-L-carnitine is an amino acid compound produced naturally within the body. Although it is related to carnitine, its chemical makeup is different. Acetyl-L-carnitine, sometimes referred to as ALC, is considered more potent than plain carnitine.

THE MIRACLE EFFECT

Acetyl-L-carnitine has proven remarkably effective for helping people with loss of memory and declining mental alertness due to age, Alzheimer's disease, or dementia. In particular, it has improved functioning in these areas:
- Logic and reason
- Verbal ability
- Long-term verbal memory
- Attentiveness
- Coordination
- Family and social interaction
- Physical activity
- Improved mood (less depression)

The secret of acetyl-L-carnitine's effectiveness is due to a cascade of chemical activities it executes within the brain. It acts as an antioxidizing agent to prevent damage done by free radicals. It protects cells and prolongs cell life by assisting in the process that supplies cells with energy. Finally, it plays a critical role in the production of acetylcholine, one of the brain's all-important chemical messengers.

HAS ACETYL-L-CARNITINE BEEN USED BEFORE?

Use of acetyl-L-carnitine supplement as an aid for memory and mental functioning is relatively new. Pioneer research, conducted primarily in Europe, dates back to the 1980s. This is not to say that the supplement is untried. Much testing has been done on human subjects, both in the form of short-term studies and in long-term studies lasting a year or more. As a result of these studies, hundreds of patients have used acetyl-L-carnitine safely and successfully.

RESEARCH FINDINGS

Acetyl-L-carnitine has been widely tested on humans. Most of the studies we reviewed showed at least moderate benefits, and no studies showed negative effects. A summary of selected studies includes these findings:

- Spagnoli and colleagues studied 130 patients with memory and mental difficulties due to severe progressive Alzheimer's disease. Half of these patients received acetyl-L-carnitine for one year, while the other half received a placebo. Patients were periodically tested on a scale of fourteen performance measures. At the end of the year, patients in both groups showed some degree of disease progression. But patients who took acetyl-L-carnitine showed much less deterioration and performed significantly better in thirteen of the fourteen measured test areas.

- A study by a University of Pittsburgh School of Medicine research team, headed by Jay Pettegrew, found that large doses of acetyl-L-carnitine may halt the progress of cognitive loss in Alzheimer's patients. When patients given 3,000 milligrams daily for one year were compared with patients who received a placebo, the former performed better on a battery of mental functioning tests. Comparison of results to those obtained at the beginning of the study revealed an even more encouraging finding. Patients who received acetyl-L-carnitine maintained mental functioning, with no significant loss.

- Acetyl-L-carnitine may delay the most severe symptoms of Alzheimer's disease, according to a 1996 report in *Neurology*. The study involved 350 patients, age fifty and up, with mild to moderate symptoms of Alzheimer's disease. Half of the patients received acetyl-L-carnitine supplement daily, while the rest received a placebo. At the end of one year, researchers noted that those who benefited most were younger individuals at the early stages of the disease. For them, acetyl-L-carnitine significantly slowed memory loss and impairment of mental functioning.

OTHER WAYS ACETYL-L-CARNITINE CAN HELP

Studies have shown that acetyl-L-carnitine supplements may also help people with non-age-related mental impairment. For example, when people with memory and mental loss due to chronic alcoholism received 2,000 milligrams of the supplement daily, they improved on a variety of mental tests.

In another study, patients with Down syndrome achieved gains in visual memory and attentiveness after taking acetyl-L-carnitine for three months.

HOW TO TAKE ACETYL-L-CARNITINE

What form does it come in? Acetyl-L-carnitine comes in capsules.

What's an effective dose? There are no government guidelines for the use of this supplement. Studies we reviewed used dosages ranging from 1,000 to 3,000 milligrams a day.

Tips for use. For best results, take in divided doses throughout the day, and do not take with food.

Are there side effects? Although acetyl-L-carnitine is considered safe and nontoxic, nausea and/or vomiting was reported by a small number of users.

WHAT ELSE CAN YOU DO?

If you're concerned with improving or protecting your mental capacities, there are two more supplement strategies to know about.

GINSENG

Numerous rodent studies show that ginseng can increase memory, learning ability, and mental functioning in lab animals. The problem is that, to date, not enough studies have been done on humans to conclusively back this up. One study, conducted on elderly patients with age-related memory problems, did not find that adding ginseng to their regular medication provided any benefit at all.

However, another study found that ginseng was extremely helpful to healthy individuals under mental and physical stress. In this study, five hundred men and women were divided into two groups. For three months, one group received a daily multivitamin and ginseng supplement while the other group received the same daily multivitamin and a placebo. At the end of the trial, ginseng-takers noted significant improvement on all eleven questions on a quality-of-life questionnaire. The group that didn't receive ginseng did not note a significant improvement on any of the eleven points.

VITAMINS C, E, AND BETA-CAROTENE

Vitamins C, E, and beta-carotene may have the ability to preserve mental functioning. A study conducted by researchers at the University of Berne, Switzerland, measured blood levels of vitamins C, E, and beta-carotene in 442 volunteers. The first measurement was done in 1971 and the second in 1993, when the volunteers ranged in age from sixty-five to ninety-four. Comparisons of the two sets of tests showed that individuals with the highest blood levels of vitamin C and beta-carotene had the least decline in memory and mental ability.

Although the study did not show the importance of vitamin E, a more recent study has suggested that vitamin E may slow the progress of Alzheimer's disease. Researchers suggest it does this by destroying free radicals and prolonging the life of individual brain cells. In a 1997 study by Sano and colleagues, patients with Alzheimer's who took 2,000 IUs of vitamin E daily for two years showed much less mental deterioration than patients who took a placebo. Since this is much above the recommended safe dosage, it is not recommended as a course of self-treatment, and should be done only with medical supervision.

CHAPTER TWENTY

Relieve

Menopause, PMS, and Other Menstrual Problems

Millions of women have discovered that natural remedies provide relief from gynecological discomforts—without the worry about long-term side effects.

Even when the female body seems to be motionless, it is constantly moving through change. In addition to the major hormonal shifts that develop during puberty and, decades later, throughout menopause, there are a welter of week-to-week changes brought about by the monthly menstrual cycle. For some women, the spikes and surges of hormones pass almost unnoticed. For others, these constant shifts cause physical and mental discomforts that make life miserable.

THE PROBLEM

What do a twenty-year-old with cramps, a thirty-five-year-old with water retention, and a fifty-year-old with night sweats have in common? Despite their diverse ages and stages of life, all can probably attribute their problems to a common cause: hormone flux.

Night sweats, hot flashes, and other symptoms of menopause have long been attributed to hormonal changes. Six or more years before periods actually cease, estrogen levels begin to decline. During this phase, known as perimenopause, women can experience all the symptoms of menopause while remaining fertile and continuing to have monthly cycles. Estrogen decline is only one piece of a large and complex puzzle. Numerous other hormones rise and fall as well, and the changes caused by their interplay, in some women, bring on the symptoms associated with menopause.

Recently, hormonal changes have been linked to difficulties during the premenopausal years as well. Cramps and painful periods, as well as the welter of uncomfortable symptoms referred to as premenstrual syndrome (PMS), are reactions to the rise and fall of an internal hormone tide.

In a study published in *The New England Journal of Medicine* in 1998, researchers from the National Institute of Mental Health found that hormone-regulating therapy significantly helped women experiencing PMS. Authors of the study suggested that it was not the hormones themselves that caused discomfort, but the women's individual sensitivity to them.

While women at the end of the reproductive cycle may suffer from too little estrogen and those at an earlier stage may suffer from a different kind of problem, the underlying cause for both is hormonal changes.

WHO SUFFERS?

Not all women suffer from cramps, irregular periods, or even PMS. And, while all women will experience menopause, not all find its symptoms uncomfortable enough to warrant treatment.

Factors associated with PMS include:

- **Age.** Premenstrual syndrome is most likely to affect women between the ages of twenty-five and forty.
- **Diet.** Women who consume large amounts of caffeine and sodium are more likely to suffer from PMS discomfort.
- **Mental or emotional turmoil.** Stress, anxiety, and depression have been associated with PMS. Researchers have pointed out that this may not be a symptom of PMS itself. Instead, the same chemical changes that trigger PMS may trigger emotional fluctuations.

Factors associated with discomfort during menopause include:

- **Age.** Studies and surveys have shown that women who go through menopause before the average age of forty-nine to fifty-two tend to have more hot flashes. In addition, women responding to a survey published in *Prevention* magazine reported more symptoms during perimenopause (the years leading up to menopause) than just after menopause.
- **Body weight.** It has long been noted that body weight seems to play a role in menopause, with thinner women having more discomfort than heavier women. One study, however, has suggested body weight may be a factor only among women who smoke.

- **Menstrual history.** Women who began menstruating before age twelve or who have a history of irregular periods are somewhat less likely to experience hot flashes.
- **Diet.** Women who eat a diet low in fat and high in grains and vegetables (especially soy products) have reported fewer and milder symptoms during menopause.

For both PMS and menopause, as well as cramps and irregular periods, these factors are *only* predictors. Each woman's body is different, and individual chemistry will ultimately determine the body's response to the ordinary phases and changes of reproductive life.

WHAT ARE THE SYMPTOMS?

Symptoms typical of PMS include:
- Fluid retention
- Abdominal bloating and/or digestive discomfort
- Constipation or diarrhea
- Breast tenderness and soreness
- Headache
- Mood swings, anxiety, irritability, or depression
- Complexion breakouts
- Increased or decreased sexual desire

Symptoms typical of menopause include:
- Hot flashes
- Night sweats
- Fatigue
- Mood swings
- Weight gain
- Loss of sexual desire

- Joint pain and/or muscle cramps
- Vaginal dryness and itching
- Urinary incontinence brought on by sneezing, coughing, etc.

Other menstrual problems. In addition to PMS and menopause, the other problems women are most likely to suffer from are severe cramping and discomfort during menstruation and irregular periods.

WHAT'S THE OUTLOOK?

If a woman is healthy and her menstrual problems aren't related to an illness, time will eventually resolve the problem. "Eventually," however, can be a long time off. There's no need to suffer in silence when natural remedies have proven both safe and effective for millions of women over the years.

WHAT YOU SHOULD KNOW

The natural remedies in this chapter can help you through life's normal changes. They aren't a way of dealing with medical disorders or infections. In addition to seeing your gynecologist for regular checkups, you should make an appointment at once if you have any of the following:

- Pain other than usual menstrual cramps, with or without fever
- Irregular bleeding
- Vaginal discharge

Symptoms like these can indicate problems such as pelvic inflammatory infection, sexually transmitted disease, (benign) fibroid cysts, and other conditions that require medical attention.

PROVEN MIRACLES

BLACK COHOSH

WHAT IS BLACK COHOSH?

A plant native to North America, black cohosh is a tall plant that takes its name not from the small white flowers adorning its stalk but from its straight dark brown root. It is the pithy white inner core of this root that, when dried and prepared, helps relieve a broad range of women's problems.

THE MIRACLE EFFECT

Black cohosh has been found especially effective for:
- Symptoms associated with premenstrual syndrome (PMS), such as tension and bloating.
- Cramps, pain, and tenderness during menstruation.
- Hot flashes, night sweats, vaginal dryness, depression, tension, and other symptoms of menopause.
- Symptoms associated with premature menopause due to hysterectomy.

Black cohosh works to combat symptoms that arise when the body's own supply of estrogen is in decline. Because estrogen declines temporarily during each monthly menstrual cycle, as well as permanently during menopause, black cohosh has been helpful to women at all stages of life.

Although the exact substances that make black cohosh so effective have not been identified, studies show that black cohosh extract has a definite estrogenic effect on the body. It works as a mild estrogen itself and, in addition, regulates and enhances estrogen produced by the body.

One reason black cohosh is so helpful during menopause may lie in its ability to suppress secretion of luteinizing hormone (LH). During menopause, sudden surges in LH are common and have been linked to hot flashes, night sweats, vaginal dryness, headaches, and other discomforts.

HAS BLACK COHOSH BEEN USED BEFORE?

Black cohosh has been used by millions of women in Europe and is now making its way back to America. We say "back" because, ironically, this miracle helper originated in North America and was known and used by Native Americans long before its export to Europe.

Black cohosh was still in use here at the turn of the century, though few knew it by its rightful name. Lydia Pinkham's Vegetable Compound, the most popular women's remedy of its day, relied on black cohosh as its main ingredient. When prescription medications replaced over-the-counter remedies as treatments of choice, black cohosh fell into disuse in America. By that time, however, it had gained popularity in Europe, where women have used it with good results for more than a century.

RESEARCH FINDINGS

Test tube studies, animal studies, and human studies have led Germany's Commission E to endorse the use of black cohosh for PMS, painful menstruation, and complaints associated with menopause.

In a study done by Düker and colleagues at the University of Göttingen, 110 women suffering a range of menopausal symptoms participated in a double-blind study of black cohosh. The group receiving the black cohosh preparation reported a significant improvement in symptoms, compared to women who received a look-alike placebo.

Another German study, conducted by Lehmann-Willenbrock and Riedel, looked at a group of women who had had hysterectomies and, as a result, were experiencing various symptoms associated with menopause. The purpose of the study was to evaluate the effects of a variety of remedies on these symptoms. The authors found that black cohosh was as effective as any of the estrogens included in the trial.

HOW TO TAKE BLACK COHOSH

What form does it come in? Concentrated extract of black cohosh is available as a tincture as well as in caplets and capsules.

What's an effective dose? If you are taking black cohosh tincture, two to four droppers, two to three times a day is usually effective. In capsule or tablet form, two a day is generally sufficient. However, since the amount of active ingredient varies from product to product, make sure to follow the manufacturer's package directions.

Tips for use. Although black cohosh is effective, its effects aren't instant. Human studies indicate that it can take up to a month for users to experience the full benefits of black cohosh extract.

Are there side effects? The only side effect reported as a result of black cohosh use has been the rare case of stomach upset. When used as directed, this herb is considered extremely safe for short-term use. Long-term use is another matter, however, since studies to evaluate the prolonged effects of black cohosh have not been done. For this reason, Germany's Commission E recommends that black cohosh should not be used for more than six months at a time.

Caution. Black cohosh should not be used by pregnant women. You should also avoid black cohosh if you are receiving any form of endocrine therapy, including birth control pills.

VITEX
(CHASTE TREE BERRY)

WHAT IS VITEX?

A shrub native to the Mediterranean, vitex agnus-castus can now be found growing throughout much of Europe as well as in the southern United States.

The plant is widely known by the popular name chaste tree. It is the fruit, or berry, of the plant that is used in herbal preparations. In researching this herb, we found it referred to as vitex, chaste tree, and agnus-cas-tus.

THE MIRACLE EFFECT

Vitex is helpful in treating a number of symptoms related to the menstrual cycle and menopause, including:

- Breast tenderness and pain
- Amenorrhea (loss of monthly periods)
- Irregular periods
- Fluid retention, tension, and discomfort resulting from PMS
- Physical discomfort, depression, and tension associated with menopause

To date, there are far more studies proving that vitex works than there are studies showing why it works so well. Current investigations show that it affects both the hypothalamus and the pituitary glands and has a hormone-regulating action. For example, German researchers have shown that it suppresses the pituitary's ability to secrete prolactin. Since an overabundance of prolactin is common in women with amenorrhea, vitex is thought to act much like the prolactin-reducing drugs usually given to correct this problem. Which substances in vitex actually suppress prolactin have yet to be established. Moreover, vitex's proven benefits extend beyond prolactin regulation, though the mechanism for these actions has yet to be identified.

HAS VITEX BEEN USED BEFORE?

Vitex has been in use for thousands of years. Homer mentioned it in *The Iliad,* and both Hippocrates and

Pliny specifically endorsed it for problems related to menstruation. Vitex got its alternate name, chaste tree berry, from ancient and medieval peoples, who believed it suppressed the libido. Monks and nuns often placed plant blossoms in their clothes to help them resist temptations of the flesh, but if this measure was effective it was largely a placebo effect. There is no evidence that vitex either decreases or increases sex drive.

In modern times, vitex has once again become valued for its ability to relieve problems related to the menstrual cycle. Extract of this herb has been available to women in Germany since the 1950s, and has recently come into use in the United States.

RESEARCH FINDINGS

Thanks to the efforts of European researchers, numerous clinical studies have documented the benefits of vitex. As early as 1979, German researchers demonstrated its benefits for women with premenstrual syndrome. A few years later, similarly positive findings for the effects of the herb on amenorrhea were published. In an impressive recent double-blind study, 175 women with PMS were given either vitex or another natural helper, vitamin B6 (see below). The test lasted through three menstrual cycles and vitex clearly out-performed B6. Approximately one-quarter of the women who tried it rated it as "excellent," while 77.1 percent reported an improvement. Lauritzen, Reuter, and Repges, the authors of the study, concluded that, compared to B6, vitex produces "a considerably more marked alleviation of typical PMS complaints, such as breast tenderness, edema, inner tension, headache, constipation, and depression."

OTHER WAYS VITEX CAN HELP

In the course of evaluating the effects of this herb on symptoms of PMS, researchers came across an unexpected finding: that vitex seems to help acne conditions. How effective it is, and whether it benefits men as well as women, remains to be thoroughly investigated, but this finding might enhance vitex's appeal to women who experience hormone-related breakouts.

HOW TO TAKE VITEX

What form does it come in? Vitex comes in tablets and capsules as well as in concentrated drops and tinctures.

What's an effective dose? Women in the PMS study described above received a daily dosage of 3.5 to 4.2 milligrams of dried extract. Another equally reputable study gave women one 175-milligram capsule daily. These vast differences are probably due to the varying standardizations of different products, and point out the importance of both choosing a reputable manufacturer and following the package instructions for that specific product.

Tips for use. Like black cohosh, the effects of vitex can take a few weeks to surface. The good news is that, unlike black cohosh, vitex is considered safe for use over extended periods of time.

Are there side effects? Although side effects are not serious, a number of women taking vitex have reported complaints such as headache, stomach upsets, and lower abdominal discomfort. In addition, some women seem to be mildly allergic to this herb and experience an itchy rash as a result of use. These side effects disappeared when use was discontinued.

Caution! If you are taking birth control pills or are being treated for an endocrine disorder, do not take this herb without consulting your doctor.

WHY *NOT* DONG QUAI?

Dong quai, also known as angelica or Chinese angelica, has long been used in Asian medicine and is currently popular in the United States. While millions of doses of this herb have been sold, we can't give it our seal of approval. Despite claims made on its behalf as a gynecological helper and overall blood "tonic," there isn't enough hard evidence to support these claims. Studies offered as proof of the herb's effectiveness often test not dong quai itself but a preparation in which dong quai is but one of several ingredients, making it impossible to judge the effect of dong quai alone. A more useful study, published in 1997, pitted dong quai against a look-alike placebo in a clinical trial on postmenopausal women. At the end of six months, neither the women nor the doctors who evaluated their symptoms, rated dong quai as any more effective than the placebo.

Serious herbal practitioners also point out that dong quai contains coumarin derivatives. While some forms of coumarins work as vasodilators and antispasmodics, these same coumarins—including at least two found in dong quai—can produce unpleasant side effects when used in concentrated doses. Writing in the journal *Science* in 1981, researchers advised against unnecessary exposure to these substances.

WHAT ELSE CAN YOU DO?

SOY: THE PREMIER PHYTOESTROGEN

In the West, 75 to 80 percent of women experience hot flashes during perimenopause and menopause. In Asia, the percentage is far smaller. The reason, researchers are now suggesting, is that traditional Chinese and Japanese diets are high in soybeans, and soybeans, in turn, are high in estrogen.

The news that phytoestrogens (estrogens made by plants) may fill in when the body's own estrogen declines has stimulated a flurry of research, and the results so far have been encouraging. In a 1995 study, women whose diet was supplemented with soy flour experienced a 40 percent reduction in hot flashes over a six-week period, while women who increased the amount of wheat flour (a weaker source of phytoestrogen) reported a 25 percent reduction.

Phytoestrogens can be found in a number of foods, including legumes such as mung beans and black beans. The problem: practicality. It is difficult to consume the daily amounts of these foods needed to realize their benefits. Recently, soy has become available as a supplement, as well as in capsule form.

Before these nutrients can be endorsed, research must be done to clarify a few key issues. First, it must be shown that soy when taken as an extract in supplement form provides the same benefits it does when consumed as food. Second, researchers suspect that phytoestrogens may stop hot flashes but fail to provide protection against osteoporosis, as prescription estrogen therapy does. A third and even more important question has to do with health risks associated with long-term use.

Many women refuse prescription estrogen therapy because it has been associated with breast cancer. Phytoestrogens are appealing because they are thought to be free of this risk—but until longer-term studies are done, this can't be guaranteed. Nevertheless, women as well as researchers are looking to soy as a way out of the estrogen-therapy dilemma, and research to date has yet to uncover any disadvantages of phytoestrogen consumption.

THE KAVA CONNECTION

Anxiety and tension are one of the most common—and unpleasant—side effects of estrogen decline. Kava, a natural tension-reliever (see chapter 1) has been proven specifically effective for reducing anxiety associated with menopause. Although there are no similar studies testing its usefulness for PMS-related tension, kava would be well worth a try.

PYRIDOXINE: ALSO KNOWN AS VITAMIN B6

Some doctors recommend B vitamins to their patients to ease the discomforts of both PMS and menopause. One reason B vitamins may help is their beneficial effect on the pituitary gland, which helps regulate ovary function and the menstrual cycle. Vitamin B6 (pyridoxine) has been found especially helpful, and research supports its benefits for women suffering from PMS.

In our discussion of vitex, we cited a study in which women receiving that herb experienced more relief than women receiving B6. However, women in both groups rated the remedies they received as "effective," and women in the B6 group had fewer side effects. Although vitex is extremely effective, B6 should not be overlooked as a source of relief.

EVERYWOMAN'S E

Vitamin E supplements have been widely recommended to help during menopause, and a number of studies conducted in the 1940s back this up. More recently, it was shown that taking vitamin E can alleviate breast tenderness and soreness associated with PMS.

GET THE MAXIMUM ON MAGNESIUM

Clinical studies have established that women who suffer from PMS often have lower levels of magnesium in their blood than women who don't have the problem. Adding magnesium supplement has been shown to help relieve symptoms such as weight gain, mood swings, and breast tenderness in many women.

WHAT ABOUT EVENING PRIMROSE OIL?

If you've been looking for something to ease your PMS, you've probably already come across products containing evening primrose oil. Over the past few years, oil from the seeds of this American wildflower have been studied in depth, and chemical analyses have pinpointed substances that, at least in theory, could well help with symptoms of PMS. The question is: Does evening primrose oil work? The answer remains in doubt. Some studies show that evening primrose supplements do benefit women with PMS, and many women swear by the herb. However, other studies show, just as convincingly, that evening primrose has no real benefit beyond a placebo effect.

CHAPTER TWENTY-ONE

Save Your Bones From

Osteoporosis

You can't avoid aging. But you can avoid developing fragile bones because of it. The remedy is already available.

Once upon a time, getting older meant developing fragile, easy-to-break bones. Especially for women. With the onset of menopause, loss of estrogen leads to rapid bone loss. This condition, known as osteoporosis, was once thought to be an inevitable part of aging. No more. By taking a few simple preventive steps, you can start taking measures today to make sure you stand tall in your golden years.

And if you're a man, don't skip this chapter. Despite the widespread attention given to women's problems with osteoporosis, men are also affected.

THE PROBLEM

As we age, a number of silent, unseen changes take place in our bodies. Falling estrogen levels in women, as well as the digestive system's decreased ability to absorb calcium as efficiently as it once did, leave the body in a state of chronic calcium deficiency.

This is a big problem because calcium is an absolutely necessary component of several body fluids. To fulfill its need for calcium, the body comes up with an ingenious solution—it pulls calcium from its own bones.

WHO SUFFERS FROM OSTEOPOROSIS?

Osteoporosis isn't a disease anyone can catch. It's a condition with well-established risks. Your chances of bone loss are influenced by such factors as:

- **Being a woman.** Both men and women can get osteoporosis. However, bone loss is more rapid and far more dramatic in women, and the consequences are usually far more serious. For most women, the acceleration begins as estrogen declines during menopause and remains in high gear for about a decade. Women who go through premature menopause as a result of hysterectomy or other procedures, are also at risk for osteoporosis.
- **Age.** Osteoporosis is age related in both men and women. Both men and women begin to lose bone from middle age onward.
- **Family history.** Researchers have found that osteoporosis has a genetic link.
- **Diet.** It's been estimated that the average American woman takes in about 574 milligrams of dietary calcium a day, while men take in 826 milligrams. For people over sixty-five, the amounts are even lower. Even the highest of these figures is well below the government's recommended guidelines.

- **Bone structure.** Some people have heavier, denser bones than others. These people are less likely to suffer from osteoporosis than people whose bones are more delicate.
- **People taking steroid drugs,** such as prednisone, for prolonged periods. People who take steroid drugs for rheumatoid arthritis, inflammatory bowel syndrome, or other diseases are at risk for osteoporosis due to this medication. (For natural aids for these disorders, see chapter 2 on Arthritis, and chapter 11 on the Digestive System.)

WHAT ARE THE SYMPTOMS OF OSTEOPOROSIS?

The most visible symptom of osteoporosis is declining stature. Stooping, due to curvature of the spine, can also occur. But the worst symptoms are hidden within the body. Under a microscope a bone with osteoporosis looks like Swiss cheese. Knocks and falls that would once have been of little consequence can now cause fractures.

WHAT'S THE OUTLOOK?

Osteoporosis is progressive unless action is taken. During and after menopause, women will have an overall average of 1 percent bone loss each year. This may not seem like much, but not all bones in the body lose mass at the same rate. Some bones—including the spine—appear to deteriorate much more quickly. This is why many people lose several inches in height and become noticeably shorter as they age.

In both men and women, severe osteoporosis often

leads to fractures. Again, women are more vulnerable than men on this score, and fractures of the hip are especially common in older women. However, an inexpensive nutrient, calcium, can bring your annual bone loss down to almost nothing (see below).

WHAT YOU SHOULD KNOW

Hormone replacement therapy, which compensates for estrogen loss, can help guard against osteoporosis. Since many feel this therapy carries risks of its own, be sure to discuss both the pros and the cons with your gynecologist before you make a decision.

PROVEN MIRACLES

CALCIUM

WHAT IS CALCIUM?

Calcium is a common mineral used for building bones and teeth. It also plays a role in transmitting nerve messages and regulating heartbeat. Many of us don't get enough calcium in the best of circumstances. And, as we grow older, our need for this mineral increases because our bodies don't absorb it as effectively as before.

THE MIRACLE EFFECT

The overwhelming majority of studies done to date show that calcium in supplement form is as effective for osteoporosis as added dietary calcium is. In both women and men regular calcium supplementation has been shown to:

- Preserve bone density
- Dramatically slow bone loss throughout the body
- Eliminate loss completely in some bones
- Reduce number of fractures

HAS CALCIUM BEEN USED BEFORE?

Calcium from dietary sources has always been an essential nutrient in the human diet. And many researchers believe that our ancestors took in far more of it than we do today. In fact, some researchers have calculated that Stone Age adults took in three to five times more calcium than a modern adult who eats a typical American diet. This is one reason why millions of doses of this supplement are sold every year.

RESEARCH FINDINGS

Unlike remedies that work for some people and not for others, calcium is a simple, easy-to-take solution that helps everyone. Here are results from just a few studies:

- More than twenty separate studies have shown the impact calcium can have on women during the post-menopausal years. For women taking calcium, the rate of loss is slowed to a near halt—just .014 percent bone loss per year.
- A placebo-controlled study tracked 118 healthy women three to six years after menopause. Women who took a placebo lost spinal bone at a rapid rate of 2 percent per year. But women who received calcium slowed spinal bone loss to just one-half of 1 percent per year.

- In another study, postmenopausal women were monitored for two years. Those who took calcium lost only one-third to one-half as much bone as women who received no calcium.

OTHER WAYS CALCIUM CAN HELP

Calcium is an indispensable nutrient and necessary throughout the life cycle. Studies suggest that it may also help overcome sleep disorders (see chapter 15 on Insomnia). In combination with vitamin D, it may offer protection against rectal cancer (see chapter 6 on Cancer).

HOW TO TAKE CALCIUM

What form does it come in? Calcium comes in tablets. Often, it is combined with magnesium or magnesium and zinc, which helps the body better use it.

What's an effective dose? Most studies we reviewed recommended a total intake of 1,000 to 1,500 milligrams of calcium per day.

Tips for use. Calcium is better used by the body when food is present in the digestive system, so take this supplement with meals.

Are there side effects? Calcium is extremely safe and nontoxic, and we did not find reports of unpleasant side effects.

WHAT ELSE CAN YOU DO?

If you're at risk for osteoporosis, there are three other things you should know about protecting your bones.

THE VITAMIN D CONNECTION

Vitamin D is necessary for proper calcium absorption. One study, done on men, suggested that lack of vitamin D may be significantly responsible for low calcium levels.

The best source of vitamin D is sunlight. However, sunlight is a prime risk factor for skin cancer, and soaking up the sun is no longer recommended. To prevent vitamin D deficiency, milk and cereals are often fortified with this vitamin. Make sure you get your recommended daily allowance (400 IUs) of this vitamin from fortified foods and/or from a vitamin supplement. Avoid megadoses, however, as too much of this vitamin can be harmful to your health.

HORMONE REPLACEMENT THERAPY

In menopausal women, hormone replacement therapy (estrogen) taken on its own helps slow bone loss. Several studies indicate that women who take both hormone replacements and calcium supplement have slower bone loss than women taking either one alone. One group of researchers has suggested that women on hormone replacement therapy need take only 800 milligrams of calcium supplement a day.

As we said before, discuss both the pros and cons of

hormone replacement therapy with your gynecologist before deciding if it's right for you.

ADD EXERCISE

Calcium is good for osteoporosis and so is exercise. The two together, experts are finding, work better than either one alone. In one study, just four hours of exercise a week, added to a calcium supplement program, was enough to produce a significant improvement over taking calcium alone. Best of all, the exercise need not be strenuous, merely weight bearing. Walking at a relaxed pace is just fine.

CHAPTER TWENTY-TWO

Relief for

Enlarged Prostate (BPH)

When studies pit the favorite prescription medication for prostate problems against the herbal remedy of choice, the results are clearcut: The herb wins by a knockout.

Men have it easy, the cliché goes. A man may not have to contend with the problems a woman's more complex reproductive system presents her with, but that doesn't mean men get off scot-free. If a man lives long enough, he will probably have an encounter with a small walnut-shaped gland known as the prostate.

THE PROBLEM

The prostate gland, part of the male reproductive system, sits between the rectum and bladder and surrounds the distal portion of the urethra. Even after a man reaches physical maturity, the prostate continues to grow. This growth is so gradual it goes unnoticed for decades. However, sometime around late middle age, problems often arise as the enlarged prostate presses in on the urethra it surrounds. Doctors refer to this condition as benign prostatic hyperplasia, or BPH for short.

WHO SUFFERS FROM BPH?

The only established risk factor for BPH is age, and the connection is a firm one. According to the National Institute of Diabetes and Digestive and Kidney Diseases, a branch of the National Institutes of Health, few men under forty experience any symptoms of BPH, but more than half of men over sixty do, and a full 90 percent of men in their seventies and eighties experience problems to some degree.

WHAT ARE THE SYMPTOMS?

Uncomfortable symptoms occur when the enlarged prostate presses against the urethra and interferes with the flow of urine. Typical symptoms of BPH include:
- Urgent need to urinate
- Need to urinate frequently, especially at night
- Partial loss of continence (leaking and/or dribbling)
- Slow, interrupted, or weak urine stream

In some cases, a man who has previously been symptom-free will be unable to urinate at all. This condition, which may be triggered by certain ingredients in nonprescription cold or allergy medications, is not as common as those listed above.

WHAT'S THE OUTLOOK?

The "benign" in benign prostatic hyperplasia means that this condition is noncancerous. BPH is *not* an early stage of cancer of the prostate; nor are men who have

BPH at increased risk for this type of cancer. It would be a mistake, however, to assume that "benign" means the condition need not be taken seriously.

Aside from the immediate discomfort of its symptoms, BPH can cause serious problems. Inability to empty the bladder completely can lead to urinary-tract infections, kidney stones, and even kidney and bladder damage. Whether or not such damage will occur is not a foregone conclusion. Doctors have noted that treatment may not be necessary if the prostate is only mildly enlarged. For many men, monitoring the condition through regular checkups is enough. In cases requiring treatment, doctors rely on prescription drugs as well as surgery to remove the excess tissue.

WHAT YOU SHOULD KNOW

Although BPH is not a risk factor for cancer of the prostate, the symptoms of BPH can resemble cancer's warning signs as well as symptoms of other diseases. For this reason, self-diagnosis is *not* an option. If you think you have BPH you're probably right—but you should get a diagnosis from your doctor to make sure.

PROVEN MIRACLES

SAW PALMETTO

WHAT IS SAW PALMETTO?

Saw palmetto, a member of the palm family, is a small, shrublike tree that grows throughout the southeastern

United States. It is the small, dark berries of the plant whose extract has proven helpful for BPH.

THE MIRACLE EFFECT

The key to understanding saw palmetto's effectiveness may have come when researchers noted that men with enlarged prostates had elevated blood levels of dihydrotestosterone (DHT for short). Since DHT, a powerful sex hormone, prompts the growth of male physical characteristics, it may well play a key role in BPH.

Lab studies suggest that saw palmetto lowers DHT in two ways, both by limiting its production and by inhibiting its binding at receptor sites. In addition, saw palmetto has an anti-inflammatory effect, which may also contribute to its effectiveness.

For men with enlarged prostates, saw palmetto's proven benefits include:
- Increased urinary flow
- Easier start of urination
- More complete urination
- Less frequent urination

HAS SAW PALMETTO BEEN USED BEFORE?

Also known as sabal and serenoa, saw palmetto was widely used for urogenital disorders in America from the turn of the century until 1950. While it fell into disuse here, it remained popular in Europe, where researchers established its effectiveness for BPH.

RESEARCH FINDINGS

Numerous studies on men with BPH have established saw palmetto as a safe and effective treatment. Over two thousand men have been involved in clinical trials in Germany alone, and saw palmetto has earned the seal of approval of Germany's Commission E.

In open studies, where all subjects receive the same treatment, saw palmetto received overall higher ratings than a standard prescription medication. Double-blind, placebo-controlled studies have also been done to determine whether saw palmetto's effect is physiological or psychological.

In 1984, 110 men suffering from BPH were divided into two groups and given a daily dosage of either saw palmetto extract or a look-alike placebo. Writing in the *British Journal of Clinical Pharmacology,* Champault and colleagues noted that after just one month, symptoms of the men receiving saw palmetto decreased measurably and far exceeded any improvements reported in the placebo group. Other studies have shown similarly favorable results.

HOW TO TAKE SAW PALMETTO

What form does it come in? Saw palmetto comes primarily in tablets and capsules.

What's an effective dose? Men in studies improved on a daily dose of 320 milligrams of standardized saw palmetto extract, the same amount recommended by Commission E. Since the product you choose may be standardized to a different strength, be sure to follow the manufacturer's package instructions.

Tips for use. Remember that saw palmetto doesn't relieve pain and discomfort in the way that aspirin does—it relieves pain by correcting the source of the problem, and this can take time. If you decide to try saw palmetto, allow a four-to-six-week trial period. This may seem like a long time, but saw palmetto actually works more quickly than most prescription medications for this condition.

Are there side effects? Saw palmetto is considered extremely safe when taken in recommended doses. It is also easy to tolerate and does not produce side effects in most people who use it. In a few rare individuals, it may produce gastric upset.

STINGING NETTLE

WHAT IS STINGING NETTLE?

The name is fierce—for good reason. Direct contact with this tall plant typically causes skin irritation and rash. Nevertheless, its leaves have been used by herbalists for centuries. Now, cutting-edge research has found that its root can relieve symptoms of BPH in men.

THE MIRACLE EFFECT

Both nettle leaves and nettle root can help the symptoms of BPH. Preparations made from the leaf increase the flow of urine. The extract made from the root is even more helpful, though researchers have not yet determined exactly why. The actions of several substances have been examined, and one or all of them may be responsible for the herb's healing effect.

In 1994 Japanese researchers found that steroidal and other components in the root significantly inhibited the enzymes that cause the prostate to grow. Another study, done on mice with artificially induced symptoms of BPH tested five different preparations, each containing an isolated substance of nettle root. Though some substances were more effective than others, none of the single-substance preparations were as effective as preparations made from a combination of nettle root substances.

HAS STINGING NETTLE BEEN USED BEFORE?

For centuries stinging nettle was used as a topical application. It's said that Roman soldiers rubbed it on their skin to produce a rash that helped keep them warm on long, cold marches. Applied directly to the scalp, its tingling effect was supposed to stimulate hair growth—an unfounded claim. In more recent times, it has been valued as an aid for urinary problems and BPH, and it is a popular remedy throughout Europe.

RESEARCH FINDINGS

Germany's Commission E, the government body in charge of evaluating claims made for phytomedicines and nutrients, has reviewed studies done on both stinging nettle leaf and root products. It has approved leaf extract as an aid in promoting urine flow and has endorsed root extract for use in treatment of BPH symptoms.

OTHER WAYS STINGING NETTLE CAN HELP

Stinging nettle has long been thought to have an anti-inflammatory effect. Research now suggests this may be true. A study appearing in *Planta Medica* in 1990 found that stinging nettle outperformed a placebo when tested on people with allergy symptoms. More recently, researchers have found evidence that stinging nettle leaf boosts the effect of anti-inflammatory drugs in people with rheumatoid arthritis (see chapter 2).

HOW TO TAKE STINGING NETTLE

What form does it come in? Stinging nettle comes in a variety of forms. Products made from the root typically come in tablets or capsules, as do leaf products. According to herbal authority Varo Tyler, tea made from the leaves, taken several times a day, can also be effective.

What's an effective dose? Dosages depend on the form and strength of the individual product. Your best way to ensure an effective dose is to purchase a standardized product from a reputable manufacturer and follow the company's package directions.

Tips for use. German authorities suggest that stinging nettle is most effective for early stages of BPH. If your case is more advanced, you may want to choose another alternative.

Side effects. Reported side effects are mild, and the chief complaint is gastrointestinal upset.

Caution! It's called stinging nettle because contact with the plant in the wild causes skin irritation. Some individuals may have a heightened sensitivity to this plant in any form, and may have an allergic reaction (rash, itching, etc.). If this happens, discontinue use at once. A study done on mice has shown that it aggravates diabetes, despite the fact that it has often been recommended as an aid for this condition. People who have diabetes or who are being treated for diabetes, as well as people taking medication for high or low blood pressure or depression, should not take stinging nettle products.

WHAT ELSE CAN YOU DO?

If you're a man with an enlarged prostate, there are a few additional strategies you may want to use.

THE GOOD NEWS ABOUT COMBINATIONS

Cutting edge research suggests that saw palmetto can be more effective when other nutrients are added. Though studies are ongoing, proven helpers so far include stinging nettle (see above) and pygeum (derived from the bark of a tropical evergreen), available in capsules and already combined with saw palmetto.

ZAP ZINC DEFICIENCY

Zinc deficiency is not at all uncommon in the United States, and older people are more at risk than younger ones. One of the consequences of zinc deficiency in men is a swollen prostate, and researchers have suggested that boosting zinc intake may be one way of dealing with BPH. In one study, taking 150 milligrams of zinc supplement daily over a two-to-four-month period improved symptoms in a significant number of men.

CHAPTER TWENTY-THREE

Treat and Heal
Skin and Scalp

Skin problems can be as diverse and irksome as those that form beneath its surface—but these natural healers have proven remarkably effective against many of them.

While you may think of your skin as mere "packaging" for the more important systems within, it is a full-fledged organ and comes with its own varied set of potential problems. It is your first line of defense against a world teeming with germs. Unfortunately, the skin is also delicate. Unlike a clam, whose hard shell protects it from injury, or an animal with a tough, shaggy hide, mankind's outer covering is a large and vulnerable organ. Learning to protect it and help it heal is fundamental to your overall good health.

THE PROBLEM

Your skin can be affected by a wide range of problems. Some, such as sunburn, chapping, and wind burn, are caused by the environment. Cuts and abrasions are also a problem, since they create an ideal breeding spot for microorganisms of all sorts. Still another set of problems occurs when the skin itself becomes the site of an infection, such as in toenail fungus.

In short, there is no one type of skin infection. But the remedies in this chapter will help take care of many of the most common problems.

WHO SUFFERS FROM SKIN PROBLEMS?

Who suffers from skin problems? Everyone! But a few factors can make you more or less vulnerable, including:

- **Individual biochemistry.** Without a doubt, some people's skin is more sensitive than others.
- **Stress.** Dermatologists have noted a new phenomenon: acne that begins in adulthood and primarily affects women. The reason isn't a rush of teenage hormones. According to Dr. Tony Chu of London's Hammersmith Hospital, the problem is stress. And stress may play a role in other skin problems as well.
- **Lifestyle factors.** Some people work at jobs that expose their skin to the sun, or make them prone to minor cuts and wounds. Even hobbies can be a factor. For example, the constant friction of toes against jogging shoes can injure toenails. This, combined with the warm, moist, airless conditions inside the shoe, creates an ideal breeding ground for toenail fungus.

WHAT ARE THE SYMPTOMS?

The infections and problems we're discussing in this chapter are mild, everyday problems whose symptoms you are already familiar with. But bear in mind that not all skin problems are of the everyday sort and some may require medical attention.

Symptoms that warrant immediate medical attention include:

- **Extreme pain, tenderness, warmth, or redness.** Minor infections always carry a degree of pain. But extreme pain and tenderness can signal that an abscess has formed or that an infection has gotten out of hand.
- **Any infection that seems to be spreading rapidly.** This is a key feature of an extremely serious streptococcal infection known as necrotizing fasciitis, or "flesh eating disease."
- **Red marks or lines trailing from the infection site.** This can be a sign of blood poisoning.
- **Small gray, black, or red scaly patches.** These may be nothing, or they may be the beginnings of skin cancers that should be removed.

WHAT'S THE OUTLOOK?

Most cuts, abrasions, and minor infections heal themselves in time. A few problems, such as acne, dandruff, and fungal infections, can be amazingly stubborn and hard to treat. The ability of the applications in this chapter to combat these problems as well as—and, in some cases, better than—expensive prescription ointments is one reason why natural remedies are gaining popularity with many people.

WHAT YOU SHOULD KNOW

If you're going to treat your own minor skin problems, it's important for you to know exactly what you're treating. If you aren't sure what your problem is, don't guess—and don't wait too long before consulting a doctor or dermatologist. This is especially true if you notice any of the problem symptoms listed above.

PROVEN MIRACLES

TEA TREE OIL

WHAT IS TEA TREE OIL?

Tea tree oil comes from the Melaleuca alternifolia, a shrubby tree native to Australia and Southeast Asia.

THE MIRACLE EFFECT

Tea tree oil, applied externally, can help control infections and reduce inflammation caused by bacteria. It has been found helpful against such common problems as toenail fungus and acne. Tea tree oil has been used for a variety of skin conditions, including:
- Acne
- Athlete's foot
- Nail fungus
- Dandruff
- Sunburn
- Skin abrasions and irritations
- Skin infections due to a variety of bacteria, fungi,

yeasts (including candida), and staphylococcus germs

Tea tree oil contains a number of antiseptic and disinfectant substances. Its effectiveness is due to the combined action of these substances, rather than to any one agent in particular.

HAS TEA TREE OIL BEEN USED BEFORE?

Tea tree oil was discovered and first widely used by the aborigines of Australia. By the early 1900s, commercial tea tree oil products, sold as disinfectants, were widely available. During World War II, every first-aid kit in the Australian army contained a bottle of tea tree oil. Interest in the oil waned with the introduction of antibiotics.

In recent years, concern about the overuse of antibiotics has revived interest in tea tree oil. It is widely used in France, especially. Solid research, dating from the mid-1990s, will undoubtedly increase its popularity.

RESEARCH FINDINGS

A great many lab studies have been done to evaluate tea tree oil's effectiveness in combating a variety of microorganisms. A few controlled human studies have also been done.

- In one trial, reported in the *Journal of Family Practice* in 1994, people with nail fungus applied tea tree oil twice a day. At the end of six months, the fungus was either partially or completely cleared up in 60 percent of patients.
- A study by Bassett and colleagues compared tea tree oil to another popular acne remedy, benzoyl

peroxide, on 124 patients with mild to moderate acne. Half of the patients used a lotion containing 5 percent benzoyl peroxide. The other half used a gel containing 5 percent tea tree oil. Both remedies significantly reduced the number of open and closed acne sores. Tea tree oil, however, had fewer side effects.

HOW TO USE TEA TREE OIL

What form does it come in? Tea tree oil comes in "pure" oil form, but you may also see it incorporated in salves, gels, and creams. No matter what form you buy, be sure to read the label. According to reports, some manufacturers mix tea tree oil with less expensive eucalyptus oil, which can cause skin irritation.

You should also check to make sure you're buying a standardized product. Tea tree oil should contain at least 30 percent terpinen-4-ol, tea tree oil's main active ingredient. Another ingredient to pay attention to is cineole, a component that can cause skin irritations. Look for a product that contains no more than 15 percent of this, and preferably less.

Tips for use. Apply externally to the affected area according to the manufacturer's package directions. Tea tree oil is not recommended for burns.

Are there side effects? A few people are allergic to tea tree oil. To be safe, apply to a small patch of skin and wait twenty-four hours before applying to a larger area. Discontinue use immediately if your condition worsens or if use causes itching and redness.

Caution! Tea tree oil can be toxic if taken internally in substantial quantities. Be sure to keep out of children's reach. Also, some reports have recommended tea tree oil for skin ailments in dogs and cats. However, animals have a tendency to lick themselves, and some cases of poisoning have been reported.

ALOE

WHAT IS ALOE?

Aloe, or aloe vera, is the gel-like substance extracted from the leaf of the aloe plant. It is not the same as aloes, a bitter juice extracted from the dried leaves of the same plant.

THE MIRACLE EFFECT

Aloe appears as an ingredient in so many skin creams and shampoos that you may have come to think of it only as a cosmetic product. That would be too bad, because the gel from the leaf of this easy-to-grow plant has true healing abilities. For centuries, aloe vera has been successfully used for a variety of skin injuries, including:

- Minor cuts, scrapes, and wounds
- Sunburn
- Mild to moderate burns
- Dermabrasion
- Frostbite
- Wind burn
- Mouth ulcers

As an aid for these problems, aloe does much more than soothe irritated skin. In fact, it's not too much of an exaggeration to say that the aloe plant gives us a first-aid kit in a leaf. A combination of active substances in aloe have been shown to carry out a number of functions essential for healing. Applying aloe to a wound or burn will:

- Reduce inflammation.
- Reduce bacteria at the wound site
- Stimulate production of collagen, the material that makes up 75 percent of our skin
- Promote wound closing and contraction
- Help wound area stay moist

HAS ALOE BEEN USED BEFORE?

Aloe is one of the oldest skin salves known to man and has been in constant use for some six thousand years. It was revered by the Egyptians and was part of every pharaoh's burial wealth. Dioscorides, a Greek physician who lived two thousand years ago, recommended it for healing wounds and blemishes. When the Spanish explored the New World in the sixteenth century, they brought aloe with them to treat cuts and soothe sunburn.

The miraculous abilities of this healing leaf have never been abandoned. But they have been given a boost by science. In the 1930s, researchers found that aloe promoted healing of burns from ultraviolet rays, X rays, and gamma rays. As news of aloe's scientifically proven healing abilities trickled down to the public, the plant became increasingly popular. It became a household word in the 1970s, and still remains so. Today aloe is routinely used by millions of people around the world.

RESEARCH FINDINGS

Aloe's undisputed reputation as a wound healer has, at times, caused it to be overlooked as a subject for research. However, some researchers have conducted systematic studies to prove that aloe does, indeed, deserve its lofty reputation.

Numerous small-animal studies have confirmed aloe's effectiveness for burns and wounds. And, as the following summaries of two important human tests indicate, aloe is one product well worth keeping on your shelf.

- A study of twenty-seven patients with moderate burns compared aloe vera to Vaseline in promoting healing. Burns treated with Vaseline took eighteen days to heal, but burns treated with aloe healed in just eleven days.
- Dermabrasion, a procedure in which the surface of the skin is literally sanded away, is a common way of minimizing acne scars and other facial blemishes. Following dermabrasion, half of a volunteer patient's face was treated with a standard wound gel. The other half of the patient's face was treated with the gel plus aloe vera. Fresh gel was applied every day for five days and the results carefully monitored. On days one and two, there was much less swelling on the aloe-treated side. On days three and four, the side treated with aloe showed less oozing and crusting. And by days five and six, healing was complete on the aloe side but not on the side treated with standard gel alone. In fact, using aloe speeded healing by three whole days!

OTHER WAYS ALOE CAN HELP

Aloe has long been valued for its soothing effect on sunburn. Recent research shows that it may also prove helpful in preventing cancer. Researchers at the University of Texas M. D. Anderson Cancer Center found that while aloe can't reverse the damage sunlight does to skin, it can do something very important. Applying aloe gel after exposure to harmful rays, Strickland and colleagues found, prevented most of the damage to the skin's immune system. Preventing this damage is a key step in preventing the development of many diseases, including cancer.

HOW TO USE ALOE

What form does it come in? Aloe comes in a variety of topical applications, including creams, gels, and ointments. Whichever product you buy, make sure it comes from a reputable manufacturer and actually contains aloe as a main ingredient.

Some beverages also contain aloe and claim you can drink your way to health. While these drinks aren't harmful, they are not necessarily helpful, either. We could find no research to support claims for the health benefits of these drinks. According to Varo Tyler, one of America's leading authorities on herbal remedies, components of aloe break down so quickly they're unlikely to last long enough in the digestive tract to be absorbed by the body.

We can't overlook one form that should be obvious: the leaf itself. If you enjoy plants, aloe is not difficult to grow. When you have a small cut, burn, or skin irritation, just snap a leaf in two and rub the inner gel on the affected area.

Tips for use. A few studies we reviewed noted that speed of healing and overall effectiveness were associated with more frequent applications. While aloe has been proven to promote healing in minor to moderate skin injuries, studies show that it may slow healing in severe burns and major wounds (such as surgical incisions).

Side effects. Remarkably, aloe gel seems to be free of side effects, and we did not find reports of allergic reactions. However, to be on the safe side, you might try a patch test first.

WHAT ELSE CAN YOU DO?

There are a lot of things you can do to protect your skin, starting with eating a healthy diet, getting plenty of exercise, and using a sunscreen to guard against sun damage. You may also want to adopt this strategy:

VITAMIN C FOR WOUNDS

If you have a cut or abrasion, don't forget the vitamin C supplements. According to studies, C helps wounds heal properly and repairs injured tissue. Since a recent survey found that many Americans don't get enough of this vitamin in dietary sources, take it in supplement form.

CHAPTER TWENTY-FOUR

Special Help for
Varicose Veins

If you have varicose veins, your doctor may already have read medical journal studies endorsing this natural miracle worker and told you about it.

Varicose veins (also known as chronic venous insufficiency) are common, and many people accept living with them as a chronic condition of life. In addition to being unsightly, they are extremely uncomfortable. On occasion, fragile distended veins can rupture and cause blood loss. In severe cases, surgery may be needed to tie off the damaged vein and let others take over its work. Fortunately, there *is* something that promotes healing in varicose veins, a natural substance that Varo Tyler, one of America's leading authorities on herbal healing, has termed "by far the most effective plant drug employed for [this] disorder."

THE PROBLEM

A varicose vein is swollen, pushed to the surface, and distended with blood. How did the vein get this way?

Researchers believe they've found the answer to this. Enzymes in the body attack and destroy the elastic tissues of the vein and weaken the strength of the walls. The weakened veins become more permeable, allowing water and solid molecules to pass through the walls. At the same time, the vein is no longer as elastic as it once was, the valves within the vein fail to work properly, and the blood is no longer moved along efficiently. Blood accumulates in the veins, causing them to become engorged and distended with the blood they can no longer move. While varicose veins can occur in a variety of sites in the body, they are most likely to affect the legs.

WHO SUFFERS FROM VARICOSE VEINS?

As health problems go, varicose veins are fairly common. Approximately 15 percent of the population will develop varicose veins at some point in their lives. Risk factors associated with varicose veins are:

- **Being a woman.** Women are much more likely to get varicose veins than men. It has been suggested that pressure on the veins during pregnancy may exacerbate a predisposition to this condition.
- **Family history.** Varicose veins seem to run in families.
- **Occupation.** Jobs that involve standing for long periods of time increase the likelihood of varicose veins. Walking doesn't have the same risk.

WHAT ARE THE SYMPTOMS?

Varicose veins are much more than a cosmetic nuisance. They pose a true health problem with symptoms that include:

- Fluid buildup and swelling in the affected area
- Aching and pain
- Sensation of heaviness or fatigue in the affected limbs
- Itching

WHAT'S THE OUTLOOK?

Varicose veins are a chronic condition with few treatment options. Wearing special elastic stockings may help some people. If the condition is severe and veins become so fragile that hemorrhage is a possibility, surgery may be necessary.

WHAT YOU NEED TO KNOW

As always, we recommend working with your doctor and getting his professional diagnosis and advice. Occasionally, a vein that bulges or comes to the surface is not a varicose vein but a symptom of a disease or condition that requires immediate medical treatment.

PROVEN MIRACLES

HORSE CHESTNUT

WHAT IS HORSE CHESTNUT?

Horse chestnut is an attractive flowering tree. While the flowers are lovely to look at, it's the large brown seed (also known as Ohio buckeye) that is beneficial to people with varicose veins.

THE MIRACLE EFFECT

Researchers believe horse chestnut owes much of its undisputed success to aescin (also spelled "escin" and "escine"), a mixture of saponins found in the seed of the plant. Numerous studies—in the lab, on animals, and in humans—have proven that aescin suppresses the specific enzymes that attack vein tissue. However, horse chestnut contains other active substances, including flavonoids, which have a proven anti-inflammatory effect.

For people with varicose veins, this means improvement not just of symptoms but of the underlying causes of the symptoms. Specifically, horse chestnut has been shown to improve the overall tone and elasticity of veins and to reduce or eliminate numerous symptoms, including:

- Fluid buildup and swelling in veins
- Leg pain and feeling of tension
- Sensation of heaviness and fatigue in legs
- Itching in affected area

HAS HORSE CHESTNUT BEEN USED BEFORE?

If you want to be the first to try horse chestnut, you're too late. A host of others have already beaten you to it. In Germany it's been an approved remedy for varicose veins and other problems with veins since 1984, when Commission E endorsed it for use. Extract of horse chestnut is also widely used in Japan, where it has been given by injection to postoperative patients to reduce inflammation following surgery.

RESEARCH FINDINGS

In addition to animal studies, numerous studies documenting the beneficial effects of horse chestnut have been done on people with varicose veins. In 1986, two double-blind placebo-controlled studies found that horse chestnut significantly improved symptoms such as swelling, blood pooling in the veins, pain, and fatigue.

One of the largest studies, by Greeske and Pohlman, involved more than five thousand patients under the care of more than eight hundred general practitioners. In the study, the doctors were asked to report patients' feedback as well as their own evaluations of the preparation's effectiveness. Horse chestnut was found so effective in reducing or completely eliminating pain, tiredness, itching, tension, and swelling in the leg that the authors concluded, "The results of this study show that rational treatment with horse chestnut extract represents an economical, practice-relevant therapeutic 'pillar,' which in comparison with compression has the additional advantage of better compliance."

The authors' comparison of horse chestnut to "compression" is a reference to a standard aid for varicose veins, elastic stockings. However, as the study points out, some patients find the stockings bothersome and often dispense with wearing them. Another study backs up Greeske and Pohlman's finding that horse chestnut is a good alternative to elasticized stockings. In an article published in *The Lancet* in 1996, Diehm and colleagues found that a twelve-week course of horse chestnut yielded comparable results to twelve weeks of compression therapy.

OTHER WAYS HORSE CHESTNUT CAN HELP

At present horse chestnut has been proven effective only for varicose veins and as an anti-inflammatory agent. However, a work published several years ago suggested that aescin may have additional uses. A lab study found that it had significant antiviral action when tested on a strain of type-A influenza. Unfortunately, this intriguing research has yet to be followed up on.

HOW TO TAKE HORSE CHESTNUT

What form does it come in? Horse chestnut seed extract comes in capsules and tablets. You'll also find horse chestnut extract listed as an ingredient in salves and ointments advertised for external use on varicose veins and/or hemorrhoids. At present, only preparations for internal use are widely endorsed by reputable herbal authorities. (See ''Are Horse Chestnut Ointments Effective?'' below.)

What's an effective dose? Studies have shown that horse chestnut works in dosages equivalent to 100 milligrams of aescin a day. Herbalist Varo Tyler sets the range for initial dosages at 90 to 150 milligrams of aescin daily.

Tips for use. If you decide to try horse chestnut, be sure to look for a brand that has standardized the amount of aescin, the plant's most active ingredient. You should also know that horse chestnut has a carry-over effect—in other words, the benefits continue to work for some time after use stops. This suggests that horse chestnut may not have to be taken on a continuous basis. Varo Tyler suggests cutting back your daily dosage by 50 percent once improvements are seen.

Are there side effects? When taken orally in recommended doses, horse chestnut is considered safe and effective. However, it does contain saponins, which can cause gastrointestinal upsets in some people.

Caution! Varicose veins are a common complication of pregnancy. Unfortunately, studies have not been done establishing that horse chestnut is safe for pregnant or breast-feeding women, so it should be avoided. Finally, the active substances in horse chestnut can interfere with other drugs and make them less effective, so if you are on any type of medication, ask your doctor before taking horse chestnut.

ARE HORSE CHESTNUT OINTMENTS EFFECTIVE?

Please note that *all* the research referenced in this chapter applies to horse chestnut taken internally. At present, there is no compelling research to support the theory that horse chestnut can be absorbed into the vein through the skin. There may be a cosmetic benefit, and bulging veins may appear to retract or shrink in size, but this is due to the astringent effects of the saponins, and can't be taken as proof that applying horse chestnut externally is as effective as taking it internally.

WHAT ELSE CAN YOU DO?

THE ABC'S OF OPC

You may have heard of OPCs, substances found in grape seed and pine bark extracts. Like horse chestnut, OPCs strengthen veins and reduce symptoms such as fluid buildup. In fact OPCs are so effective they're becoming a treatment of choice in France. Unlike horse chestnut, which primarily works on veins, OPC strengthens arteries as well, so instead of including a discussion of it here, we've included it in chapter 5 on Blood Vessels. If you suffer from varicose veins, you'll want to learn more about this wonderful helper.

REMEMBER RUTIN

The recent interest in horse chestnut and OPC has overshadowed earlier research done on rutin, a flavonoid. As early as 1946, rutin was shown to have a strengthening effect on capillaries, and a study from 1971 found it helpful for varicose veins. More research should be done on this promising but overlooked nutrient.

GLOSSARY

Amino acid. A nitrogen-bearing organic compound that plays a vital role in building muscle and making protein. There are more than twenty different amino acids.

Antioxidant. Any nutrient or chemical that neutralizes free radicals (see below). By intervening in this way, antioxidants prevent free radicals from damaging healthy cells.

Bioflavonoid. See **flavonoid,** below.

Carcinogen. A substance that harms cells and leads to the formation of cancer. A few carcinogens are potent enough to cause problems through a single exposure. More often, problems arise through long-term exposure to various carcinogens.

Carotenoid. Carotenoids are the plant pigments found in red, yellow, and orange vegetables and fruits. There are more than six hundred members of the carotene family, but not all of them are equally beneficial.

Commission E. A famous German government panel that evaluates herbal remedies and judges their usefulness. Commission E does not set up or run studies itself. Instead, it gathers and reads available data. Based on its findings, various remedies are either approved or not approved for use. Although Commission E has no official power outside of Germany, it is useful because it is one of the few reputable review boards that systematically studies and evaluates information on herbal remedies.

Double-blind study. A highly reliable method of testing the effectiveness of specific remedies. In a double-blind study, volunteers receive either the "real" medication being evaluated or a look-alike placebo (see below). Neither volunteers nor those who administer and supervise the study know who has received which substance until the study is complete and the final data have been gathered and analyzed.

Effective. When a supplement is deemed "effective," it does not mean that it will work for every person every single time. Not even the most "effective" medicines on earth can achieve that. Researchers and doctors designate a remedy effective when it has a significant effect on a significant number of people. To be considered effective, a substance must alleviate most or all of the troublesome symptoms and must do so for a majority of people, not just for isolated cases.

Flavonoid. Also known as bioflavonoids, flavonoids are vitaminlike plant substances. There are literally hundreds of flavonoids, though very few of them are known by their technical names.

Free radical. Harmful, cell-damaging molecules that get into our bodies in a variety of ways. There are numerous types of free radicals, but all have an unpaired oxygen atom. Because of this, they seek to "kidnap" an atom from a healthy cell. This damages the cell and sets the stage for disease.

Gram. One gram is equal to 1,000 milligrams. Abbreviation: g.

In vitro study. See **lab study,** below.

IU. IU stands for International Unit, a measurement designation. Although this term is gradually being phased out, you will still see it on some supplement labels. There is no fixed measure for an IU, and an IU of one supplement is different from an IU of another supplement. Here are the most common IU equivalents:

1 IU of Vitamin A = 0.3 micrograms
1 IU of Vitamin D = 0.025 micrograms
1 IU of Vitamin E = 0.67 milligrams

Lab study. Also known as an *in vitro* study, this is an analysis or test performed in a petri dish. Lab studies work with cell cultures, often to test the effectiveness of a substance on living cells before going on to animal and/or human testing.

Microgram. One thousandth of a milligram. Abbreviation: mcg.

Milligram. One-thousandth of a gram. Abbreviation: mg.

OPCs. A class of flavonoids (see above). OPCs (short for oligomeric proanthocyanidins) are found in such plant products as pine bark and grape seed extracts.

Phyto-. This prefix simply means "plant." Thus, "phytomedicine" refers to a remedy made from plants, and "phytoestrogen" refers to estrogen derived from a plant.

Placebo. A "dummy" pill or capsule used in a study. The purpose is to give some people in a clinical trial the active ingredient being tested, while others receive this harmless look-alike.

Standardized product. A product that has been chemically analyzed and is guaranteed to contain a specific amount of an active ingredient (or ingredients) in each and every dose. Standardization is especially important in products made from plants, because the chemical components may vary from plant to plant and from crop to crop.

REFERENCES

The following books and articles provide further information about the subjects discussed in this book. They are available at many libraries and medical research libraries throughout the country. Where material was used from the Internet, the URL is also given.

INTRODUCTION

Beecher, H. "The Powerful Placebo." *Journal of the American Medical Association* 159 (1955): 1602–06.

Campion, E. "Why Unconventional Medicine?" *New England Journal of Medicine* 328: 4 (January 28, 1993).

Eisenberg, D., R. Kessler, C. Foster et al. "Unconventional Medicine in the United States—Prevalence, Costs, and Patterns of Use." *New England Journal of Medicine* 328:4 (January 28, 1993).

Mitchell, S. "Healing Without Doctors." *American Demographics Magazine* (July 1993).

Porter, R. *The Greatest Benefit To Mankind.* New York: Norton, 1997.

Smith, T. "Alternative Medicine." *British Medical Journal* 287 (1983): 307–08.

Tyler, V. *The Honest Herbal.* Binghamton: Pharmaceutical Products Press, 1993.

CHAPTER ONE: Anxiety

Achterrath-Tuckerman, U. et al. "Pharmacological Investigations with Compounds of Chamomile. V.: Investigations on the Spasmolytic Effect of Compounds of Chamomile and Kamillosan on the Isolated Guinea Pig Ileum." *Planta Medica* 39 (1980): 38–50.

American Psychiatric Association: *Diagnostic and Statistical Manual of Mental Disorders (DSM-IV),* 4th ed. American Psychiatric Association Press, 1994.

Bone, K. "Kava—a Safe Herbal Treatment for Anxiety." *British Journal of Phytotherapy* 3:4 (1993/94): 147–53.

Davies, L. et al. "Kava: Pyrones and Resin: Studies in GABAa, GABAb and Benzodiazepine Binding Sites in the Rodent Brain." *Pharmacological Toxicology* 71 (1992): 120–26.

Duffield, P. and D. Jamieson. "Development of Tolerance to Kava in Mice." *Clinical and Experimental Journal of Pharmacological Physiology* 18 (August 1991): 571–78.

Habersang, S. et al. "Pharmacological Studies with Compounds of Chamomile IV: Studies on Toxicity of (-)-α-bisabolol." *Planta Medica* 39 (1979): 115–23.

Ikram, M. "Medicinal Plants as Hypercholesterolemic Agents." *Journal of the American Medical Association* 30 (1980): 278–82.

Jamieson, D., P. Duffield, D. Cheng and A. Duffield. "Comparison of the Central Nervous System Activity of the Aqueous and Lipid Extract of Kava." *Archives of International Pharmacodynamic Therapy* 301 (September–October 1989): 66–80.

Kinzler, E., J. Kromer and E. Lehmann. "Effect of a Special Kava Extract in Patients with Anxiety—'Tension'—and Excitation States of Non-psychotic Genesis." *Arzneimittelforschung* 41 (June 1991): 584–88.

Mann, C. and E. Staba. "The Chemistry, Pharmacology, and Commercial Formulations of Chamomile," 235–80 in L. Craker and J. Simon, eds. *Herbs, Spices and Medicinal Plants: Recent Advances in Botany, Horticulture and Pharmacology.* Phoenix: Oryx Press, 1986.

Mathews, J. et al. "Effects of the Heavy Usage of Kava on Physical Health: Summary of a Pilot Survey in an Aboriginal Community." *Medical Journal of Australia* 148 (6 June 1988): 548–55.

Meyer, H. "Pharmacology of Kava," 133–40 in B. Holmsteadt and N. Kline, eds. *Ethnopharmacological Search for Psychoactive Drugs.* Philadelphia: Raven Press, 1979.

Newall, C., L. Anderson and J. D. Phillipson. *Herbal Medicines.* Pharmaceutical Press, 1996.

Schelosky, L. et al. "Kava and Dopamine Antagonism." *Journal of Neurology, Neurosurgery and Psychiatry* 58:5 (1995): 639–40.

Seitz, U., A. Schüle and J. Gleitz. "3H-Monoamine Uptake Inhibition Properties of Kava Pyrones." *Planta Medica* 63 (December 1997): 548–49.

Singh, Y. "Effects of Kava on Neuromuscular Transmission and Muscle Contractility." *Journal of Ethnopharmacology* 7 (May 1983): 267–76.

———."Kava: An Overview." 37 *Journal of Ethnopharmacology* (August 1992): 13–45.

Suss, R. and P. Lehmann. "Hematogenous Contact Eczema Caused by Phytogenic Drugs Exemplified by Kava Root Extract." *Hautarzt* 47 (June 1996): 459–61.

Tyler, V. *The Honest Herbal.* 3d ed. Binghamton: Pharmaceutical Products Press, 1993.

———.*Herbs of Choice.* Binghamton: Pharmaceutical Products Press, 1994.

Volz, H. and M. Kieser. "Kava-kava Extract WS 1490 Versus Placebo in Anxiety Disorders: A Randomized Placebo-Controlled 25-Week Outpatient Trial." *Pharmacopsychiatry* 30 (January 1997): 1–5.

Warnecke, G. "Psychosomatic Dysfunctions in the Female Climacteric: Clinical Effectiveness and Tolerance of Kava Extract WS 1490." *Fortschritte der Medizin* 190 (10 February 1991): 119–22.

CHAPTER TWO: Arthritis

Altman R. et al. "Capsaicin Cream 0.025% as Monotherapy for Osteoarthritis: A Double-Blind Study." *Seminars in Arthritis and Rheumatism* 23:Supplement 3 (June 1994): 25–33.

Balch, J. and P. Balch. *Prescription for Nutritional Healing.* Wayne: Avery, 1997.

Briffa, J. "Glucosamine Sulphate in the Treatment of Osteoarthritis." *International Journal of Alternative and Complementary Medicine* 15 (October 1997): 15–16.

Cameron, E. and L. Pauling. *Cancer and Vitamin C.* Philadelphia: Camino Books, 1993.

Chellem, J. "Hot Peppers Lead to Even Hotter Research on Arthritis and Other Conditions." *The Nutrition Reporter* 153 (1995).

Clark, C., C. Richards and R. Iozzo. "Post-Translational Alterations in Newly Synthesized Cartilage Pro-teoglycans Induced by the Glut-amine 6-diazo-5-oxo-l-norleucine." *Biochemistry Journal* 273 (1991): 283–88.

Cleland, L. and M. James. "Rheumatoid Arthritis and the Balance of Dietary N-6 and N-3 Essential Fatty Acids." *British Journal of Rheumatology* 36 (May 1997): 513–14.

"Cod Liver Oil and Arthritis." *Prevention* (April 1990).

Crolle, G. and D'Este, E. "The Basic Treatment of Osteoarthrosis." *Current Medical Research and Opinion* 7 (1980): 104.

Crubasik, S., W. Enderlein, R. Bauer and W. Grabaer. "Evidence For Antirheumatic Effectiveness of Herbs Uriticae Dioicae in Acute Arthritis: A Pilot Study." *Phytomedicine* 4:2 (1997): 105–08.

D'Ambrosio, E., B. Casa, R. Bompani et al. "Glucosamine Sulphate: A Controlled Clinical Investigation in Arthrosis." *Pharmatherapeutica* 2 (1981): 504.

Deal C. "The Use of Topical Capsaicin in Managing Arthritis Pain: A Clinician's Perspective." *Seminars in Arthritis and Rheumatism* 23: Supplement 3 (June 1994): 48–52.

Drovanti, A., A. Bignamini and A. Rovati. "Therapeutic Activity of Oral Glucosamine Sulfate in Osteo-arthritis: A Placebo-Controlled Double-Blind Investigation." *Clinical Therapeutics* 3:4 (1980).

Dyerberg, J. *Philosophical Transactions of the Royal Society of London* 294 (1981): 373.

Edmonds, S. et al. "Putative Analgesic Activity of Repeated Oral Doses of Vitamin E in the Treatment of Rheumatoid

Arthritis." *Annals of Rheumatic Diseases* 56 (November 1997).

Ellis C. et al. "A Double-Blind Evaluation of Topical Capsaicin in Pruritic Psoriasis." *Journal of the American Academy of Dermatology* 29 (September 1993): 438–42.

Fischer, M., K. Forster, L. Rovati and I. Setnikar. "Glucosamine Sulfate in Osteoarthritis of the Knee." *Osteoarthritis and Cartilage* 2 (1994): 51–59.

Fortin, P., R. Lew, M. Liang et al. "Validation of a Meta-analysis: The Effects of Fish Oil in Rheumatoid Arthritis." *Journal of Clinical Epidemiology* 48:11 (November 1995): 1379–90.

Fusco, B. et al. "Preventive Effect of Repeated Nasal Applications of Capsaicin in Cluster Headache." *Pain* 59 (December 1994): 321–25.

Gottleib, M. "Conservative Management of Spinal Osteoarthritis with Glucosamine Sulfate and Chiropractic Treatment." *Journal of Manipulative Physiological Therapy* 20:6 (July/August 1997): 400–14.

Griffith, H. W. *Complete Guide to Vitamins, Minerals & Supplements.* Tucson: Fisher Books, 1988.

Halliwell, B. et al. "Biologically Significant Scavenging of the Myeloperoxidase-Derived Oxidant Hypochlorous Acid by Ascorbic Acid: Implications for Antioxidant Protection in the Inflamed Rheumatoid Joint." *FEBS Letter* 213 (9 March 1987): 15–17.

Hatch, G. "Asthma, Inhaled Oxidants, and Dietary Antioxidants." *American Journal of Clinical Nutrition* 61:3 (March 1993): 625S–30S.

Infei, C., D. Frankling, J. Garrison et al. "Ten Great Medical Advances of 1996." *Hippocrates* 11:1 (1997): 54–59. http://www.medscape.com/time/hippocrates/public/about.hippocrates.html

Karzel, K. and R. Domenjoz. "Effects of Hexosamine Derivatives and Uronic Acid Derivatives on Glycosaminoglycane Metabolism of Fibroblast Cultures." *Pharmacology* 5 (1971): 337–45.

Kerrigan, D. C., M. Todd and P. O'Riley. "Knee Osteoarthritis and High-Heeled Shoes." *The Lancet* 351 (1998): 1399–401.

Kim, J. and H. Conrad. "Effects of D-Glucosamine Concentration on the Kinetics of Mucopolysaccharide Biosynthesis in Cultured Chick Embryo Vertebral Cartilage." *Journal of Biological Chemistry* 249:10 (25 May 1974): 3091–97.

Kinsella, J. *Food Technology* 40 (February 1986): 89.

Knapp, H. et al. *New England Journal of Medicine* 314 (10 April 1986): 937.

Kremer, J., D. Lawrence, R. Stocker et al. "Effects of High-Dose Fish Oil on Rheumatoid Arthritis After Stopping Nonsteroidal Antiinflammatory Drugs. Clinical and Immune Correlates." *Arthritis and Rheumatism* 38:8 (August 1995): 1107–14.

Kromhout, D. et al. *New England Journal of Medicine* 312 (9 May 1985): 1205.

Lopez, A. "Double-Blind Clinical Evaluation of the Relative Efficacy of Ibuprofen and Glucosamine Sulphate in the Management of Osteoarthrosis of the Knee in Out-Patients." *Current Medical Research and Opinion* 8 (1982): 145.

Lorenz, R. et al. *Circulation* 67:3 (March 1983): 504.

Lunec, J. B. "The Determination of Dehydroascorbic Acid and Ascorbic Acid in the Serum and Synovial Fluid of Patients with Rheumatoid Arthritis." *Free Radical Research Communications* 1:1 (1985): 31–39.

Mathias B. et al. "Topical Capsaicin for Chronic Neck Pain." *American Journal of Physical Medicine & Rehabilitation* 74 (January/February 1995): 39–44.

Mayell, M. *Off the Shelf Natural Health.* New York: Bantam, 1995.

McAlindon, T. and D. Felson: "Nutrition: Risk Factors for Osteoarthritis." *Annals of the Rheumatic Diseases* 56 (July 1997): 397–402.

McCarty, M. "Glucosamine For Wound Healing." *Medical Hypotheses* 47:4 (October 1996): 273–75.

Muller-Fasbender, H., G. Bach, W. Haase, L. Rovati and I.

Setnikar. "Glucosamine Sulfate Compared to Ibuprofen in Osteoarthritis." *Osteoarthritis and Cartilage* 2 (1994): 61–69.

Nakazawa, K. et al. "The Therapeutic Effect of Chondroitin Polysulphate in Elderly Atherosclerotic Patients." *Journal of International Medical Research* 6:3 (1978): 217.

Nutrition Reviews 43 (September 1985): 268.

Pujalte, J., E. Llavore, Ylescupidez. "The Basic Treatment of Osteoarthrosis." *Current Medical Research and Opinion* 7 (1980): 110.

Quillan, P. *Healing Nutrients.* New York: Vintage Books, 1989.

Ramm, S. and C. Hansen. "Brennesselblatter-Extrakt Bei Arthrose Und Rheumatoider Arthritis." *Therapiewoche* 28 (1996): 3–6.

Reicheltl, A., K. Forster, M. Fischer, L. Rovati and I. Setnikar. "Efficacy and Safety of Intra-Muscular Glucosamine Sulfate in Osteoarthritis of the Knee: A Randomized, Placebo-Controlled, Double-Blind Study." *Drug Research* 44(I): 1 (1994).

Roden, L. "Effect of Hexosamines on the Synthesis of Chondroitin Sulphuric Acid in Vitro." *Arkiv for Kemi Band* 10:23 (1956).

Rovati, L. "Clinical Research in Osteoarthritis: Design and Results of Short-Term and Long-Term Trials with Disease-Modifying Drugs." *Journal of Tissue Reaction* xiv:5 (1992): 243–51.

Sato, M. et al. "Quercitin, a Bioflavonoid, Inhibits the Induction of Interleukin 8 and Monocyte Chemoattractant Protein-1 Expression by Tumor Necrosis Factor-Alpha in Cultured Human Synovial Cells." *Journal of Rheumatology* 24 (September 1977): 1680–84.

Schnitzer T. et al. "Topical Capsaicin Therapy for Osteoarthritis Pain: Achieving a Maintenance Program." *Seminars in Arthritis and Rheumatism* 23: Supplement 3 (June 1994): 34–40.

Setnikar, I., C. Giacchetti and G. Zanolo. "Pharmacokinetics of

Glucosamine in the Dog and in Man." *Drug Research* 36 (I): 4 (1986).

Setnikar, I., R. Palumbo, S. Canali and G. Zanolo. "Pharmacokinetics of Glucosamine in Man." *Drug Research* 43 (II):10 (1993).

Setnikar, R., M. Cereda, A. Pacini and L. Revel. "Antireactive Properties of Glucosamine Sulfate." *Drug Research* 41(1):2 (1991).

Simopoulus, A. and J. Robinson. *The Omega Plan.* New York: Harper Collins, 1998.

Srivastava, K. "Effect of Onion and Ginger Consumption on Platelet Thromboxane Production in Humans." *Prostaglandins, Luekotrienes and Essential Fatty Acids* 35 (1989): 183–85.

Srivastava, K. et al. "Ginger and Rheumatic Disorders." *Med Hypoth* 29 (1989): 25–28.

Talent, J. and R. Gracy. "Pilot Study of Oral Polymeric N-acetyl-d-glucosamine as a Potential Treatment for Patients with Osteoarthritis." *Clinical Therapy* 18:6 (November/December 1996): 1184–90.

Tamkins, T. "Fish Oil Eases Pain in Arthritis Patients." Medical Tribune News Service, 11 September 1995.

Tapadinhas, M., I. Rivera and A. Bignamini. "Oral Glucosamine Sulphate in the Management of Arthrosis: Report on a Multi-Center Open Investigation in Portugal." *Pharmatherapeutica* 3 (1982): 157.

Theodosakis, J., with B. Fox and B. Adderly: *The Arthritis Cure: The Medical Miracle That Can Halt, Reverse, and May Even Cure Osteoarthritis.* New York: St. Martins, 1997.

Vaz A. "Double-Blind Clinical Evaluation of the Relative Efficacy of Ibuprofen and Glucosamine Sulphate in the Management of Osteoarthrosis of the Knee in Out-Patients." *Current Medical Research and Opinion* 8 (1982): 145–49.

"Vitamins Slow Progression of Osteoarthritis." *International Health News* 71 (November 1997). http://vvv.com/healthnews/

Will, J. and T. Byers. "Does Diabetes Mellitus Increase the Requirement for Vitamin C?" *Nutrition Reviews* 54:7 (July 1996): 193–202.

Woodcock, B. et al. "Beneficial Effect of Fish Oil on Blood Viscosity in Peripheral Vascular Disease." *British Medical Journal* 288 (25 February 1984): 592.

Yongyudh, V. "Double-Blind Evaluation of Intra-Articular Glucosamine in Outpatients With Gonarthrosis." *Clinical Therapeutics* 3:5 (1981).

CHAPTER THREE: Asthma and Allergies

Aderele, W., S. Ette, O. Oduwole and S. Ikpeme. "Plasma Vitamin C (Ascorbic Acid) Levels in Asthmatic Children." *Afr J Med Sci* 14:3–4 (September–December 1985): 115–20.

Atkins, R. *Dr. Atkins' Vita-Nutrient Solution.* New York: Simon & Schuster, 1998.

Bernstein, W., T. Khasthir, A. Khastgir et al. "Lack of Effectiveness of Magnesium in Chronic Stable Asthma. A Prospective, Randomized, Double-Blind, Placebo-Controlled, Crossover Trial in Normal Subjects and in Patients with Chronic Stable Asthma." *Archives of Internal Medicine* 155:3 (13 February 1995): 271–76.

Bielory, L. and R. Gandhi. "Asthma and Vitamin C." *Annals of Allergy* 73:2 (August 1994): 89–96.

Bucca, C. et al. New York Academy of Sciences 16 (9–12 February 1992): 16.

Bucca, C., G. Rolla, A. Oliva and J. Farina. "Effect of Vitamin C on Histamine Bronchial Responsiveness of Patients with Allergic Rhinitis." *Annals of Allergy* 65:4 (October 1990): 311–14.

Burr, M. et al. "Food-allergic Asthma in General Practice." *Human Nutrition, Applied Nutrition* 39:5 (October 1985): 349–55.

Cohen H., I. Neuman and H. Nahum. "Blocking Effect of Vitamin C in Exercise-Induced Asthma." *Archives of Pediatric and Adolescent Medicine* 151:4 (April 1997): 367–70.

Della Loggia, R., E. Ragazzi, A. Tubaro et al. "Anti-Inflammatory Activity of Benzopyrones That Are Inhibitors of Cyclo- and Lipo-Oxygenase." *Pharmacol Res Commun* 20 (1988): S91–S94.

Fantidis, P., J. Cacho, M. Marin et al. "Intracellular (Polymorphonuclear) Magnesium Content in Patients with Bronchial Asthma Between Attacks." *J R Soc Med* 88:8 (August 1995): 441–45.

Fedoseev, G., A. Emelianov, K. Malakauska et al. "The Therapeutic Potentials of Magnesium Sulfate in Bronchial Asthma." *Ter Arkh* 63:12 (1991): 27–29.

Hatch, G. "Asthma, Inhaled Oxidants, and Dietary Antioxidants." *American Journal of Clinical Nutrition* 61:3 (March 1995): 625S–30S.

Hill, J., A. Mickelwright, S. Lewis and J. Britton. "Investigation of the Effect of Short-Term Change in Dietary Magnesium Intake in Asthma." *European Respiratory Journal* 10:10 (October 1997): 2225–29.

Johnston, C. et al. *Journal of the American Dietetic Association* 92:8 (August 1992): 988–89.

Koepke, J. et al. "Inhaled Metabisulfate Sensitivity." *Annals of Allergy* 54 (March 1985): 213.

McKinney, M. *Medical Tribune* (5 June 1997): 6.

Middleton, E. "Quercetin Inhibits Lipopolysaccharide-induced Expression of Endothelial Cell Intracellular Adhesion Molecule 1." *International Archives of Allergy and Immunology* 107 (1995): 435–36.

Miric, M. and M. Haxihiu. "Effect of Vitamin C on Exercise-Induced Bronchoconstriction." *Plucne Bolesti* 43: 1–2 (January–June 1991): 94–97.

Pelikan, Z. et al. "Bronchial Response to the Food Ingestion Challenge." *Annals of Allergy* 58 (March 1987): 164.

Pletsityi, K., S. Vasipa, T. Davydova and V. Fomina "Vitamin E: Immunocorrecting Effect in Bronchial Asthma Patients." *Vopr Med Khim* 41:4 (July–August 1995): 33–36.

Reidenberg, M. "Essential Drugs and Who Model List: Addressing New Issues. Report of a Workshop Focusing on the Report of the World Health Organization Expert Committee on the Use of Essential Drugs." *Clinical Pharmacology and Therapeutics* 59 (1996): 62–71.

Skotnicki, A., M. Jablonski, J. Musial and J. Swadzba. "The Role of Magnesium in the Pathogenesis and Therapy of Bronchial Asthma." *Przegl Lek* 54:9 (1997): 630–33.

Soutar, A., A. Seaton and K. Brown. "Bronchial Reactivity and Dietary Antioxidants." *Thorax* 52:2 (February 1997): 166–70.

Troisi R., W. Willett, S. Weiss et al. "A Prospective Study of Diet and Adult-Onset Asthma." *Am J Respir Crit Care Med* 151:5 (May 1995): 1401–08.

Weiss, S. Ciba Foundation Symposium 206 (1977): 244–57.

Welton A., L. Tobias, C. Fiedler-Nagy et al. "Effect of Flavonoids on Arachidonic Acid Metabolism." *Prog Clin Biol Res* 213 (1986): 231–42.

CHAPTER FOUR: Bladder Infections

Avorn, J., M. Monane et al. "Reduction of Bacteriuria and Pyuria After Ingestion of Cranberry Juice." *Journal of the American Medical Association* 271 (1994): 751–54.

Barney, P. *Clinical Applications of Herbal Medicine.* Pleasant Grove: Woodland Publishing, 1996.

Bomser, J., D. Madhavi, K. Singletary and M. Smith. "In Vitro Anticancer Activity of Fruit Extracts from Vaccinium Species." *Planta Medica* 62 (June 1996): 212–16.

"Breakthroughs: Cranberry Therapy." *Discover Magazine* (August 1994).

Fleet, J. "New Support for a Folk Remedy: Cranberry Juice Reduces Bacteriuria and Pyuria in Elderly Women." *Nutrition Review* 271 (May 1994): 168–70.

"Flushing Out Trouble." Wire Networks and Rodale Press, 1997. http://www.prevention.com/healing/vitamin/bladder-infections/more1.html.

Fowler, J. "Urinary Tract Infections in Women." *Urological Clinics of North America* 13:4 (1986): 673–83.

Monane, M. and J. Avorn. "Cranberry Juice and Urinary Tract Infections." *Healthline* (August 1994). http://www.healthline.com

Murray, M. and J. Pizzorno. *The Encyclopedia of Natural Medicine.* Rocklin: Prima, 1991.

Ofek, I. et al. "Anti-Escherichia Coli Adhesion of Cranberry and Blueberry Juices." *New England Journal of Medicine* 324 (1991): 1599.

Scmidt, D. and A. Sabota: "An Examination of the Anti-Adherence Activity of Cranberry Juice on Urinary and Nonurinary Bacterial Isolates." *Microbios* 55 (1988): 173–81.

Zafriri, D., I. Olek et al. "Inhibitory Activity of Cranberry Juice on Adherence of Type 1 and Type P Fimbriated Escherichia Coli to Eucaryotic Cells." *Antimicrobial Agents in Chemotherapy* 271 (January 1989): 92–98.

CHAPTER FIVE: Blood Vessels

Bagchi, D., A. Garg, R. Krohn et al. "Oxygen Free Radical Scavenging Abilities of Vitamins C and E, and a Grape Seed Proanthocyanidin Extract In Vitro." *Res Commun Mol Pathol Pharmacol* 95:2 (February 1997): 179–89.

Brevetti, Gregorio et al. "Effect of Propionyl-l-carnitine on Quality of Life in Intermittent Claudication." *American Journal of Cardiology* 79 (March 15 1997): 777–80.

Challem, J. "A Critical Look at the Flavonoids and Some Sound Recommendations. The Real Story Behind French Pine Bark, Grape Seed Extract, Green Tea, and Citrus." *Nutrition Reporter* 153 (1996). www.jrthorns.com/Challem/Look–at–Flavonoids.html

Delacrois P. "A Double Blind Study of Endotelon in Chronic Venous Insufficiency." *La Revue de Médecine* 27 (1981): 28–31.

Doutremepuich J., A. Barbier, F. Lacheretz. "Effect of Endotelon (Procyanidolic Oligomers) on Experimental Acute

Lymphedema of the Rat Hindlimb." *Lymphology* 24:3 (September 1991): 135–39.

Drubaix I., L. Robert, M. Maraval and A. Robert. "Synthesis of Glycoconjugates by Human Diseased Veins: Modulation by Procyanidolic Oligomers." *Int J Exp Pathol* 78:2 (April 1997): 117–21.

Facino, R. et al. "Free Radical Scavenging Action and Anti-Enzyme Activities of Procyanidines From Vitis Vinifra a Mechanism for Their Capillary Protective Action." *Arzneimittle-Forsch* 44 (1994): 592–601.

Feine-Haake, G. "A New Therapy for Venous Diseases." *Zeitschrift für Allgemeinmedizin* 839 (30 June 1975).

Gabor M. "Biochemical, Cellular, and Medicinal Properties in Plant Flavonoids." 1–15 in *Biology and Medicine*. City: Liss, Inc., 1988.

Gomez Trillo J. "Varicose Veins of the Lower Extremities, Symptomatic Treatment With a New Vasculotrophic Agent." *Prensa Med Mex* 38 (1973): 293–96.

Henriet, J. "Veno-Lymphatic Insufficiency: 4,729 Patients Undergoing Hormonal and Procyanidol Oligomer Therapy." *Phebologie* 46 (1993): 313–25.

Kakegawa, H., et al. *Chem. Pharm. Bull* 33:5079 (1985): 5.

Kuttan, R., P. Donnelly and N. Di Ferrante. "Collagen Treated With Catechin Becomes Resistant to the Action of Mammalian Collagenase." *Experientia* 37 (1981): 221.

Lagrue G., F. Olivier-Martin, A. Grillot. "Study of the Effects of Procyanidol Oligomers on Capillary Resistance in Hypertension and in Certain Nephropathies." *Sem Hop* 57: 33–36 (18–25 September 1981): 1399–401.

Le Bars, P., M. Katz, N. Berman et al. "A Placebo-Controlled, Double-Blind, Randomized Trial of an Extract of Ginkgo Biloba for Dementia." *Journal of the American Medical Association* 278 (1997): 1327–32.

Maffei F. et al. "Free Radicals Scavenging Action and Anti-Enzyme Activities of Procyanidines from Vit is Vinifera: A

Mechanism for Their Capillary Protective Action." *Arznei-mittel-Forschung* 44 (May 1994): 592–601.

Masquelier, J., M. Dumon, J. and Dumas, J. "Stabilisation du Collagene par des Oligomeres Procyanidoliques." *Acta Therapeutics* 7 (1981): 101–05.

Masquelier J., J. Michaud, J. Laparra, M. Dumon. "Flavonoids and Pygnogenols." *Int J Vitam Nutr Res* 49:3 (1979): 307–311.

Michiels, C., T. Arnould, A. Houbiob and J. Remacle. "A Comparative Study of the Protective Effect of Different Phlebotonic Agents on Endothelial Cells in Hypoxia." *Phlebologie* 44:3 (July–October 1991): 779–86.

Pizzorno, J. and M. Murray. *A Textbook of Natural Medicine,* New Canaan: John Bastyr College Publications, 1985.

Robert, A., N. Groult, C. Six and L. Robert. "The Effect of Procyanidolic Oligomers on Mesenchymal Cells in Culture II—Attachment of Elastic Fibers to the Cells." *Pathol Biol* 38:6 (June 1990): 601–07.

Robert, L., G. Godeau, C. Gavignet-Jeannin et al. "The Effect of Procyanidolic Oligomers on Vascular Permeability. A Study Using Quantitative Morphology." *Pathol Biol* 38:6 (June 1990): 608–16.

Tixier, J., G. Godeau, A. Robert, and W. Hornbeck. "Evidence by In Vivo and In Vitro Studies That Binding of Pycnogenols to Elastin Affects Its Rate of Degradation by Elastases." *Biochem. Pharm* 33 (1984): 3933–39.

Zafirov D. et al. "Antiexudative and Capillaritonic Effects of Procyanidines Isolated from Grape Seeds (V. Vinifera)." *Acta Physiologica et Pharmacologica Bulgarica* 16 (1990): 50–54.

CHAPTER SIX: Cancer

Adlercreutz, H., H. Markkannen and S. Watanabe. "Plasma Concentrations of Phyto-Oestrogens in Japanese Men." *Lancet* 342:8881 (1993): 1209–10.

Ahmad, N., D. Feyes, A. Nieminen et al. "Green Tea Constituent

Epigallocatechin-3-Gallate and Induction of Apoptosis and Cell Cycle Arrest in Human Carcinoma Cells.'' *Journal of the National Cancer Institute* 89:24 (December 1997): 1881–86.

Aidoo A., L. Lyn-Cook, S. Lensing and W. Warner. ''Ascorbic Acid (Vitamin C) Modulates the Mutagenic Effects Produced by an Alkylating Agent In Vivo.'' *Environ Mol Mutagen* 24:3 (1994): 220–28.

Anonymous. ''The Effect of Vitamin E and Beta-Carotene on the Incidence of Lung Cancer and Other Cancers in Male Smokers. The Alpha-Tocopherol, Beta-Carotene Cancer Prevention Study Group.'' *New England Journal of Medicine* 330:15 (14 April 1994): 1029–35.

Baldwin, C. et al. ''What Pharmacists Should Know About Ginseng.'' *Pharm J* 237 (1986): 583–86.

Ben-Amotz, A. and Y. Levy. ''Bioavailability of a Natural Isomer Mixture Compared With Synthetic All-TransBeta-Carotene in Human Serum.'' *American Journal of Clinical Nutrition* 63:5 (May 1996): 729–33.

Bespalov, V., V. Aleksandrov, V. Davydov et al. ''Inhibition of Mammary Gland Carcinogenesis Using a Tincture From Biomass of Ginseng Tissue Culture.'' *Biull Eksp Biol Med* 115:1 (January 1993): 59–61.

Bespalov, V., V. Davydov, A. Limarenko et al. ''The Inhibition of the Development of Experimental Tumors of the Cervix Uteri and Vagina by Using Tinctures of the Cultured-Cell Biomass of the Ginseng Root and Its Germanium-Selective Stocks.'' *Biull Eksp Biol Med* 116:11 (November 1993): 534–36.

Blot, W., J. Li, P. Taylor et al. ''The Linxian Trials: Mortality Rates by Vitamin-Mineral Intervention Group.'' *American Journal of Clinical Nutrition* 62:6 Supplement (December 1995): 1424–26.

Brody, J. ''In Vitamin Mania, Millions Are Taking a Gamble on Their Health.'' *New York Times* 26 October 1997.

Caso-Marasco, A., R. Vargas-Ruiz, A. Salas-Villagomez and C.

Begona Infante. "Double-Blind Study of a Multivitamin Complex Supplemented With Ginseng Extract." *Drugs Exp Clin Res* 22:6 (1996): 323–29.

Castillo, M., E. Perkins, J. Campbell et al. "The Effects of the Bioflavonoid Quercetin on Squamous Cell Carcinoma of Head and Neck Origin." *American Journal of Surgery* 158:4 (October 1989): 351–55.

Challem, J. "A Critical Look at the Flavonoids and Some Sound Recommendations. The Real Story Behind French Pine Bark, Grape Seed Extract, Green Tea, and Citrus." *Nutrition Reporter* 153, (1996). www.jrthorns.com/Challem/Look–at–Flavonoids.html

————."Is Beta-Carotene Bad, Or Just the Studies? Let's Not Throw Away the Baby with the Bath Water . . ." *Nutrition Reporter* 153 (1996). www.jrthorns.com/Challem/beta-carotene.html

Chen, H. and A. Tappel. "Protection by Vitamin E, Selenium, Trolox C, Ascorbic Acid Palmitate, Acetylcysteine, Coenzyme Q, Beta-Carotene, Canthaxanthin, and (+)-Catechin Against Oxidative Damage to Liver Slices Measured by Oxidized Heme Proteins." *Free Radical Biology and Medicine* 16 (1994): 437–44.

Clark, L., G. Combs, B. Turnbull et al. "Effects of Selenium Supplementation for Cancer Prevention in Patients with Carcinoma of the Skin. A Randomized Controlled Trial. Nutritional Prevention of Cancer Study Group." *Journal of the American Medical Association* 276:4 (25 December 1996): 1957–63.

Combs, A., J. Choe, D. Truong and K. Folkers. "Reduction by Coenzyme Q10 of the Acute Toxicity of Adriamycin in Mice." *Res Commun Chem Pathol Pharmacol* 18:3 (November 1977): 565–68.

Cozzi, R., T. Aglitti, V. Gatta et al. "Ascorbic Acid and Beta-Carotene as Modulators of Oxidative Damage." *Carcinogenesis* 18:1 (January 1997): 223–28.

D'Avanzo, B., E. Ron, C. Vecchia et al. "Selected Micronutrient

Intake and Thyroid Carcinoma Risk." *Cancer* 79 (1997): 2186–92.

Diplock A. "Antioxidants and Disease Prevention." *Molecular Aspects of Medicine* 15 (1994): 295–376.

Dovinova, I. "Alpha-Lipoic Acid—a Natural Disulfide Cofactor and Antioxidant With Anticarcinogenic Effects." *Ceska Slov Farm* 45:5 (September 1996): 237–41.

Drake, I., M. Davies, N. Maostone et al. "Ascorbic Acid May Protect Against Human Gastric Cancer by Scavenging Mucosal Oxygen Radicals." *Carcinogenesis* 17:3 (March 1996): 559–62.

Duda, R., B. Taback, B. Kessel et al. "Ps2 Expression Induced by American Ginseng in Mcf-7 Breast Cancer Cells." *Annals of Surgical Oncology* 3:6 (November 1996): 515–20.

Ferguson, L. "Antimutagens as Cancer Chemoprotective Agents in the Diet." *Mutat Res* 307:1 (1 May, 1994): 395–410.

Fleet, J. "Dietary Selenium Repletion May Reduce Cancer Incidence in People at High Risk Who Live in Areas with Low Soil Selenium." *Nutr Rev* 55:7 (July 1997): 277–79.

Fujiki, H., S. Yoshizawa, T. Horiuchi et al. "Anticarcinogenic Effects of (-)-Epigallocatechin Gallate." *Preventative Medicine* 21:4 (July 1992): 503–09.

Garewal, H. and S. Schantz. "Emerging Role of Beta-Carotene and Antioxidant Nutrients in Prevention of Oral Cancer." *Arch Otolaryngol Head Neck Surg* 121: 2 (February 1995): 141–44.

Gartner, C., W. Stahl and H. Sies. "Lycopene Is More Bioavailable From Tomato Paste Than From Fresh Tomatoes." 66:1 *American Journal of Clinical Nutrition* (July 1997) 116–22.

Gaziano J., E. Johnson, R. Russell et al. "Discrimination in Absorption or Transport of Beta-Carotene Isomers After Oral Supplementation With Either All-Trans- or 9-Cis-Beta-Carotene." *American Journal of Clinical Nutrition* 61:6 (June 1995): 248–52.

Giavannucci, E., A. Ascherio, E. Rimm, M. Stampfer et al. "Intake of Carotenoids and Retinol in Relation to Risk of Prostate Cancer.'' *Journal of the National Cancer Institute* 87:23 (6 December 1996): 1767–76.

Giles, G. and P. Ireland. ''Diet, Nutrition and Prostate Cancer.'' *International Journal of Cancer* 10 Supplement (1997).

Greenwald, P. ''Colon Cancer Overview.'' *Cancer* 70:5 Supplement (1 September 1992): 1206–15.

Gridley G., J. McLaughlin, G. Block. ''Vitamin Supplement Use and Reduced Risk of Oral and Pharyngeal Cancer.'' *American Journal of Epidemiology* 135:10 (15 May 1992): 1083–92.

Griffith, H. W. *Complete Guide to Vitamins, Minerals & Supplements.* Tucson: Fisher Books, 1988.

Gutteridge, J. and B. Halliwell. ''The Measurement and Mechanism of Lipid Peroxidation in Biological Systems.'' *Trends Biochem Sci* 15 (1990): 129–35.

Hall, A. ''Liarozole Amplifies Retinoid-Induced Apoptosis in Human Prostate Cancer Cells.'' *Anticancer Drugs* 7:3 (7 May 1996): 312–20.

Hazuka, M., J. Edwards-Prasa, F. Newman et al. ''Beta-Carotene Induces Morphological Differentiation and Decreases Adenylate Cyclase Activity in Melanoma Cells in Culture.'' *Journal of the American College of Nutrition* 9:2 (April 1990): 143–49.

Heinonen, O., D. Albanes, J. Virtamo et al. ''Prostate Cancer and Supplementation With Alpha-Tocopherol and Beta-Carotene: Incidence and Mortality in a Controlled Trial.'' *J Natl Cancer Inst* 90:6 (18 March 1998): 440–46.

Helzlsouer, K., A. Alberg, E. Norkus et al. Prospective Study of Serum Micronutrients and Ovarian Cancer.'' *Journal of the National Cancer Institute* 88:1 (January 1996): 32–37.

Hirano, T. K. Abe, M. Goto and K. Oka. ''Citrus Flavone Tangeretin Inhibits Leukaemic Hl-60 Cell Growth Partially Through Induction of Apoptosis With Less Cytotoxicity on Normal Lymphocytes.'' *British Journal of Cancer* 72:6 (December 1995): 1380–88.

Hirose, M., T. Hoshiya, K. Akagi et al. ''Inhibition of Mammary

Gland Carcinogenesis by Green Tea Catechins and Other Naturally Occurring Antioxidants in Female Sprague-Dawley Rats Pretreated With 7,12-Dimethylbenz[alpha]anthracene." *Cancer Letters* 83:1–2 (15 August 1994): 149–56.

Imai, K. et al. "Cancer-Preventive Effects of Drinking Green Tea Among a Japanese Population." *Preventive Medicine* 26 (November/December 1997): 769–75.

Ingles, S., et al. "Plasma Tocopherol and Prevalence of Colorectal Adenomas in a Multiethnic Population." *Cancer Research* 58 (15 February 1998): 661–66.

Ip, C., D. Lisk and G. Stoewsand. "Mammary Cancer Prevention by Regular Garlic and Selenium-Enriched Garlic." *Nutr Cancer* 17:3 (1992): 279–86.

Kao T., W. Meyer and J. Post. "Inhibitory Effects of Ascorbic Acid on Growth of Leukemic and Lymphoma Cell Lines." *Cancer Lett* 70:1–2 (15 June 1993): 101–06.

Katiyar S., N. Korman, H. Mukhtar and R. Agarwal. "Protective Effects of Silymarin Against Photocarcinogenesis in a Mouse Skin Model." *Journal of the National Cancer Institute* 89:8 (16 April 1997): 556–66.

Key, T., P. Silcocks, G. Davey et al. "A Case-Control Study of Diet and Prostate Cancer." *British Journal of Cancer* 76:5 (1997): 678–87.

Kim, J., D. Germolec and M. Luster. "Panax Ginseng as a Potential Immunomodulator: Studies in Mice." *Immunopharmacology and Immunotoxicology* 12:2 (1990): 257–76.

Kokawa, T., K. Shiota, K. Oda et al. "Coenzyme Q10 in Cancer Chemotherapy—Experimental Studies on Augmentation of the Effects of Masked Compounds, Especially in the Combined Chemotherapy With Immunopotentiators." *Gan To Kagaku Ryoho* 10:3 (March 1983): 768–74.

Knekt, P., A. Aromaa, J. Maatela. "Vitamin E and Cancer Prevention." *American Journal of Clinical Nutrition* 53:1 Supplement (January 1991): 283–86.

Knekt, P. et al. "Dietary Flavonoids and the Risk of Lung Cancer and Other Malignant Neoplasms.'' *American Journal of Epidemiology* 146 (1 August 1997): 223–30.

Kuo, S., H. Morehouse and C. Lin. ''Effect of Antiproliferative Flavonoids on Ascorbic Acid Accumulation in Human Colon Adenocarcinoma Cells.'' *Cancer Lett* 116:2 (24 June 1997): 131–37.

Lamm, D., D. Riggs, J. Shriver et al. ''Megadose Vitamins in Bladder Cancer: A Double-Blind Clinical Trial.'' *J Urol* 151:1 (January 1994): 21–26.

Levy, J., E. Bosin, B. Feldman et al. ''Lycopene Is a More Potent Inhibitor of Human Cancer Cell Proliferation Than Either Alpha-Carotene or Beta-Carotene.'' *Nutr Cancer* 24:3 (1995): 257–66.

Li, W. ''Preliminary Observations on Effect of Selenium Yeast on High Risk Populations With Primary Liver Cancer.'' *Chung Hua Yu Fang I Hsueh Tsa Chih* 26:5 (September 1992): 268–71.

Li, X. and X. Wu. ''Effects of Ginseng on Hepatocellular Carcinoma in Rats Induced by Diethylnitrosamine—A Further Study.'' *Journal of Tongji Medical University* 11:2 (1991): 73–80.

Liberti, L. and A. Der Marderosian. ''Evaluation of Commercial Ginseng Products.'' *Journal of Pharmaceutical Sciences* 67 (1978): 1487–89.

Liu, T., S. Soong, N. Wilson et al. ''A Case Control Study of Nutritional Factors and Cervical Dysplasia.'' *Cancer Epidemiol Biomarkers Prev* 2:6 (November–December 1993): 525–30.

Lockwood, K., S. Moesgaard and K. Folkers. ''Partial and Complete Regression of Breast Cancer in Patients in Relation to Dosage of Coenzyme Q10.'' *Biochem Biophys Res Commun* 199:3 (30 March 1994): 1504–1508.

Lockwood, K., S. Moesgaard, T. Hanioka and K. Folkers. ''Apparent Partial Remission of Breast Cancer in 'High Risk' Patients Supplemented With Nutritional Antioxidants, Essential

Fatty Acids and Coenzyme Q10." *Mol Aspects Med* 15 Supplement (1994): 231–40.

Lockwood, K., S. Moesgaard, S. Yamamoto and K. Folkers. "Progress on Therapy of Breast Cancer With Vitamin Q10 and the Regression of Metastases." *Biochem Biophys Res Commun* 212:1 (6 July 1995): 172–77.

Lou, H., R. Wu and Y. Fu. "Relation Between Selenium and Cancer of Uterine Cervix." *Chung Hua Chung Liu Tsa Chih* 17:2 (March 1995): 112–14.

Lubawy, W., R. Dallam, L. Hurley. "Protection Against Anthramycin-Induced Toxicity in Mice by Coenzyme Q10." *Journal of the National Cancer Institute* 64:1 (January 1980): 105–09.

Maramag, C., M. Menon, K. Balaji et al. "Effect of Vitamin C on Prostate Cancer Cells In Vitro: Effect on Cell Number, Viability, and DNA Synthesis." *Prostate* 32:3 (1 August 1997): 188–95.

Matsunaga, H., M. Katano, H. Yamamoto et al. "Studies on the Panaxytriol of Panax Ginseng C. A. Meyer. Isolation, Determination and Antitumor Activity." *Chem Pharm Bull* (Tokyo) 37:5 (May 1989): 1279–81.

Meyskens, F. "Strategies for Prevention of Cancer in Humans." *Oncology* 6:2 Supplement (February 1992): 15–24.

Mikhail M., P. Palan, J. Basu et al. "Decreased Beta-Carotene Levels in Exfoliated Vaginal Epithelial Cells in Women With Vaginal Candidiasis." *Am J Reprod Immunol* 32:3 (October 1994): 221–25.

Morton, M., P. Chan and C. Cheng et al. "Lignans and Isoflavonoids in Plasma and Prostatic Fluid in Men: Samples From Portugal, Hong Kong, and the United Kingdom." *Prostate* 32:2 (1 July 1997): 122–28.

Nano, J., D. Czerucka, F. Menguy and P. Rampal. "Effect of Selenium on the Growth of Three Human Colon Cancer Cell Lines." *Biol Trace Elem Res* 20:1–2 (April–May 1989): 31–43.

Newall, C., L. Anderson and J. D. Phillipson. *Herbal Medicines:*

A Guide For Healthcare Professionals. Philadelphia: Pharmaceutical Press, 1996.

Nomura, A., G. Stemmermann, J. Lee and N. Craft. "Serum Micronutrients and Prostate Cancer in Japanese Americans in Hawaii." *Cancer Epidemiol Biomarkers Prev* 6:7 (July 1997): 487–91.

O'Fallon, J. and B. Chew. "The Subcellular Distribution of Beta-Carotene in Bovine Corpus Luteum." *Proc Soc Exp Biol Med* 177 (1984): 406–11.

Oishi, K., O. Yoshida and F. Schroeder. "The Geography of Prostate Cancer and Its Treatment in Japan." *Cancer Survey* 23 (1995): 267–80.

Omenn, G., G. Goodman, M. Thornquist et al. "Risk Factors for Lung Cancer and for Intervention Effects in CARET, Thebeta-Carotene and Retinol Efficacy Trial." *Journal of the National Cancer Institute* 88:21 (6 November 1996): 1550–59.

Packer, L., E. Witt and H. Tritschler. "Alpha-Lipoic Acid as a Biological Antioxidant." *Free Radical Biology and Medicine* 19:2 (August 1995): 227–50.

Pagliacci, M., M. Smacchia, G. Migliorati et al. "Growth-Inhibitory Effects of the Natural Phyto-Oestrogen Genistein in Mcf-7 Human Breast Cancer Cells." *European Journal of Cancer* 30A:11 (1994): 1675–82.

"Personal Behaviors Are What Really Matters When It Comes to Avoiding Cancer According to the American Cancer Society." PRNewswire (22 March 1997).

Petkov, V. and A. Mosharrof. "Effects of Standardized Ginseng Extract on Learning, Memory and Physical Capabilities." *American Journal of Chinese Medicine* 15:1–2 (1987): 19–29.

Rayman, M. "Dietary Selenium: Time to Act Low Bioavailability in Britain and Europe Could Be Contributing to Cancers, Cardiovascular Disease, and Subfertility." *British Medical Journal* 314 (8 February 1997): 387–88.

Rayman M., F. Abou-Shakra, N. Ward and C. Redman. "Comparison of Selenium Levels in Pre-Eclamptic and Normal Pregnancies." *Biol Trace Element Res* 55 (1996): 9–20.

Rhee, Y., J. Ahn and J. Choe. "Inhibition of Mutagenesis and Transformation by Root Extracts of Panax Ginseng In Vitro." *Planta Medica* 57:2 (April 1991): 125–28.

Ribaya-Mercado J., M. Garmyn, B. Gilchrest and R. Russell. "Skin Lycopene Is Destroyed Preferentially Over Beta-Carotene During Ultraviolet Irradiation in Humans." *J Nutr* 125:7 (July 1995): 1854–59.

Rui, H. "Research and Development of Cancer Chemopreventive Agents in China." *Journal of Cell Biochemistry* 27 Supplement (1997): 7–11.

Salikhova, R., N. Umnova, M. Fomina and G. Poroshenko. "An Antimutagenicity Study of Bioginseng." *Izv Akad Nauk Ser Biol* (January–February 1994): 48–55.

Scott R., A. MacPherson and R. Yates. "Selenium Supplementation in Sub-Fertile Human Males." in P. Fischer, M. L'Abbé, K. Cockell and R. Gibson, eds. *Trace Elements in Man and Animals-9 (TEMA 9)* NRC Research Press, 1997.

Shamberger, R., S. Tytko and C. Willis. "Antioxidants and Cancer. Part vi. Selenium and Age-Adjusted Human Cancer Mortality." Archives of Environmental Health 31:5 (September–October 1976): 231–35.

Sies, H., W. Stahl, A. Sundquist. "Antioxidant Functions of Vitamins. Vitamins E and C, Beta-Carotene, and Other Carotenoids." *Annals of the New York Academy of Sciences* 669 (30 September 1992): 7–20.

Simone, C. et al. "Nutritional and Lifestyle Modification to Augment Oncology Care: An Overview." *Journal of Orthomolecular Medicine* 12:4 (Fourth Quarter 1997): 197–206.

Simone, C. and R. Good. *Cancer and Nutrition.* Wayne: Avery, 1992.

Singh, J., A. Rivenson, M. Tomita et al. "Bifidobacterium Longum, A Lactic Acid-Producing Intestinal Bacterium Inhibits Colon Cancer and Modulates the Intermediate Biomarkers of Colon Carcinogenesis.'' *Carcinogenesis* 18:4 (April 1997): 833–41.

Slattery M., T. Abbott and J. Overall. ''Dietary Vitamins A, C, and E and Selenium as Risk Factors for Cervical Cancer.'' *Epidemiology* 1:1 (January 1990): 8–15.

Smigel, K. ''Vitamin E Reduces Prostate Cancer Rates in Finnish Trial: U.S. Considers Follow-up.'' *Journal of the National Cancer Institute* 90 (18 March 1998): 416–17.

Stahl, W. and H. Sies. ''Lycopene: A Biologically Important Carotenoid for Humans?'' *Arch Biochem Biophys* 336:1 (1 December 1996): 1–9.

Statland, B. ''Nutrition and Cancer.'' *Clin Chem* 38:8 B Part 2 (August 1992): 1587–94.

Stenson, J. ''Beta-Carotene Shows Promise for Prostate Cancer.'' *Medical Tribune News Service* (June 19, 1997).

Stephens, F. ''Phytoestrogens and Prostate Cancer: Possible Preventive Role.'' *Medical Journal of Australia* 167 (4 August 1997): 138–40.

Sun, X., T. Matsumoto, H. Kiyohara et al. ''Cytoprotective Activity of Pectic Polysaccharides From the Root of Panax Ginseng.'' *Journal of Ethnopharmacology* 1 (31 January 1991): 101–07.

Sundstrom, H., H. Korpela, L. Viinikka and A. Kauppila. ''Serum Selenium and Glutathione Peroxidase, and Plasma Lipid Peroxides in Uterine, Ovarian or Vulvar Cancer, and Their Responses to Antioxidants in Patients With Ovarian Cancer.'' *Cancer Lett* 24:1 (24 August 1984): 1–10.

Sweetman, S., J. Strain and V. McKelvey-Martin. ''Effect of Antioxidant Vitamin Supplementation on DNA Damage and Repair in Human Lymphoblastoid Cells.'' *Nutr Cancer* 27:2 (1997): 122–30.

Tamkins, T. ''Vitamin A May Fight Melanoma.'' Reuters (22 September 1997).

Taylor, P., B. Li, S. Dawsey et al. ''Prevention of Esophageal Cancer: The Nutrition Intervention Trials in Linxian, China.

Linxian Nutrition Intervention Trials Study Group." *Cancer Research* 54:7 Supplement (1 April 1994): 2029–31.

Toma, S., P. Losardo, M. Vincent and R. Palumbo. "Effectiveness of Beta-Carotene in Cancer Chemoprevention." *European Journal of Cancer Prevention* 4:3 (June 1995): 213–24.

Umnova, N., T. Michurina, N. Smirnova et al. "Study of Antimutagenic Properties of Bio-Ginseng in Mammalian Cells In Vitro And In Vivo." *Biull Eksp Biol Med* 111:5 (May 1991): 507–09.

Van Poppel, G. "Epidemiological Evidence for Beta-Carotene in Prevention of Cancer and Cardiovascular Disease." *European Journal of Clinical Nutrition* 50 Supplement 3 (July 1996): 57–61.

Wakabayashi, C., H. Hasegawa, J. Murata and I. Saiki. "In Vivo Antimetastatic Action of Ginseng Protopanaxadiol Saponins Is Based on Their Intestinal Bacterial Metabolites After Oral Administration." *Oncology Research* 9:8 (1997): 411–17.

Wald N., J. Boreham, J. Hayward and R. Bulbrook. "Plasma Retinol, Beta-Carotene and Vitamin E Levels in Relation to the Future Risk of Breast Cancer." *British Journal of Cancer* 49:3 (March 1984): 321–24.

Wassertheil-Smoller, S., S. Romney, J. Rosett-Wylie et al. "Dietary Vitamin C and Uterine Cervical Dysplasia." *American Journal of Epidemiology* 114:5 (November 1981): 714–24.

White, E., J. Shannon and R. Patterson. "Relationship Between Vitamin and Calcium Supplement Use and Colon Cancer." *Cancer Epidemiol Biomarkers Prev* 6:10 (6 October 1997): 769–74.

Xiaoguang, C., L. Hongyan, L. Xiaohong et al. "Cancer Chemopreventive and Therapeutic Activities of Red Ginseng." *Journal of Ethnopharmacology* 60:1 (February 1998): 71–78.

Yamanaka, N., T. Kato, K. Nishida et al. "Elevation of Serum Lipid Peroxide Level Associated With Doxorubicin Toxicity and Its Amelioration by [Dl]-Alpha-Tocopheryl Acetate or Coenzyme Q10 in Mouse (Doxorubicin, Toxicity, Lipid Peroxide, Tocopherol, Coenzyme Q10).'' *Cancer Chemother Pharmacol* 3:4 (1979): 223–27.

Yu, S., Y. Zhu and W. Li. "Protective Role of Selenium Against Hepatitis B Virus and Primary Liver Cancer in Qidong." *Biol Trace Elem Res* 56:1 (January 1997): 117–24.

Yun, T. and S. Choi. "Preventive Effect of Ginseng Intake Against Various Human Cancers: A Case-Control Study on 1987 Pairs." *Cancer Epidemiol Biomarkers Prev* 4:4 (June 1995): 401–08.

Yun, T., Y. Yun and I. Han. "Anticarcinogenic Effect of Long-Term Oral Administration of Red Ginseng on Newborn Mice Exposed to Various Chemical Carcinogens." *Cancer Detection and Prevention* 6:6 (1983): 515–25.

Yun, Y., H. Moon, Y. Oh et al. "Effect of Red Ginseng on Natural Killer Cell Activity in Mice With Lung Adenoma Induced by Urethan and Benzo(a)pyrene." *Cancer Detect Prev* 1 Supplement (1987): 301–09.

Zhang, D., T. Yasuda, Y. Yu et al. "Ginseng Extract Scavenges Hydroxyl Radical and Protects Unsaturated Fatty Acids From Decomposition Caused by Iron-Mediated Lipid Peroxidation." *Free Radic Biol Med* 20:1 (1996): 145–60.

Zhao, X. "Antisenility Effect of Ginseng-Rhizome Saponin." *Chung Hsi I Chieh Ho Tsa Chih* 10:10 (October 1990): 586–89.

Zheng W., K. Anderson, L. Kushi et al. "A Prospective Cohort Study of Intake of Calcium, Vitamin D, and Other Micronutrients in Relation to Incidence of Rectal Cancer Among Postmenopausal Women." *Cancer Epidemiol Biomarkers Prev* 7:3 (March 1998): 221–25.

Ziglar, W. *Whole Foods* 2:4 (1979): 48–53.

CHAPTER SEVEN: Cholesterol and Triglycerides

Adler, A. and B. Holub. "Effect of Garlic and Fish-Oil Supplementation on Serum Lipid and Lipoprotein Concentrations in Hypercholesterolemic Men." *American Journal of Clinical Nutrition* 65:2 (February 1997): 445–50.

Agarwal, K. "Therapeutic Actions of Garlic Constituents." *Med Res Rev* 16:1 (January 1996): 111–24.

Arora R., S. Arora S and R. Gupta. "The Long-Term Use of Garlic in Ischemic Heart Disease—An Appraisal." *Atherosclerosis* 40:2 (October 1981): 175–79.

Atkins, R. *Dr. Atkins' Vita-Nutrient Solution.* New York: Simon & Schuster, 1998.

Berthold, H., T. Sudhop and K. Bergmann. "Garlic Powder and Plasma Lipids and Lipoproteins: A Multicenter, Randomized, Placebo-Controlled Trial." *Journal of the American Medical Association* 279 (8 June 1998): 1900–02.

Binaghi P., G. Cellina, G. Lo Cicero et al. "Evaluation of the Cholesterol-Lowering Effectiveness of Pantethine in Women in Perimenopausal Age." *Minerva Med* 81:6 (June 1990): 475–79.

Bordia, A. "Effect of Garlic on Blood Lipids in Patients With Coronary Heart Disease." *American Journal of Clinical Nutrition* 34:10 (October 1981): 2100–03.

Bordia T., N. Mohammed, M. Thomson, M. Ali. "An Evaluation of Garlic and Onion as Antithrombotic Agents." *Prostaglandins, Leukotrienes and Essential Fatty Acids* 54:3 (March 1996): 183–86.

Borets V., M. Lis, V. Pyrochkin et al. "Therapeutic Efficacy of Pantothenic Acid Preparations in Ischemic Heart Disease Patients." *Vopr Pitan* 2 (March–April 1987): 15–17.

Challem, J. "Vitamin E: High-Doses Reduce the Risk of Heart Attack." *Nutrition Reporter* 153 (May 1996).

Ernst, E. "Garlic and Blood Lipids." *British Medical Journal* 291 (1985): 139.

———. "Cardiovascular Effects of Garlic (Allium Satvium): A Review." *Pharmatherapeutica* 8 (1987): 83–89.

Fulder, S. "Garlic and the Prevention of Cardiovascular Disease." *Cardiology in Practice* 7 (1989): 30–35.

Fuller, C. et al. "Effects of Increasing Doses of Alpha-Tocopherol in Providing Protection of Low-Density Lipoprotein

From Oxidation." *American Journal of Cardiology* 81 (15 January 1998): 231–33.

Gey, K., H. Stahelin and P. Ballmer. "Essential Antioxidants in Cardiovascular Diseases—Lessons for Europe." *Ther Umsch* 51:7 (July 1994): 475–82.

Ghatak, A., M. Brar, A. Agarwal et al. "Oxy Free Radical System in Heart Failure and Therapeutic Role of Oral Vitamin E." *International Journal of Cardiology* 57:2 (6 December 1996): 119–27.

Glanze, W., ed. *The Signet/Mosby Medical Encyclopedia.* New York: Signet, 1987.

Gridley, G. et al. "Vitamin Supplement Use and Reduced Risk of Oral and Pharyngeal Cancer." *American Journal of Epidemiology* 135 (1992): 1083–92.

Guivernau, M., N. Meza, P. Barja and O. Roman. "Clinical and Experimental Study on the Long-Term Effect of Dietary Gamma-Linolenic Acid on Plasma Lipids, Platelet Aggregation, Thromboxane Formation, and Prostacyclin Production." *Prostaglandins, Leukotrienes and Essential Fatty Acids* 51:5 (November 1994): 311–16.

Harris. W. "Fish Oils in Hypertriglyceridemia: a Dose-response study." *American Journal of Clinical Nutrition* 51 (1990): 399–406.

———. "N-3 Fatty Acids and Serum Lipoproteins: Human Studies." *American Journal of Clinical Nutrition* 65:5 Supplement (May 1997): 1645S–1554S.

He, G. "Effect of the Prevention and Treatment of Atherosclerosis of a Mixture of Hawthorn and Motherworn." *Chung Hsi I Chieh Ho Tsa Chih* 10:6 (June 1990): 361, 326.

Holzgartner H., U. Schmidt, U. Kuhn. "Comparison of the Efficacy and Tolerance of a Garlic Preparation Vs. Bezafibrate. *Arzneimittelforschung* 42:12 (December 1992): 1473–77.

"Hyperlipidemia" Health Answers, Orbis Broadcast Group, Interactive Media, 1997.
http://www.healthanswers.com/database/ami/converted/003493.html

http://www.healthanswers.com/database/ami/converted/000403.html

Ide, N., A. Nelson and B. Lau. "Aged Garlic Extract and Its Constituents Inhibit Cu(2+)-Induced Oxidative Modification of Low Density Lipoprotein." *Planta Medica* 63:3 (June 1997): 263–64.

Jain A., R. Vargas, S. Gotzkowsky and F. McMahon. "Can Garlic Reduce Levels of Serum Lipids? A Controlled Clinical Study." *American Journal of Medicine* 94:6 (June 1993): 632–35.

Kenzelmann R., F. Kade. "Limitation of the Deterioration of Lipid Parameters by a Standardized Garlic-Ginkgo Combination Product. A Multicenter Placebo-Controlled Double-Blind Study." *Arzneimittelforschung* 43:9 (September 1993): 978–81.

Knekt, P., et al. *American Journal of Clinical Nutrition* 53 (1991): 2835–65.

LaCour, B., P. Molgaard and Z. Yi. "Traditional Chinese Medicine in Treatment of Hyperlipidaemia." *Journal of Ethnopharmacolog* 46:2 (May 1995): 125–29.

LaRosa, J. "Triglycerides and Coronary Risk in Women and the Elderly." *Archives of Internal Medicine* 157 (12 May 1997): 961–68.

Lau, B. et al. "Allium Sativum (Garlic) and Atherosclerosis: A Review." *Nutrition Research* 3 (1983): 119–28.

———. "Effect of an Odor-Modified Garlic Preparation on Blood Lipids." *Nutrition Research* 7 (1987): 139–49.

Leaf, A. "Omega-3 Fatty Acids and Prevention of Ventricular Fibrillation." *Prosta Leuko Essen Fatty Acid* 52 (1995): 197–98.

Maggi, E., E. Marchesi, V. Ravetta et al. "Low-Density Lipoprotein Oxidation in Essential Hypertension." *J Hypertens* 11:10 (October 1993): 1103–11.

Marquié G., T. Menouar T, M. Pieraggi et al. "Prevention of Preatheromatous Lesions in Sand Rats by Treatment With a

Nutritional Supplement." *Arzneimittelforschung* 46:6 (June 1996): 610–14.

Morcos, N. "Modulation of Lipid Profile by Fish Oil and Garlic Combination." *Journal of the National Medical Association* 89:10 (October 1997): 673–78.

Nityanand, S., J. Srivastava JS and O. Asthana. "Clinical Trials With Gugulipid. A New Hypolipidaemic Agent." *J Assoc Physicians India* 37:5 (May 1989): 323–28.

Paige, J., R. Liao and R. Hajjar. "Effect of a High Omega-3 Fatty Acid Diet on Cardiac Contractile Performance in Oncorhynchus Mykiss." *Cardiovascular Research* 31:2 (February 1996): 249–62.

Phelps, S. and W. Harris. "Garlic Supplementation and Lipoprotein Oxidation Susceptibility." *Lipids* 28:5 (May 1993): 475–77.

Plotnik, G. et al. "Effect of Antioxidant Vitamins on the Transient Impairment of Endothelium-Dependent Brachial Artery Vasoactivity Following a Single High-Fat Meal." *Journal of the American Medical Association* 278 (26 November 1997): 1682–86.

Ponte, E., D. Cafagna and M. Balbi. "Cardiovascular Disease and Omega-3 Fatty Acids." *Minerva Med* 88:9 (September 1997): 343–53.

Pyzh, M., N. Gratsianskii, G. Areshev and S. Kulakova. "Dietary Effect of Omega-3 Polyunsaturated Fatty Acid Supplementation on Blood Fatty Acids, Lipid and Lipoproteins in Patients With Ischemic Heart Disease." *Kardiologiia* 33:5 (1993): 21–26.

Shanthi, S, K. Parasakthy, P. Deepalakshmi and S. Devaraj. "Hypolipidemic Activity of Tincture of Crataegus in Rats." *Indian J Biochem Biophys* 31:2 (April 1994): 143–46.

Steiner, M., A. Khan, D. Holbert and R. Lin. "A Double-Blind Crossover Study in Moderately Hypercholesterolemic Men That Compared the Effect of Aged Garlic Extract and Placebo Administration on Blood Lipids." *American Journal of Clinical Nutrition* 64:6 (December 1996): 866–70.

Stephens, N. et al. "Randomised Controlled Trial of Vitamin E Levels in Relation to the Future Risk of Breast Cancer." *Lancet* 347 (23 March 1996): 781–86.

————."Anti-Oxidant Therapy for Ischaemic Heart Disease: Where Do We Stand." *Lancet* 349 (14 June 1997) 1710–11.

"Symposium on the Chemistry, Pharmacology and Medical Applications of Garlic." *Cardiology in Practice* 7 (1989): 1–15.

Tamkins, T. "Fish Ditches 'Bad' Cholesterol." Reuters (14 November 1997).

Wald, N. et al. "Plasma Retinol, Beta-carotene and Vitamin E Levels in Relation to the Future Risk of Breast Cancer." *British Journal of Cancer* 49 (1984): 321–24.

Zak, A., M. Zeman and D. Vitkova. "Comparison of the Effects of Omega-3 Polyunsaturated Fatty Acids and Olbetam (Acipimox) in the Treatment of Hypertriglyceridemia." *Cas Lek Cesk* 133:24 (22 December 1994): 755–58.

CHAPTER EIGHT: Colds, Coughs, and Other Upper Respiratory Infections

Adetumbi, M. and B. Lau. "Allium Satvium (Garlic)—A Natural Antibiotic." *Medical Hypothesis* 12 (1983): 227–37.

Afifi, A. et al. "High dose Ascorbic Acid in the Management of Thalassaemia Leg Ulcers—A Pilot Study." *British Journal of Dermatology* 92 (1975): 339.

Al-Nakib, W., P. Higgins, I. Barrow, G. Batstone and D. Tyrrell. "Prophylaxis and Treatment of Rhinovirus Colds With Zinc Gluconate Lozenges." *Journal of Antimicrob Chemotherapy* 20:6 (December 1987): 893–901.

Anderson, R. et al. "The Effects of Increasing Weekly Doses of Ascorbate on Certain Cellular and Humoral Immune Functions in Normal Volunteers." *American Journal of Clinical Nutrition* 33 (1980): 71.

Anderson, T. *Nutrition Today* 12 (1977): 6.

Atkins, R. *Dr. Atkins' Vita-Nutrient Solution.* New York: Simon and Schuster, 1998.

Bauer, R. "Echinacea Drugs: Effects and Active Ingredients." *Z Arztl Frotbild* 90:2 (April 1996): 111–15.

Bauer, R., P. Remiger, K. Jurcic and H. Wagner. *Zeitschrift für Phytoptherapie* 10 (1989): 43–48.

Bauer, R. and H. Wagner. "Echinacea Species as Potential Immunostimulatory Drugs." *Economic and Medicinal Plant Research* 5 (1991): 253–321.

Braunig B. et al. "Echinacea Purpurea Radix for Strengthening the Immune Response in Flulike Infections." *Z Phytotherapie* 13 (1992): 7–13.

Bucca, C. et al. "Effect of Vitamin C on Transient Increase of Bronchial Responsiveness in Conditions Affecting the Airways." New York Academy of Sciences 16 (9–12 February 1992): 16.

Bundesanzeiger (2 March 1989).

Cameron, E. and A. Campbell. "The Orthomolecular Treatment of Cancer. Ii. Clinical Trial of High Dose Ascorbic Acid Supplements in Advanced Human Cancer." *Chemical-Biological Interactions* 9 (1974): 285–315.

Cameron, E. et al. "Ascorbic Acid and Cancer: A Review." *Cancer Research* 39 (1979): 663–81.

Carr, A. et al. "Vitamin C and the Common Cold: a Second MZ Cotwin Control Study." *Acta Geneticae et Gemellologiae* 30 (1981): 249.

Chandra, R. "Excessive Intake of Zinc Impairs Immune Responses." *Journal of the American Medical Association* 252 (September 1984): 1443.

Delaha, E. and V. Garagusi. "Inihibition of Microbacterial Cell Growth by Garlic Extract (Allium Sativum)." *Antimicrobial Agents and Chemotherapy* 27 (1985): 485–86.

Denyer, C., P. Jackson, D. Loakes et al. "Isolation of Antirhinoviral Sesquiterpenes From Ginger (Zingiber Officinale)." *Journal of Natural Products* 57: 5 (May 1994): 658–62.

Duchateau, J. et al. *Journal of the American Medical Association* 70 (May 1981): 1001.

Duke, J. *The Green Pharmacy.* Emmaus: Rodale Press, 1997.

Esanau, V. "Research in the Field of Antiviral Chemotherapy Performed in the Stefan S. Nicolau Institute of Virology." *Virologie* 53:4 (October–December 1984): 281–93.

Fraser, R. et al. *American Journal of Clinical Nutrition* 33 (1980): 839.

Garland, M. and K. Hagemeyer. "The Role of Zinc Lozenges in Treatment of the Common Cold." *Annals of Pharmacotherapy* 32:1 (January 1998): 63–69.

Godfrey, J., S. Conant, D. Smith, J. Turco et al. "Zinc Gluconate and the Common Cold: A Controlled Clinical Study." *Journal of Internal Medicine Research* 20:3 (June 1992): 234–46.

Godfrey, J., N. Godfrey and S. Novick. "Zinc for Treating the Common Cold: Review of All Clinical Trials Since 1984." *Alternative Ther Health Med* 2:6 (November 1996): 63–72.

Haas, H. *Arzneipflanzenkunde*. Bonn: Wissenschaftsverlag, 1991.

Hallfish, J. *American Journal of Clinical Nutrition* 60 (1994): 100–05.

Hatch, G. "Asthma, Inhaled Oxidants, and Dietary Antioxidants." *American Journal of Clinical Nutrition* 61:3 (March 1995): 625S–630S.

Hemila, A. "Vitamin C Intake and Susceptibility to the Common Cold." *British Journal of Nutrition* 77:1 (January 1997): 59–72.

Hemila, H. "Vitamin C and the Common Cold." *British Journal of Nutrition* 67:1 (January 1992): 3–16.

———. "Does Vitamin C Alleviate the Symptoms of the Common Cold?—A Review of Current Evidence." *Scandinavian Journal of Infectious Diseases* 26:1 (1994): 1–6.

———. "Vitamin C and Common Cold Incidence: A Review of Studies With Subjects Under Heavy Physical Stress." *International Journal of Sports Medicine* 17:5 (July 1996): 379–83.

———. "Vitamin C Supplementation and Common Cold Symptoms: Problems With Inaccurate Reviews." *Nutrition* 12:11/12 (November/December 1996): 804–09.

———. "Vitamin C Intake and Susceptibility to Pneumonia." *Pediatric Infectious Disease Journal* 16:9 (1997): 836–37.

———. "Vitamin C Supplementation and the Common Cold—Was Linus Pauling Right or Wrong?" *International Journal of Vitamin and Nutritional Research* 67:5 (1997): 329–35.

Hemila, H. and Z. Herman. "Vitamin C and the Common Cold: A Retrospective Analysis of Chalmers' Review." *Journal of the American College of Nutrition* 14:2 (April 1995): 116–23.

Hobbs C. *The Echinacea Handbook*. City: Eclectic Medical Publication, 1989.

———. "Echinacea: A Literature Review." *Herbalgram* 30 (1994): 33–47.

Houghton, P. "Echinacea." *Pharmaceutical Journal* 253 (1994): 342–43.

Hughes, B. et al. "Antiviral Constituents From Allium Sativum." *Planta Medica* 55 (1989): 114.

Klenner, F. *Journal of Applied Nutrition* 23 (1971): 61–88.

Lansdown, A., et al. *Lancet* 347 (1996): 706–07.

Levine, G. et al. "Ascorbic Acid Reverses Endothelial Vasomotor Dysfunction in Patients With Coronary Artery Disease." *Circulation* 93:6 (15 March 1996): 1107–13.

Liberman, S. and N. Bruning. *The Real Vitamin & Mineral Book*. Avery: Avery Publishing, 1990.

Lloyd, J. "A Treatise on Echinacea." Lloyd Brothers, 1924.

McClain, C. *Journal of the American College of Nutrition* 9:5 (1990): 545.

McKinney, M. "Vitamin C Helps Reduce Asthma After Exercise." *Medical Tribune* (5 June 1997): 6.

Melchart, D., K. Linde, F. Worku, L. Sarkady et al. "Results of Five Randomized Studies on the Immunomodulatory Activity of Preparations of Echinacea." *Journal of Alternative and Complementary Medicine* 1:2 (Summer 1995): 145–60.

Mose, J. "Effect of Ehinacin on Phagocytosis and Natural Killer Cells." *Med. Welt* 34 (1983): 1463–67.

Mossad, S., M. Macknin, S. Medendorp and P. Mason. "Zinc Gluconate Lozenges for Treating the Common Cold. A Randomized, Double-Blind, Placebo-Controlled Study." *Annals of Internal Medicine* 125:2 (15 July 1996): 81–88.

Newall, C., L. Anderson and J. D. Phillipson. *Herbal Medicines: A Guide For Healthcare Professionals.* Philadelphia: Pharmaceutical Press, 1996.

Nutrition Review 40:7 (July 1990): 286–87.

Roesler, J., et al. "Application of Purified Polysaccharides From Cell Cultures of the Plant Echinacea Purpurea to Mice Mediates Protection Against Systemic Infections With Listeria Monocytogenes and Candida Albicans." *International Journal of Immunopharmacology* 13 (1991): 27–37.

Pauling, L. *Medical Tribune* (24 March 1976): 18.

Rogers, S. et al. *International Clinical and Nutrition Review* 10 (1990): 253–58.

Sazawal, S. et al. "Zinc Supplementation" *New England Journal of Medicine* 333 (1995): 839–44.

Schoneberger, D. "The Influence of Immune Stimulating Effects of Pressed Juice From Echinacea Purpurea on the Course and Severity of Colds." *Forum Immunologie* 8 (1992): 2–12.

Simon, J. "Vitamin C and Cardiovascular Disease: A Review." *Journal of the American College of Nutrition* 11:2 (1992): 107–25.

Taylor, T. et al. "Ascorbic Acid Supplementation in the Treatment of Pressure-Sores." *Lancet* (1974): 544.

Tragni, E. et al. "Evidence From Two Classic Irritation Tests for an Anti-Inflammatory Action of a Natural Extract, Echinacina B." *Food Chem Toxicol* 23 (1985): 317–19.

Tsai, Y., L. Cole, L. Davis et al. "Antiviral Properties of Garlic: In Vitro Effects on Influenza B, Herpes Simplex and Coxsackie." *Planta Medica* 51 (October 1985): 460–61.

Tubaro A. et al. "Anti-Inflammatory Activity of a Polysaccharide Fraction of Echinacea Angustiforia Root." *Journal of Pharm Pharmacol* 39 (1987): 567–69.

Tyler, V. *The Honest Herbal.* 3rd ed. Binghamton: Pharmaceutical Products Press, 1993.

————. *Herbs of Choice.* Binghamton: Pharmaceutical Products Press, 1994.

Wagner, H., H. Stuppner et al. "Immunologically Active Polysacchharides of Echinacea Purpurea Cell Culture." *Phytochemistry* 27 (1988): 119.

Weber, N., D. Anderson, J. North et al. "In Vitro Virucidal Effects of Allium Sativum (Garlic) Extract and Compounds." *Planta Medica* 58:5 (October 1992): 417–23.

Weismann, K., J. Jakobsen, J. Weismann, U. Hammer et al. "Zinc Gluconate Lozenges for Common Cold. A Double-Blind Clinical Trial." *Danish Medical Bulletin* 37:3 (June 1990): 279–81.

CHAPTER NINE: Depression

American Psychiatric Association: *Diagnostic and Statistical Manual of Mental Disorders, 4th ed. (DSM-IV)* Washington: American Psychiatric Association Press, 1994.

Baureithel, K., K. Buter, A. Engesser et al. "Inhibition of Benzodiazepine Binding In Vitro by Amentoflavone, a Constituent of Various Species of Hypericum." *Acta Helv* 72:3 (1997): 153–57.

Bladt, S. and H. Wagner. "Inhibition of MAO by Fractions and Constituents of Hypericum Extract." *Journal of Geriatric Psychiatry and Neurology* 7. Supplement 1 (October 1994): S57–S59.

Brody, Jane. "An Herb May Be a Gentle Remedy for Mild Depression." *New York Times* 10 September 1997.

Campbell, S. and P. Murphy. "Extraocular Circadian Phototransduction in Humans." *Science* 279 (16 January 1998): 396–99.

Cocchi, R. "Antidepressive Properties of L-Glutamine. Preliminary Report." *Acta Psychiatrica of Belgium* 76 (1976): 658–66.

Couldwell, W., R. Gopalakrishna, D. Hinton et al. "Hypericin: A Potential Antiglioma Therapy." *Neurosurgery* 35:5 (November 1994): 993.

Cracchiolo, C. "Hypericum Perforatum and Hypericum Augustifolia." v.2.02a, (August 1997). http://www.primenet.com/~camilla.

Cuthoys, N. et al. *Annual Review of Nutrition* 15 (1995): 133–59.

Ernst, E. "St.-John's-wort as Antidepressive Therapy." *Fortschritte der Medizin* 113:25 (10 September 1995): 354–55.

Golsch, S., E. Vocks, J. Rakoski et al. "Reversible Increase in Photosensitivity to UV-B Caused by St.-John's-wort Extract." *Hautarzt* 48:4 (April 1997): 249–52.

Hansgen, K., J. Vesper and M. Ploch. "Multicenter Double-Blind Study Examining the Antidepressant Effectiveness of the Hypericum Extract LI 160." *Journal of Geriatric Psychiatry and Neurology* 7. Supplement 1 (October 1994): S15–S18.

Harrer, G., W. Hubner and H. Podzuweit. "Effectiveness and Tolerance of the Hypericum Extract LI 160 Compared to Maprotiline: A Multicenter Double-Blind Study." *Journal of Geriatric Psychiatry and Neurology* 7. Supplement 1 (October 1994): S24–S28.

Hobbs, C. "St.-John's-wort, Hypericum Perforatum L." *Herbalgram* 18/19 (1989): 24–33.

Hubner, W., S. Lande and H. Podzuweit. "Hypericum Treatment of Mild Depression With Somatic Symptoms." *Journal of Geriatric Psychiatry and Neurology* 7: Supplement 1 (October 1994): S12–S14.

Kako, M. et al. "Studies of Sheep Experimentally Poisoned With Hypericum Perforatum." *Veterinary and Human Toxicology* 35:4 (August 1993): 298–300.

Linde, K., G. Ramirez, C. Mulrow et al. "St.-John's-wort for Depression—An Overview and Meta-Analysis of Randomized Clinical Trials." *British Medical Journal* 313:7052 (3 August 1996): 253–58.

Martinez, B., S. Kasper, S. Ruhrmann and H. Moller. "Hypericum in the Treatment of Seasonal Affective Disorders." *Journal of Geriatric Psychiatry and Neurology* 7: Supplement 1 (October 1994): S29–S33.

Meruelo, D., G. Lavie and D. Lavie. ''Therapeutic Agents With Dramatic Antiretrovital and Little Toxicity at Effective Doses: Aromatic Polycyclic Diones Hypericin and Pseudohypericin.'' Proceedings of the National Academy of Science [USA] 85:14 (July 1988): 5230–34.

Muldner, H. and M. Zoller. ''Antidepressive Effect of a Hypericum Extract Standardized to an Active Hypericine Complex: Biochemical and Clinical Studies.'' *Arzneimittelforschung* 37:1 (January 1987): 10–13.

Newall, Carol, L. Anderson and J. D. Phillipson. *Herbal Medicines.* Philadelphia: The Pharmaceutical Press, 1996.

Nordfors, M. and P. Hartvig. ''St.-John's-wort Against Depression in Favor Again.'' *Lakartidningen* 94:25 (18 June 1997): 2365–67.

Oren, D. and M. Terman. ''Tweaking the Human Circadian Clock With Light.'' *Science* 279 (16 January 1998): 333–34.

Perovic S. and W. Muller. ''Pharmacological Profile of Hypericum Extract. Effect on Serotonin Uptake by Postsynaptic Receptors.'' *Arzneimittelforschung* 45:11 (November 1995): 1145–48.

Schlich, D. F. Brauckmann and N. Schenk. ''Treatment of Depressive Conditions With Hypericum.'' *Psychology* 13 (1987): 440–44.

Schmidt, U. and H. Sommer. ''St.-John's-wort Extract in the Ambulatory Therapy of Depression. Attention and Reaction Ability Are Preserved.'' *Fortschritte der Medizin* 111:19 (10 July 1993): 339–42.

Schubert, H. and P. Halama. ''Depressive Episode Primarily Unresponsive to Therapy in Elderly Patients: Efficacy of Ginkgo Biloba (Egb 761) in Combination With Antidepressants.'' *Geriatr Forschrit* 3 (1993): 45–53.

Schulz, H. and M. Jobert. ''Effects of Hypericum Extract on the Sleep EEG in Older Volunteers.'' *Journal of Geriatric Psychiatry and Neurology* 7: Supplement 1 (October 1994): S39–S43.

Shipochliev, T. "Uterotonic Action of Extracts From a Group of Medicinal Plants." *Vet Med* Nauki 18:4 (1981): 94–98.

Sommer, H. and G. Harrer. "Placebo-Controlled Double-Blind Study Examining the Effectiveness of an Hypericum Preparation in 105 Mildly Depressed Patients." *Journal of Geriatric Psychiatry and Neurology* 7: Supplement 1 (October 1994): S9–S11.

Suzuki, O. et al. "Inhibition of Monoamine Oxidase by Hypericin." *Planta Medica* 50 (1984): 272–74.

Taylor, R., N. Manandhar, J. Hudson and G. Towers. "Antiviral Activities of Nepalese Medicinal Plants." *Journal of Ethnopharmacology* 52:3 (5 July 1996): 157–63.

Thiede, H. and A. Walper. "Inhibition of MAO and COMT by Hypericum Extracts and Hypercin." *Journal of Geriatric Psychiatry and Neurology* 7:Supplement 1 (October 1994): S54–S56.

Vorbach, E., W. Hubner and K. Arnoldt. "Effectiveness and Tolerance of the Hypericum Extract LI 160 in Comparison With Imipramine: Randomized Double-Blind Study With 135 Outpatients." *Journal of Geriatric Psychiatry and Neurology* 7:Supplement 1 (October 1994): S19–S23.

Wichtel, M. *Herbal Drugs and Phytopharmaceuticals.* Gainesville: CRC Press/ Scientific Publishers, 1994.

Witte, B., G. Harrer, T. Kaptan et al. "Treatment of Depressive Symptoms With a High Concentration of Hypericum Preparation. A Multicenter Placebo-Controlled Double-Blind Study." *Fortschrift Med* 113:28 (10 October 1995): 404–08.

Woelk, H., G. Burkard and J. Grunwald. "Benefits and Risks of Hypericum Extract LI 160: Drug Monitoring Study With 3250 Patients." *Journal of Geriatric Psychiatry and Neurology* 7:Supplement 1 (October 1994): S34–S38.

Zhang, W., D. Hinton, A. Surnock and W. Couldwell. "Malignant Glioma Sensitivity to Radiotherapy, High-Dose Tamoxifen, and Hypericin: Corroborating Clinical Response In Vitro: Case Report." *Neurosurgery* 38:3 (March 1996): 587–60, 590–91.

CHAPTER TEN: Diabetic Damage

Anderson, R., N. Cheng and N. Bryden. "Elevated Intakes of Supplemental Chromium Improve Glucose and Insulin Variables in Individuals With Type 2 Diabetes." *Diabetes* 46:11 (November 1997): 1786–91.

Bennett, P., S. Haffner, B. Kasiske et al. "Screening and Management of Microalbuminuria in Patients With Diabetes Mellitus: Recommendations to the Scientific Advisory Board of the National Kidney Foundation From an Ad Hoc Committee of the Council on Diabetes Mellitus of the National Kidney Foundation." *American Journal of Kidney Disease* 25: 1 (1995): 107–12.

Braus, P. "Selling Drugs." *American Demographics* (January 1998).

Cahn, J. and M. Borzeix. "Administration of Procyanidolic Oligomers in Rats. Observed Effects on Changes in the Permeability of the Blood-Brain Barrier." *Sem Hop* 59 (1983): 2031–34.

Cefalu, W. "Treatment of Type II Diabetes: What Options Have Been Added to Traditional Methods?" *Postgraduate Medicine* 99:3 (March 1996): 109–19, 122.

Challem, J. "Alpha-Lipoic Acid: Quite Possibly the 'Universal' Antioxidant." *Nutrition Reporter* 153 (July 1996).

Estrada, D., H. Ewart. T. Tsakiridis et al. "Stimulation of Glucose Uptake by the Natural Coenzyme Alpha-Lipoic Acid/Thioctic Acid: Participation of Elements of the Insulin Signaling Pathway." *Diabetes* 45:12 (December 1996): 1798–804.

Feine-Haake, G. "A New Therapy for Venous Diseases." *Zeitschrift für Allgemeinmedizin* 839 (30 June 1975).

Fox, G. and Z. Sabovic. "Chromium Picolinate Supplementation for Diabetes Mellitus." *Journal of Family Practice* 46:1 (January 1998): 83–86.

Gomez Trillo J. "Varicose Veins of the Lower Extremities, Symptomatic Treatment With a New Vasculotrophic Agent." *Prensa Med Mex* 38 (1973): 293–96.

Guillausseau, P. "Preventive Treatment of Diabetic Microangiopathy: Blocking the Pathogenic Mechanisms." *Diabete Metab* 20:2 Part 2 (1994): 219–28.

Henriet, J. "Veno-Lymphatic Insufficiency: 4,729 Patients Undergoing Hormonal and Procyanidol Oligomer Therapy." *Phebologie* 46 (1993): 313–25.

Kahler, W., B. Kuklinski, B. Ruhlman and C. Plotz. "Diabetes Mellitus—A Free Radical-Associated Disease. Results of Adjuvant Antioxidant Supplementation." *Z Gesamte Inn Med* 48:5 (May 1993): 223–32.

Klein, W. "Treatment of Diabetic Neuropathy With Oral Alpha-Lipoic Acid." *MMW Munch Med Wochenschr* 117:22 (30 May 1975): 957–58.

Krolewski, A., L. Laffel, M. Krolewski et al. "Glycosylated Hemoglobin and the Risk of Microalbuminuria in Patients With Insulin-Dependent Diabetes Mellitus." *New England Journal of Medicine* 332 (11 May 1995): 1251–55.

Low, P., K. Nickander and H. Tritschler. "The Roles of Oxidative Stress and Antioxidant Treatment in Experimental Diabetic Neuropathy." *Diabetes* 46 Supplement 2 (September 1997): 38–42.

Nickander, K., B. McPhee, P. Low and H. Tritschler. "Alpha-Lipoic Acid: Antioxidant Potency Against Lipid Peroxidation of Neural Tissues In Vitro and Implications for Diabetic Neuropathy." *Free Radical Biology & Medicine* 21:5 (1996): 631–39.

Nishikawa, T., M. Omura, T. Iizuka et al. "Short-Term Clinical Trial of 1-(1-[4-(3-Acetylaminopropoxy)-Benzoyl]-4-Piperidyl)-3, 4-Dihydro-2(1h)-Quinolinone in Patients With Diabetic Nephropathy. Possible Effectiveness of the Specific Vasopressin V1 Receptor Antagonist for Reducing Albuminuria in Patients With Non-Insulin-Dependent Diabetes Mellitus." *Arzneimittelforschung* 46:9 (September 1996): 875–78.

Packer, L., E. Witt and H. Tritschler. "Alpha-Lipoic Acid as a

Biological Antioxidant.'' *Free Radical Biology & Medicine* 19 (1995): 227–50.

Passwater, A. and C. Kandawswami. *Pycnogenol: The Super Protectant Nutrient.* New Canaan: Keats Publishing, 1994.

Pedrini M., S. Levey, J. et al. The Effect of Dietary Protein Restriction on the Progression of Diabetic and Nondiabetic Renal Diseases: A Meta-Analysis. *Annals of Internal Medicine* 124:7 (1996): 627–32.

Robert, L. et al. ''The Effect of Procyanidolic Oligomers on Vascular Permeability. A Study Using Quantitative Morphology.'' *Pathol Biol* 38 (1990): 608–16.

Rona, Z. ''Treating Peripheral Neuropathy.'' *Toronto Star* (2 August 1998).

Senft, V. and J. Kohout. ''Is Chromium an Essential or a Toxic Element?'' *Cas Lek Cesk* 135:5 (6 March 1996): 150–53.

Toba, K., Y. Ouchi, M. Akishita et al. ''Improved Skin Blood Flow and Cutaneous Temperature in the Foot of a Patient With Arteriosclerosis Obliterans by Vasopressin V1 Antagonist (Opc21268). A Case Report.'' *Angiology* 46:11 (November 1995): 1027–33.

Whiteman, M., H. Trtischler and B. Halliwell. ''Protection Against Peroxynitrite-Dependent Tyrosine Nitration and Alpha 1-Antiproteinase Inactivation by Oxidized and Reduced Lipoic Acid.'' *FEBS Letters* 379:1 (22 January 1996): 74–76.

Yamada, K., H. Nakano, M. Nishimura and S. Yoshida. ''Effect of Avp.vl-Receptor Antagonist on Urinary Albumin Excretion and Renal Hemodynamics in Niddm Nephropathy: Role of Avp.vl-Receptor.'' *Journal of Diabetes Complications* 9:4 (October–December 1995): 326–29.

Ziegler, D. and F. Gries. ''Alpha-Lipoic Acid in the Treatment of Diabetic Peripheral and Cardiac Autonomic Neuropathy.'' *Diabetes* 46 Supplement 2 (September 1996): 62–66.

Ziegler, D., M. Hanefeld, K. Ruhnau et al. ''Treatment of Symptomatic Diabetic Peripheral Neuropathy With the Anti-Oxidant Alpha-Lipoic Acid. A 3-Week Multicenter Randomized

Controlled Trial (Aladin Study)." *Diabetologia* 38:12 (December 1995): 1425–33.

Ziegler, D., H. Schatz, F. Conrad et al. "Effects of Treatment With the Antioxidant Alpha-Lipoic Acid on Cardiac Autonomic Neuropathy in Niddm Patients. A 4-Month Randomized Controlled Multicenter Trial (Dekan Study) Deutsche Kardiale Autonome Neuropathie." *Diabetes Care* 20:3 (March 1997): 369–73.

CHAPTER ELEVEN: The Digestive System

Adetumbi, M. and B. Lau. "Allium Sativum (Garlic)—A Natural Antibiotic." *Med Hypoth* 12 (1983): 227–37.

Aldoori, W., E. Giovannucci, E. Rimm et al. "Use of Acetaminophen and Nonsteroidal Anti-Inflammatory Drugs: A Prospective Study and the Risk of Symptomatic Diverticular Disease in Men." *Archives of Family Medicine* 7 (May–June 1998): 255–60.

Ashraf, W., F. Park, J. Lof and E. Quigley. "Effects of Psyllium Therapy on Stool Characteristics, Colon Transit and Anorectal Function in Chronic Idiopathic Constipation." *Aliment Pharmacol Ther* 9:6 (December 1995): 639–47.

Baker, M. "Licorice and Enzymes Other Than 11 Beta-Hydroxysteroid Dehydrogenase: An Evolutionary Perspective." *Steroids* 59:2 (February 1994): 136–41.

Bengmark, S. and B. Jeppsson. "Gastrointestinal Surface Protection and Mucosa Reconditioning." *J Parenter Enteral Nutr* 19:5 (September–October 1995): 410–15.

Berkow, R. et al. *The Merck Manual of Medical Information*. Whitehouse Station: Merck & Co., 1997.

Bogdanov, I. *Digest* (1982): 3–19.

Bone M., D. Wilkinson and J. Young et al. "Ginger Root—A New Antiemetic. The Effect of Ginger Root on Postoperative Nausea and Vomiting After Major Gynecological Surgery." *Anaesthesia* 45:8 (August 1990): 669–71.

Bundesanzeiger (30 November 1985).

Bundesanzeiger (13 March 1986).

Bundesanzeiger (15 May 1986).

Burton, R. and V. Manninen. "Influence of a Psyllium-Based Fibre Preparation on Faecal and Serum Parameters." *Acta Medica Scandinavica* 668 Supplement (1982): 91–94.

Canganella, F., S. Paganini, M. Ovidi et al. "A Microbiology Investigation on Probiotic Pharmaceutical Products Used for Human Health." *Microbiol Res* 152:2 (July 1997): 171–79.

Christensen, E., E. Juhl and N. Tygstrup. "Treatment of Gastric Ulcer. The Randomized Clinical Trials From 1964 to 1974 and Their Impact." *American Journal of Gastroenterology* 69:3 (March 1978): 272–82.

Dehpour, A., M. Zolfaghari, T. Samadian and Y. Vahedi. "The Protective Effect of Liquorice Components and Their Derivatives Against Gastric Ulcer Induced by Aspirin in Rats." *J Pharm Pharmacol* 46:2 (February 1994): 148–49.

European Heart Journal 19 (1998): 387–94.

Galitskii L., O. Barnaulov, B. Zaretskii et al. "Effect of Phytotherapy on the Prevention and Elimination of Hepatotoxic Responses in Patients with Pulmonary Tuberculosis, Carriers of Hepatitis B Virus Markers." *Probl Tuberk* 4 (1997): 35–38.

"Gastrointestinal Blues." Science News Online. 6 November 1996.
http://www.sciencenews.org/sn–arch/11–9–96/bob2.htm

Graham, H. and E. Graham. "Inhibition of Aspergillus Parasiticus Growth and Toxic Production by Garlic." *Journal of Food Safety* 8 (1987): 101–08.

Grontved, A., T. Brask, J. Kambskard and E. Hentzer. "Ginger Root Against Seasickness. A Controlled Trial on the Open Sea." *Acta Otolaryngol* 105: 1–2 (January–February 1988): 45–49.

Guslandi, M. "Ulcer-Healing Drugs and Endogenous Prostaglandins." *Int J Clin Pharmacol Ther Toxicol* 23 (1985): 398–402.

Hills, J. and P. Aasronson. "The Mechanism of Action of Peppermint Oil on Gastrointestinal Smooth Muscle. An Analysis

Using Patch Clamp Electrophysiology and Isolated Tissue Pharmacology in Rabbit and Guinea Pig." *Gastroenterology* 101:1 (July 1991): 55–65.

Hilton E., H. Isenberg, P. Alperstein et al. "Ingestion of Yogurt Containing Lactobacillus Acidophilus as Prophylaxis for Andidal Vaginitis." *Annals of Internal Medicine* 116:5 (1 March 1992): 353–57.

Hotz, J. and K. Plein. "Effectiveness of Plantago Seed Husks in Comparison With Wheat Bran on Stool Frequency and Manifestations of Irritable Colon Syndrome With Constipation." *Med Klin* 89:12 (15 December 1994): 645–51.

Hughes, V. et al. "Microbiologic Characteristics of Lactobacillus Products Used for Colonization of the Vagina." *Obstetrics and Gynecology* 75:2 (1990): 244.

Joshi, D. et al. "Gastrointestinal Actions of Garlic Oil." *Phytotherapy Research* 1 (1987): 140–41.

Kabir A., Y. Aiba Y, A. Takagi et al. "Prevention of Helicobacter Pylori Infection by Lactobacilli in a Gnotobiotic Murine Model." *Gut* 41:1 (July 1997): 49–55.

Kocian, J. "Lactobacilli in the Treatment of Dyspepsia Due to Dysmicrobia of Various Causes." *Vnitr Lek* 40:2 (February 1994): 79–83.

Liu, J., G. Chen, H. Ye et al. "Enteric-Coated Peppermint-Oil Capsules in the Treatment of Irritable Bowel Syndrome: A Prospective, Randomized Trial." *Journal of Gastroenterology* 32:6 (December 1997): 765–68.

Longstreth, G., D. Fox, L. Youkeles et al. "Psyllium Therapy in the Irritable Bowel Syndrome. A Double-Blind Trial." *Annals of Internal Medicine* 95:1 (July 1981): 53–56.

May, B., H. Kuntz, M. Keiser and S. Kohler. "Efficacy of a Fixed Peppermint Oil/Caraway Oil Combination in Non-Ulcer Dyspepsia." *Arzneimittelforschung* 46:12 (December 1996): 1149–53.

Meyer K., J. Schwartz, D. Crater and B. Keyes. "Zingiber Officinale (Ginger) Used to Prevent 8-Mop Associated Nausea." *Dermatol Nurs* 7:4 (August 1995): 242–44.

Midolo, P., J. Lambert, R. Hull et al. "In Organic Acids and Lactic Acid Bacteria." *Journal of Applied Bacteriology* 79:4 (October 1995): 475–79.

Mishina, D., Greenstein, R., et al. "On the Etiology of Crohn Disease. Proceedings of The National Academy of Sciences" 93 (3 September 1996): 9816.

Morgan, A., W. McAdam, C. Pacsoo et al. "Cimetidine: An Advance in Gastric Ulcer Treatment?" *British Medical Journal* 2:6148 (11 November 1978): 1323–26.

Mowrey, D. *The Scientific Validation of Herbal Medicine.* New Canaan: Keats, 1986.

Mowrey, D. and D. Clayson. "Motion Sickness, Ginger and Psychophysics." *Lancet* I (1982): 655–57.

Nadar, T. and M. Pillai. "Effect of Ayurvedic Medicines on Beta-Glucuronidase Activity of Brunner's Glands During Recovery From Cysteamine-Induced Duodenal Ulcers in Rats." *Indian J Exp Biol* 27:11 (November 1989): 959–62.

Newall, C., L. Anderson and J. D. Phillipson. *Herbal Medicines: A Guide for Healthcare Professionals.* Philadelphia: Pharmaceutical Press, 1996.

Niebyl, J. "Drug Therapy During Pregnancy." *Curr Opin Obstet Gynecol* 4:1 (February 1992): 43–47.

Nieman, C. *Chemist and Druggist* 177 (1962): 741–45.

Phillips S., R. Ruggier and S. Hutchinson. "Zingiber Officinale (Ginger)—An Antiemetic for Day Case Surgery." *Anaesthesia* 48:8 (August 1993): 715–17.

Rani B., N. Khetarpaul. "Probiotic Fermented Food Mixtures: Possible Applications in Clinical Anti-Diarrhea Usage." *Nutr Health* 12:2 (1998): 97–105.

Rath, H., Sartor, B. et al. "Normal Luminal Bacteria, Especially Bacteroides Species, Mediate Chronic Colitis, Gastritis, and Arthritis in Hla-B27/Human (2 Microglobulin Transgenic Rats." *The Journal of Clinical Investigation* 98 (August 1996): 1.

Salminen S., E. Isolauri and T. Onnela. "Gut Flora in Normal and Disordered States." *Chemotherapy* 1995 41:Supplement 1 (1995): 5–15.

Salminen S., E. Isolauri and E. Salminen. "Clinical Uses of Probiotics for Stabilizing the Gut Mucosal Barrier: Successful Strains and Future Challenges." *Antonie Van Leeuwenhoek* 70:2 (October 1996): 347–58.

Singh, J., A. Rivenson, M. Tomita et al. "Bifidobacterium Longum, a Lactic Acid-Producing Intestinal Bacterium Inhibits Colon Cancer and Modulates the Intermediate Biomarkers of Colon Carcinogenesis." *Carcinogenesis* 18:4 (April 1997): 833–41.

Smalley, J., W. Klish, M. Campbell and M. Brown. "Use of Psyllium in the Management of Chronic Nonspecific Diarrhea of Childhood." *J Pediatr Gastroenterol Nutr* 1:3 (1982): 361–63.

Smyrnov, V., S. Reznyk and I. Sorokulov. "The Highly Effective Biological Preparation Biosporin." *Lik Sprava* 5–6 (May–June 1994): 133–38.

Sorokulova I., V. Beliavskaia, V. Masycheva and V. Smirnov. "Recombinant Probiotics: Problems and Prospects of Their Use for Medicine and Veterinary Practice." *Vestn Ross Akad Med Nauk* 3 (1997): 46–49.

Stevens J., P. VanSoest, J. Robertson and D. Levitsky. "Comparison of the Effects of Psyllium and Wheat Bran on Gastrointestinal Transit Time and Stool Characteristics." *J Am Diet Assoc* 88:3 (March 1988): 323–26.

Strus, M. "The Significance of Lactic Acid Bacteria in Treatment and Prophylaxis of Digestive Tract Disorders." *Postepy Hig Med Dosw* 51:6 (1997): 605–19.

Thompson, W. "A Strategy for Management of the Irritable Bowel." *American Journal of Gastroenterology* 81:2 (February 1986): 95–100.

Tyler, V. *Herbs of Choice*. Binghamton: Pharmaceutical Products Press, 1994.

Utsunomiya, T., M. Kobayashi, R. Pollard and F. Suzuki. "Glycyrrhizin, an active Component of Licorice Roots, Reduces

Morbidity and Mortality of Mice Infected With Lethal Doses of Influenza Virus." *Antimicrob Agents Chemother* 41:3 (March 1997): 551–56.

CHAPTER TWELVE: Headaches

Anderson, D., P. Jenkinson, R. Dewdney et al. "Chromosomal Aberrations and Sister Chromatid Exchanges in Lymphocytes and Urine Mutagenicity of Migraine Patients: A Comparison of Chronic Feverfew Users and Matched Nonusers." *Human Toxicology* 7:2 (March 1988): 145–52.

Awang, D. "Feverfew Fever—A Headache for the Consumer." *Herbalgram* 29 (1993): 34–36, 66.

Berry, M. "Feverfew." *Pharm J* 253 (1994): 806–08.

Facchinetti, F., P. Borella, G. Sances et al. "Magnesium Prophylaxis of Menstrual Migraine: Effects on Intracellular Magnesium." *Headache* 31:5 (May 1991): 298–301.

Facchinetti, F., P. Borella, G. Sances, L. Fioroni. "Oral Magnesium Successfully Relieves Premenstrual Mood Changes." *Obstetrics and Gynecology* 78:2 (August 1991): 177–181.

Foltz-Gray, D. "Move Over Aspirin: Seven Herbs to Stock Up On—And to Keep You Out of the Doctor's Office." *Prevention* 49 (1 November, 1997): 97–98.

Gallai, V., P. Sarchielli, P. Morucci and G. Abbritti. "Red Blood Cell Magnesium Levels in Migraine Patients." *Cephalalgia* 13:2 (April 1993).

Göbel, H., G. Schmidt and D. Soyka. "Effect of Peppermint and Eucalyptus Oil Preparations on Neurophysiological and Experimental Algesimetric Headache Parameters." *Cephalalgia* 14:3 (June 1994): 228–34.

Johnson, E., N. Kadam, D. Hylands and P. Hylands. "Efficacy of Feverfew as Prophylactic Treatment of Migraine." *British Medical Journal* (Clinical Research Edition) 291:6495 (31 August 1985): 569–73.

Loesche, W., A. Mazurov, T. Voyno-Yasenetskaya et al. "Feverfew—An Antithrombotic Drug?" *Folia Haematol Int Mag Klin Morphol Blutforsch* 115:1–2 (1988): 181–84.

Mauskop, A. and B. Altura. "Role of Magnesium in the Pathogenesis and Treatment of Migraines." *Clinical Neuroscience* 5:1 (1998): 24–27.

Mauskop, A., B. Altura, R. Cracco and B. Altura. "Chronic Daily Headache—One Disease or Two? Diagnostic Role of Serum Ionized Magnesium." *Cephalalgia* 41:1 (February 1994): 24–28.

———."Intravenous Magnesium Sulfate Relieves Cluster Headaches in Patients With Low Serum Ionized Magnesium Levels." *Headache* 35:10 (November–December 1995): 597–600.

———."Intravenous Magnesium Sulfate Rapidly Alleviates Headaches of Various Types." *Headache* 36:3 (March 1996): 154–160.

———."Intravenous Magnesium Sulphate Relieves Migraine Attacks in Patients With Low Serum Ionized Magnesium Levels: A Pilot Study." *Clin Sci* 89:6 (December 1996): 633–36.

"Migraines: Management and Treatment." *Midlife Woman* 6 (1 April 1997): 7ff.

Mishima, K., T. Takeshima, T. Shimomura et al. "Platelet Ionized Magnesium, Cyclic Amp, and Cyclic Gmp Levels in Migraine and Tension-Type Headache." *Headache* 37:9 (October 1997): 561–64.

Milne, R., B. More and B. Goldberg. *An Alternative Medicine Definitive Guide to Headaches.* Tiburon:Future Medicine, 1996.

Murphy, J., S. Heptinstall, J. Mitchell. "Randomized Double-Blind Placebo-Controlled Trial of Feverfew in Migraine Prevention." *Lancet* 2:8604 (23 July 1988): 189–92.

Murray, M. "Migraine: The Ultimate Headache." 22 Contemporary Women's Issues Database (1 March 1997): 23–24.

National Headache Foundation Factsheet; http://www.headaches.org/facts.html

Opavsky, J. "Magnesium and Its Combination With Cinnarizine

in the Long-Term Treatment of Headache." *Acta Univ Palacki Olomuc Fac Med* 131 (1991): 157–64.

Peikert, A., C. Wilimzig and R. Köhne-Volland. "Prophylaxis of Migraine With Oral Magnesium: Results From a Prospective, Multi-Center, Placebo-Controlled and Double-Blind Randomized Study." *Cephalalgia* 16:4 (June 1996): 257–63.

Ramadan N., H. Halvorson, A. Vande-Linde. "Low Brain Magnesium in Migraine." *Headache* 29:7 (July 1989): 416–19.

———."Low Brain Magnesium in Migraine." *Headache* 29:9 (October 1989): 590–93.

Rodriguez, E. et al. "The Role of Sesquiterpene Lactones in Contact Hypersensitivity to Some North and South American Species of Feverfew." *Contact Dermatitis* 3 (1977): 155–62.

Sarchielli, P., G. Coata, C. Firenze et al. "Serum and Salivary Magnesium Levels in Migraine and Tension-Type Headache. Results in a Group of Adult Patients." *Cephalalgia* 12:1 (February 1992): 21–27.

Schoenen, J., J. Sianard-Gainko and M. Lenaerts. "Blood Magnesium Levels in Migraine." *Cephalalgia* 11:2 (May 1992): 97–99.

Taubert, K. "Magnesium in Migraine. Results of a Multicenter Pilot Study." *Fortschritte der Medizin* 112:24 (30 August 1994): 328–30.

Tyler, V. *The Honest Herbal.* City: Pharmaceutical Products Press, 1994.

CHAPTER THIRTEEN: Heart Disease and Coronary Artery Disease

Al Makdessi, S., H. Sweidan, S. Mullner and R. Jacob. "Myocardial Protection by Pretreatment With Crataegus Oxyacantha: An Assessment by Means of the Release of Lactate Dehydrogenase by the Ischemic and Reperfused Langendorff Heart." *Adzneimittelforschung* 46:1 (January 1996): 25–27.

Azuma, J. et al. "Usefulness of Taurine in Chronic Congestive Heart Failure and its Prospective Application." *Japanese Circulation Journal* 56:1 (1992): 95–99.

Baggio, E., R. Gandini, A. Plancher et al. "Italian Multicenter Study on the Safety and Efficacy of Coenzyme Q10 as Adjunctive Therapy in Heart Failure (Interim Analysis). The CoQ10 Drug Surveillance Investigators." *Clinical Investigation* 71:8 Supplement (1993): 145–49.

————."Italian Multicenter Study on the Safety and Efficacy of Coenzyme Q10 as Adjunctive Therapy in Heart Failure. CoQ10 Drug Surveillance Investigators." *Mol Aspects Med* 15 Supplement (1994): 287–94.

Bahorun, T., B. Gressier, F. Trotin et al. "Oxygen Species Scavenging Activity of Phenolic Extracts From Hawthorn Fresh Plant Organs and Pharmaceutical Preparations." 46:11 (November 1996): 1086–89.

Bertelli, A. and G. Ronca. "Carnitine and Coenzyme Q10: Biochemical Properties and Functions, Synergism and Complementary Action." *Int J Tissue React* 12:3 (1990): 183–86.

Bordia, A. "The Effect of Vitamin C on Blood Lipids, Fibrinolytic Activity and Platelet Adhesiveness in Patients with Coronary Artery Disease." *Atherosclerosis* 35 (1980): 181.

Bosma, H., M. Marmot, H. Hemingway et al. "Low Job Control and Risk of Coronary Heart Disease in Whitehall Ii (Prospective Cohort)." *British Medical Journal* 31:4 (22 February 1997): 558–65.

Brody, J. *New York Times* (26 October 1997).

Bundesanzeiger (3 January 1984).

Bundesanzeiger (5 May 1988).

Chapman, R. et al. *Cardiovascular Research* 27 (1993): 358–63.

Chatterjee, S., E. Koch, H. Jaffy and T. Krzeminski. "In Vitro and In Vivo Studies on the Cardioprotective Action of Oligomeric Procyanidins in a Crataegus Extract of Leaves and Blooms." *Arzneimittelforschung* 47:7 (July 1997): 821–25.

Cordova, C. et al. "Influence of Ascorbic Acid on Platelet Aggregation in Vitro and in Vivo." *Atherosclerosis* 41 (1982): 15.

Cortes, E., M. Gupta, C. Chou C. et al. "Adriamycin Cardiotoxicity: Early Detection by Systolic Time Interval and Possible Prevention by Coenzyme Q10." *Cancer Treatment Report* 62 (1978): 887–91.

Crawford, R. "Proposed Role for a Combination of Citric Acid and Ascorbic Acid in the Production of Dietary Iron Overload: A Fundamental Cause of Disease." *Biochem Mol Med* 54:1 (February 1995): 1–11.

Davini, A., F. Cellerini and P. Topi. "Coenzyme Q10: Contractile Dysfunction of the Myocardial Cell and Metabolic Therapy." *Minerva Cardioangiology* 40:11 (November 1992): 449–53.

Digiesi, V., C. Cantini and B. Brodbeck. "Effect of Coenzyme Q10 on Essential Hypertension." *Curr Ther Res* 47 (1990): 841–45.

Digiesi, V., F. Cantini, A. Oradei et al. "Coenzyme Q10 in Essential Hypertension." *Molec Aspects Med* 15 Supplement (1994): 257–63.

Ely, J. et al. "Hemorrhagic Stroke in Human Pretreated With Coenzyme Q10: Exceptional Recovery as Seen in Animal Models." *Journal of Orthomolecular Medicine* 13:2 (Second Quarter 1998): 105–09.

Fallest-Strobl, P. et al. "Homocysteine: A New Risk Factor for Atherosclerosis." *American Family Physician* 56 (15 October 1997): 1607–12.

Fitzpatrick, D., S. Hirschfield and R. Coffey. "Endothelium-Dependent Vasorelaxing Activity of Wine and Other Grape Products." *American Journal of Physiology* 265:H (August 1993): 774–78.

Folkers, K. and R. Simonsen. "Two Successful Double-Blind Trials With Coenzyme Q10 (Vitamin Q10) on Muscular Dystrophies and Neurogenic Atrophies." *Biochim Biophys Acta* 1271:1 (24 May 1995): 281–86.

Folkers, K., J. Wolaniuk, R. Simonsen et al. "Biochemical Rationale and the Cardiac Response of Patients With Muscle Disease to Therapy With Coenzyme Q10." Proceedings of the National Academy of Sciences 82 (1985): 4531–16.

Fujioka, T., Y. Sakamoto, and G. Mimura. "Clinical Study of Cardiac Arrhythmias Using a 24-Hour Continuous Electro-cardiographic Recorder (5th Report)—Antiarrhythmic Action of Coenzyme Q10 in Diabetics." *Tohoku Journal of Experimental Medicine* 141 Supplement (1983): 453–63.

Haglund, K. *Medical News* (26 May 1984): 3.

Harris, T., R. Ballard-Barbasch and J. Madans. "Overweight, Weight Loss, and Risk of Coronary Heart Disease in Older Women. The Nhanes I Epidemiologic Follow-Up Study." *American Journal of Epidemiology* 137:12 (15 June 1993): 1318–27.

Harris, T., L. Launer, J. Madans and J. Feldman. "Cohort Study of Effect of Being Overweight and Change in Weight on Risk of Coronary Heart." *British Medical Journal* 314:7097 (21 June 1997): 1791–94.

He, G. "Effect of the Prevention and Treatment of Atherosclerosis of a Mixture of Hawthorn and Motherworn." *Chung Hsi I Chieh Ho Tsa Chih* 10:6 (June 1990): 361, 326.

Herrera, M. and M. Deitel. "Cardiac Function in Massively Obese Patients and the Effect of Weight Loss." *Canadian Journal of Surgery* 34:5 (October 1991): 431–34.

Hobbs, C. "Hawthorn for the Heart." *Let's Live Magazine* (1996). Also available at: http://www.healthy.net/library/articles/hobbs/hawthll.htm

Hobbs, C. and S. Foster. "Hawthorn—A Literature Review." *Herbalgram* 22 (1990): 19–33.

Horsey, J., B. Livesley and J. Dickerson. "Ischaemic Heart Disease and Aged Patients: Effects of Ascorbic Acid on Lipoproteins." *Journal of Human Nutrition* 35:1 (February 1981): 53–58.

Iwamoto, M. et al. "Klinische Wirkung von Cratagutt bei Herzekrangkungen Ischamisher und/oder Hypertensiver Genese." *Planta Medica* 42 (1981): 1–16.

Jia, X., R. Emerick and H. Kayongo-Male. "Biochemical Interactions Among Silicon, Iron and Ascorbic Acid in the Rat." *Biol Trace Elem Res* 59: 1–3 (Winter 1997): 123–32.

Judy, W., J. Hall, W. Dugan et al. "Coenzyme Q10 Reduction Of Adriamycin Cardiotoxicity." 231–41 in K. Folkers and Y. Yamamura, eds. *Biomedical and Clinical Aspects of Coenzyme Q,* vol. 4, New York: Elsevier, 1984.

Kamikawa, T., A. Kobayashi, T. Yamashita et al. "Effects of Coenzyme Q10 on Exercise Tolerance in Chronic Stable Angina Pectoris." *American Journal of Cardiology* 56 (1985): 247–51.

Kobayashi, A. et al. *Japanese Circulation Journal* 56 (January 1992): 86–94.

Kucharska, J., A. Gvozdjakova, M. Snircova et al. "Determination of Coenzyme Q10 and Alpha-Tocopherol Levels in Patients With Cardiopathies of Unknown Origin: Perspectives in Diagnosis." *Bratisl Lek Listy* 97:6 (June 1996): 351–54.

Landbo, C. and T. Almdal. "Interaction Between Warfarin and Coenzyme Q10." *Ugeskr Laeger* 160:22 (25 May 1998): 3226–27.

Langsjoen, P., K. Folkers and P. Langsjoen. "Long-Term Efficacy and Safety of Coenzyme Q10 Therapy for Idiopathic Dilated Cardiomyopathy." *American Journal of Cardiology* 65 (1990): 521–23.

———."A Six-year Clinical Study of Therapy of Cardiomyopathy With Coenzyme Q10." *Int J Tissue React* 12:3 (1990): 169–71.

Langsjoen, P., K. Folkers, K. Lyson et al. "Effective and Safe Therapy With Coenzyme Q10 for Cardiomyopathy." *Klin Wochenschr* 66 (1988): 583–90.

Langsjoen P., K. Folkers, P. Langsjoen, and R. Willis. "Treatment of Essential Hypertension With Coenzyme Q10." *Molec Aspects Med* 15:Supplement (1994): 265–72.

Langsjoen P., K. Folkers and S. Vadhanavikit. "Effective Treatment With Coenzyme Q10 of Patients With Chronic Myocardial Disease." *Drugs Exptl Clin Res* 11 (1985): 577–79.

Leuchtgens, H. "Crataegus Special Extract Ws 1442 in NYHA-II Heart Failure. A Placebo-Controlled Randomized Double-

Blind Study.'' *Frotschrittle der Medizin* 111: 20–21 (20 July 1993): 352–54.

Levine, G., B. Frei, S. Koulouris et al. ''Ascorbic Acid Reverses Endothelial Vasomotor Dysfunction in Patients With Coronary Artery Disease.'' *Circulation* 93:6 (15 March 1996): 1107–13.

Manson, J., et al. *Circulation* 85 (1992):865.

Manson, J., G. Colditz, M. Stampfer et al. ''A Prospective Study of Obesity and Risk of Coronary Heart Disease in Women.'' *New England Journal of Medicine* 322: 13 (29 March 1990): 882–89.

Marshall, M. ''Varicose Vein Drugs—New Attempts at Objectivation of the Effects of Therapy.'' *Fortschrittle der Medizin* 102:29 (16 August 1984): 772.

Moghadasian, M. et al. ''Homocysteine and Coronary Artery Disease.'' *Archives of Internal Medicine* 157 (10 November 1997): 2299–308.

Morisco, C., B. Trimarco and M. Condorelli. ''Effect of Coenzyme Q10 Therapy in Patients With Congestive Heart Failure: A Long-Term Multicenter Randomized Study.'' *Clinical Investigator* 71:8 Supplement (1993): 134–36.

Mortensen, S. ''Perspectives on Therapy of Cardiovascular Diseases With Coenzyme Q10 (Ubiquinone).'' *Clinical Investigator* 71:8 Supplement (1993): 116–23.

Mortensen, S., S. Vadhanavikit, U. Baandrup and K. Folkers. ''Long-Term Coenzyme Q10 Therapy: A Major Advance in the Management of Resistant Myocardial Failure.'' *Drugs Exptl Clin Res* 11 (1985): 581–93.

Newall, C., L. Anderson and J. D. Phillipson. *Herbal Medicines: A Guide for Healthcare Professionals.* London: Pharmaceutical Press, 1996.

Nishima, Y., S. Sugiyama, M. Yokoya et al. ''The Effects of a High Dose of Ascorbate on Ischemia-Reperfusion-Induced Mitochondrial Dysfunction in Canine Hearts.'' *Heart Vessels* 7:1 (1992): 18–23.

Popping, S., H. Rose, I. Ionescu et al. ''Effect of a Hawthorn

Extract on Contraction and Energy Turnover of Isolated Rat Cardiomyocytes." *Arzneimittelforschung* 45:11 (November 1995): 1157–61.

Rath, M. *Journal of Applied Nutrition* 48 (1996): 22–33.

Reitz, V. et al. *American Journal of Cardiology* (March 1990): 755–60.

Rodale, J. *The Hawthorn Berry for the Heart.* Emmaus: Rodale Press, 1971.

Schmidt, U., U. Kuhn, M. Ploch and W. D. Hübner. "Efficacy of the Hawthorn (Crataegus) Preparation LI 132 in 78 Patients With Chronic Congestive Heart Failure Defined as NYHA Functional ClassII." *Phythomedicine* 1 (1994): 17–24.

Simon, J., E. Hudes and W. Browner. "Serum Ascorbic Acid and Cardiovascular Disease Prevalence in U.S. Adults." *Epidemiology* 9:3 (May 1998): 316–21.

Sinatra, S. "Refractory Congestive Heart Failure Successfully Managed With High Dose Coenzyme Q10 Administration." *Mol Aspects Med* 18 Supplement (1997): 299–305.

Solzbach, U., B. Hornig, M. Jeserich and H. Just. "Vitamin C Improves Endothelial Dysfunction of Epicardial Coronary Arteries in Hypertensive Patients." *Circulation* 96:5 (2 September 1997): 1513–19.

Trout, D. "Vitamin C and Cardiovascular Risk Factors." *American Journal of Clinical Nutrition* 53:1 Supplement (January 1991): 322–25.

Weber, C., A. Bysted and G. Holmer. "Coenzyme Q10 in the Diet—Daily Intake and Relative Bioavailability." *Mol Aspects Med* 18 Supplement (1997): 251–54.

Weihmayr, T. and E. Ernst. "Therapeutic Effectiveness of Crataegus." *Frotschritte de Medizin* 114:1–2 (20 January 1996): 27–29.

Weikl, A., K. Assmus, A. Neukum-Schmidt et al. "Crataegus Special Extract WS 1442. Assessment of Objective Effectiveness in Patients With Heart Failure (NYHA II)." *Frotschritte der Medizin* 114:24 (30 August 1996): 291–96.

CHAPTER FOURTEEN: Homocysteine

American Heart Association: "High Homocysteine Concentrations in Blood Warn of Increased Heart Attack Risk in Young Women." (15 July 1997).
http://www.americanheart.org/Whats–News/
AHA–News–Releases /974566.html

Arnesen, E. "Serum Total Homocysteine and Coronary Heart Disease." *International Journal of Epidemiology* 24 (1995):704–09.

Atkins, R. *Dr. Atkins' Vita-Nutrient Solution.* New York: Simon & Schuster, 1998.

Boushey, C., S. Beresford et al. "A Quantitative Assessment of Plasma Homocysteine as a Risk Factor for Vascular Disease. Probable Benefits of Increasing Folic Acid Intakes." *Journal of the American Medical Association* 274 (4 October 1995): 1049–57.

Challem, J. "The B-Vitamins and Heart Disease." *Nutrition Reporter* 153 (1995). http://www.jrthorns.com/challem

Fallest-Strobl, P, et al. "Homocysteine: A New Risk Factor for Atherosclerosis." *American Family Physician* 56 (15 October 1997): 1607–12.

Griffith, H. *The Complete Guide to Vitamins, Minerals and Supplements.* Tucson: Fisher Books, 1988.

"High Homocysteine Concentration Raises Risk of Carotid Stenosis in Elderly." *Medical Sciences Bulletin* (March 1995).

"The Homocysteine Saga: B6, B12, and Folate." *Medical Sciences Bulletin* (April 1994).

Hultberg B., M. Berglund, A. Andersson and A. Frank. "Elevated Plasma Homocysteine in Alcoholics." *Alcohol Clin Exp Res* 17:3 (1993): 687–89.

"Lowering Blood Homocysteine With Folic Acid Based Supplements: Meta-Analysis of Randomised Trials." *British Medical Journal* 316:21 (1998): 894–98.

Magaziner, A. "Homocysteine: A New Risk Factor for Heart Disease." http://www.healthy.net/pan/chg/faim/newslet/96–01/ homocyst.htm

McCully, K. "Vascular Pathology of Homocysteinemia: Implications for the Parthogenesis of Arteriosclerosis." *American Journal of Pathology* 56 (July 1969): 111–28.

McCully, K. "Chemical Pathology of Homocysteine. I. Atherogenesis." *Annals of Clinical and Laboratory Science* 23 (November–December 1993): 477–93.

McCully, K. and S. Kilmer. "Homocysteine, Folate, Vitamin B-6, and Cardiovascular Disease." *Journal of the American Medical Association* 279 (4 February 1998): 392–93.

Moghadasian, M. et al. "Homocysteine and Coronary Artery Disease." *Archives of Internal Medicine* 157 (10 November 1997): 2299–308.

Nygard, O. et al. "Coffee Consumption and Plasma Total Homocysteine: the Hordaland Homocysteine Study." *American Journal of Clinical Nutrition* 65 (1997): 136–43.

Rimm, Eric B., et al. "Folate and Vitamin B-6 From Diet and Supplements in Relation to Risk of Coronary Heart Disease Among Women." *Journal of the American Medical Association* 279 (4 February 1998): 359–64.

Selhub J. et al. "Association Between Plasma Homocysteine Concentrations and Extracranial Carotid-artery Stenosis." *New England Journal of Medicine* 332 (1995): 286–91.

Stampfer M. and W. Willett. "Homocysteine and Marginal Vitamin Deficiency: The Importance of Adequate Vitamin Intake." *Journal of the American Medical Association* 270 (1993): 2726–27.

Ubbink J. "Vitamin B-12, Vitamin B-6, and Folate Nutritional Status in Men with Hyperhomocysteinemia." *American Journal of Clinical Nutrition* 57 (January 1993): 47–53.

CHAPTER FIFTEEN: Insomnia

American Institute of Preventative Medicine: "Insomnia." http://www.healthy.ney/hwlibrarybooks/healthyself/womens/insomnia.htm HealthWorld Online, 1996.

Aoyagi, N., R. Kimura and T. Murata. "Studies on *Passiflora incarnata* Dry Extract. I. Isolation of Maltol and Ethylmaltol

and Pharmacological Action of Maltol and Ethylmaltol."
Chemical and Pharmaceutical Bulletin 22 (1974): 1008–13.

Balderer, G. and A. Borbely. "The Effect of Valerian on Human
Sleep." *Psychopharmacology* 87 (1985): 406–09.

Bundesanzeiger (30 November 1985).

Bundesanzeiger (March 1990).

Campbell, S. et al. "Alleviation of Sleep Maintenance Insomnia
With Timed Exposure to Bright Light." *Journal of the American Geriatrics Society* 41 (August 1993): 829–36.

Duke, J. *The Green Pharmacy.* Emmaus: Rodale, 1997.

"Experts: Melatonin Hormone Unproven as Sleep Aid." AP (4
September 1997).

Foreman, J. "So, You're Stuck in Sleep-Loss Hell." *Boston
Globe* (17 September 1997).

Hoffman, D. "Passion Flower *Passiflora incarnata.*"
http://www/healthy.net./hwlibrarybooks/hoffman/materiamed-
ica/passion. htm HealthWorld Online, 1996.

Houghton, P. "The Biological Activity of Valerian and Related
Plants." *Journal of Ethnopharmacology* 327 (February/
March 1988): 121–42.

"Insomnia and Valerian Root (Valeriana Officinalis)."
http://www.eurohost.com/docwelln/vr.html Center for Health,
1996.

Jadrnak, J. "Filling in the Gaps on Melatonin." *Albuquerque
Journal* (2 February 1998).

Kamura, R. et al. "Central Depressant Effects of Maltol Analogs
in Mice." *Chemical and Pharmaceutical Bulletin* 28 (1980):
2570–79.

Lawrence Review of Natural Products (May 1988).

Leathwood, P. and E. Chauffard. "Quantifying the Effects of
Mild Sedatives." *Journal of Psychiatric Research* 17 (1983):
115–22.

———."Aqueous Extract of Valerian Reduces Latency to Fall
Asleep in Man." *Planta Medica* 54 (1985): 144–48.

Leathwood, P., F. Chauffard, E. Heck and R. Munoz-Box.
"Aqueous Extract of Valerian Root (Valeriana Officinalis L.)

Improves Sleep Quality in Man." *Pharmacological and Biochemical Behavior* 17 (July 1982): 65–71.

Leathwood, P. et al. "Aquenous Extract of Valerian Root Improves Sleep Quality in Man." *Pharmacology and Biochemical Behavior* 17 (1982): 65–71.

Lieberman, S. and N. Bruning. *The Real Vitamin and Mineral Book.* Tucson: Avery, 1990.

Lindahl, O. and L. Lindwall. "Double-Blind Study of a Valerian Preparation." *Pharmacological and Biochemical Behavior* 327 (April 1989): 1065–66.

Mann, Denise: "Jury Still Out on Melatonin." *New York Times* (3 March 1997).

Mayell, M. *Off-the-Shelf Natural Health.* New York: Bantam, 1995.

Mills, S. *The Dictionary of Modern Herbalism,* San Francisco: Thorsons, 1985.

Natural Products Research Consultants: "Nature's Answer to Insomnia and Anxiety." Seattle, Washington, 1998. http://www.cats-claw.com/products/val-lab.html

Newall, C., L. Anderson and J. D. Phillipson. *Herbal Medicines.* London: Pharmaceutical Press, 1996.

Nicholls, J. "Pasicol, an Antibacterial and Antifungal Agent Produced by *Passiflora* Plant Species." *Antimicrobial Agents and Chemotherapy* 3 (1973): 110–17.

Reichenberg-Ullman, J. and R. Ullman. "Sleep Easy." http://www.healthy.net/hwlibraryarticles/rbullman/sleepeas.htm HealthWorld Online, 1996.

Reynolds, J., ed. *Martindale: The Extra Pharmapcopoeia,* 29th ed. London: Pharmaceutical Press, 1989.

Sakamoto, T., Y. Mitani and K. Nakajima. "Psychotropic Effects of Japanese Valerian Root Extract." *Chemical Pharmaceutical Bulletin* 40 (March 1992): 758–61.

Schulz, H. and M. Jobert. "Effects of Hypericum Extract on the Sleep EEG in Older Volunteers." *Journal of Geriatric Psychiatry and Neurology* 7:Supplement 1 (October 1994): S39–S43.

Schulz, H., C. Stolz and J. Muller. "The Effect of Valerian Extract on Sleep Polygraphy in Poor Sleepers: A Pilot Study." *Pharmacopsychiatry* 27 (July 1994): 147–51.

Speroni, E. and A. Minghetti. "Neuropharmacological Activity of Extracts From *Passiflora Incarnata.*" *Planta Medica* 54 (1988): 488–91.

Tyler, V. *The Honest Herbal.* 3d ed. Binghamton: Pharmaceutical Products Press, 1993.

———.*Herbs of Choice.* Binghamton: Pharmaceuticals Products Press, 1994.

Warner, D. "Seniors: Helping the Elderly Sleep Like Babies." *Detroit News* (7 February 1997).

Willard, T. "Insomnia: Wake Up to Ten Simple Solutions." http://www.healthy.net/hwlibraryarticles/hfn/sleep.htm HealthWorld Online, 1996.

Willard, Terry. *Herbs and their Clinical Uses.* Mohomet: Wild Rose College of Natural Healing Ltd., 1996.

Zand, J. "Natural Medicine for Insomnia." http://www.healthy.net/hwlibraryarticles/zand/insomnia.htm Healthy.Net, 1996.

CHAPTER SIXTEEN: Kidney Stones

Bundesanzeiger (14 April 1984).

Chodera, A. et al. *Acta Poloniae Pharmeceutica* 42 (1985): 199–204.

Coe, F., et al. "Diet and Calcium: The End of an Era?" *Annals of Internal Medicine* 126 (1 April 1997): 553–55.

Curhan, G. et al. "A Prospective Study of Dietary Calcium and Other Nutrients and the Risk of Symptomatic Kidney Stones." *New England Journal of Medicine* 328 (25 March 1993): 833–38.

———."Comparison of Dietary Calcium with Supplemental Calcium and Other Nutrients as Factors Affecting the Risk of Kidney Stones in Women." *Annals of Internal Medicine* 126 (1 April 1997): 497–504.

Curhan, G. and S. Curhan. "Dietary Factors and Kidney Stone Formation." *Comprehensive Therapy* 20:9 (1994): 485–89.

Editors of *Prevention* Magazine Health Books: "Kidney Stones" in *Vitamin Prescriptions for Healing*. Emmans, Pa.: Rodale Press, 1997.

Grieve, M. *A Modern Herbal,* 1931. http://www.botanical.com/botanical/mgmh/g/golrod26.html.

Kemp, N. and Don, B. "Kidney Stones: Metabolic Evaluation and Diagnosis." http://www.healthline.com Kidney Health, 1994.

"Kidney Stones: Myth and Fact." *UC Berkeley Wellness Letter* (March 1998).

"Magnesium May Counterbalance Calcium." http://www.prevention.com/healing/vitamin/kidneys/more2.html; Wire Networks and Rodale Press, 1997.

McMurdo, M., P. Davey, M. A. Elder et al. "A Cost-Effectiveness Study of the Management of Intractable Urinary Incontinence by Urinary Catheterisation or Incontinence Pads." *Journal of Epidemiology and Community Health* 46 (1992): 222–26.

"Protection with Potassium Power." http://www.prevention.com/healing/vitamin/kidneys/more2.html; Wire Networks and Rodale Press, 1997.

Reznicek, G. et al. *Planta Medica* 58 (1992): 94–98.

Tyler, V. *Herbs of Choice*. Binghamton: Pharmaceutical Products Press, 1994.

"Vitamin B6 Provides Anti-Oxalate Protection." http://www.prevention.com/healing/vitamin/kidneys/more2.html; Wire Networks, Inc. and Rodale Press, 1997.

CHAPTER SEVENTEEN: Liver

Albrecht, M. "Therapy of Toxic Liver Pathologies With Legalon." *Zeitschrift für Klinischen Medizin* 47:2 (1992): 87–92.

American Liver Foundation: http://gi.ucsf.edu/ALF.

Atkins, R. *Dr. Atkins' Vita-Nutrient Solution*. New York: Simon & Schuster, 1998.

Bundesanzeiger (13 March 1986).

Buzzelli, G. "A Pilot Study on the Liver Protective Effect of Silybin-Phosphatidycholine Complex (IdB1016) in Chronic Active Hepatitis." *International Journal of Pharmacological Therapy and Toxicology* 31 (1993): 456–60.

Duke, J. *The Green Pharmacy*. Emmaus, Pa.: Rodale, 1997.

Ferenci, P. et al. "Randomized Controlled Trial of Silymarin Treatment in Patients With Cirrhosis of the Liver." *Journal of Heptatology* 9 (July 1989): 105–13.

Flora, K., M. Hahn, H. Rosen and K. Brenner. "Milk Thistle (Silybum marianum) for the Therapy of Liver Disease." *American Journal of Gastroenterology* 93 (February 1998): 139–43.

Griffith, H. W. *Complete Guide to Symptoms, Illness, and Surgery*. New York: Putnam Berkley, 1995.

Hikino, H., Y. Kiso et al. "Antihepatoxic Actions of Flavanlignans From Silybum Marianum Fruits." *Planta Medica* 50 (1984): 248–50.

Kiesewetter, E. "Results of Two Double-Blind Studies on the Effect of Silymarin in Chronic Hepatitis." *Leber Magen Darm* 7 (1977): 318–23.

Lawrence Review of Natural Products (March 1988).

Leng-Peschlow, E. and A. Strenge-Hesse. *Zeitschrift für Phytotherapie* 12 (1991): 162–74.

Muzes, G. "Effect of the Bioflavonoid Silymarin on the In Vitro Activity and Expression of Superoxide Dismutase (SOD) Enzyme." *Acta Physiologia Hungaria* 78 (1991): 3–9.

Palasciano, G. "The Effect of Silymarin on Plasma Levels of Malon-Dialdehyde in Patients Receiving Long-Term Treatment With Psychotropic Drugs." *Current Therapeutic Research* 55:5 (May 1994): 537–45.

Sonnenbichler, J. and I. Zetl. *Planta Medica* Supplement A580 (1992).

Szilard, S. "Protective Effect of Legalon in Workers Exposed to

Organic Solvents." *Acta Medica Hungaria* 45:2 (1988): 249–56.

Tyler, V. *Herbs of Choice.* Binghamton: Pharmaceutical Products Press, 1994.

Valenzuela, A. et al. "Selectivity of Silymarin on the Increase of Glutathione in Different Tissues of the Rat." *Planta Medica* 55 (October 1989): 420–22.

Velussi, M. et al. *Current Therapeutic Research* 53:5 (May 1993): 533–45.

Zi, X., H. Mukhtar and R. Agarwal. "Novel Cancer Chemoprotective Effects of a Flavonoid Antioxidant Silymarin: Inhibition of mRNA Expression of an Edogenous Tumor Promoter TNF-Alpha." *Biochemical and Biophysical Research Communication* 239 (9 October 1997): 334–39.

CHAPTER EIGHTEEN: Male Sexuality and Fertility

Atkins, R. *Dr. Atkins' Vita-Nutrient Solution.* New York: Simon and Schuster, 1998.

Bahrke, M. and W. Morgan. "Evaluation of the Ergogenic Properties of Ginseng." *Sports Medicine* 18:4 (October 1994): 229–48.

Baldwin, C. et al. "What Pharmacists Should Know About Ginseng." *Pharm* J 237 (1986): 583–86.

Banerjee, U. and J. Izquierdo. "Antistress and Antifatigue Properties of Panax Ginseng: Comparison with Piracetam." *Acta Physiol Lat Am* 32: 4 (1982): 277–85.

Behne, D., H. Weiler and A. Kyriakopoulos. "Effects of Selenium Deficiency on Testicular Morphology and Function in Rats." *J Reprod Fertil* 106 (1996): 291–97.

Bundesanzeiger (14 August 1987).

Bundesanzeiger (1 February 1990).

Caso-Marasco, A., R. Vargas-Ruiz, A. Salas-Villagomez and C. Begona-Infante. "Double-Blind Study of a Multivitamin Complex Supplemented With Ginseng Extract." *Drugs Exp Clin Res* 22:6 (1996): 323–29.

Choi, H., D. Seong and K. Rha. "Clinical Efficacy of Korean

Red Ginseng for Erectile Dysfunction." *International Journal of Impotence Research* 7:3 (September 1995): 181–86.

Engels, H. and J. With. "No Ergogenic Effects of Ginseng (Panax Ginseng C.a. Meyer) During Graded Maximal Aerobic Exercise." *J Am Diet Assoc* 97:10 (October 1997): 1110–15.

Fahim, M., Z. Fahim, J. Harman et al. "Effect of Panax Ginseng on Testosterone Level and Prostate in Male Rats." *Archives of Andrology* 8:4 (June 1982): 261–63.

Grabek, M., A. Swies and A. Borzecki. "The Influence of Selenium on the Reproduction of Rats." *Ann Univ Mariae Curie Sklodowska* 46 (1991): 103–05.

Griffith, H. W. *Complete Guide to Vitamins, Minerals & Supplements.* Tucson: Fisher Books, 1988.

Herold, E., J. Mottin and Z. Sabry. "Effect of Vitamin E on Human Sexual Functioning." *Archives of Sexual Behavior* 8:5 (1979): 397–403.

Kessopoulou, E., H. Powers, K. Sharma et al. "A Double-Blind Randomized Placebo Crossover Controlled Trial Using the Antioxidant Vitamin E to Treat Reactive-Oxygen-Species-Associated Male Infertility." *Fertility and Sterility* 64:4 (October 1995): 825–31.

Kim, C., H. Choi, C. Kim et al. "Influence of Ginseng on Mating Behavior of Male Rats." *American Journal of Chinese Medicine* 4:2 (Summer 1976): 163–68.

"Male Infertility" Mayo Clinic (6 February 1997). http://www.mayohealth.org/mayo/9702/htm/male–inf.htm

Moilanen, J. and O. Hovatta. "Excretion of Alpha-Tocopherol Into Human Seminal Plasma After Oral Administration." *Andrologia* 27:3 (May–June 1995): 133–36.

Newall, C., L. Anderson and J. D. Phillipson. *Herbal Medicines: a Guide for Healthcare Professionals.* Pharmaceutical Press, 1996.

Petkov, V. and A. Mosharrof. "Effects of Standardized Ginseng Extract on Learning, Memory, and Physical Capabilities."

American Journal of Chinese Medicine 15:1–2 (1987): 19–29.

Salvati, G., G. Genovesi, L. Marcellini et al. "Effects of Panax Ginseng C.a. Meyer Saponins on Male Fertility." *Panminerva Ped* 38:4 (December 1996): 249–54.

Scott, R., A. MacPherson and R. Yates. "Selenium Supplementation in Subfertile Human Males." In P. Fischer, M. L'AlAbbé, K. Cockell and R. Gibson, eds. *Trace Elements in man and Animals-9 (Tema 9)* Ottawa: NRC Research Press, 1997.

Sies, H., W. Stahl, A. Sundquist. "Antioxidant Functions of Vitamins. Vitamins E and C, Beta-Carotene, and Other Carotenoids." *Annals of the New York Academy of Sciences* 669 (30 September 1992): 7–20.

Suleiman, S., M. Ali, Z. Zaki et al. "Lipid Peroxidation and Human Sperm Motility: Protective Role of Vitamin E." *J Androl* 17:5 (October 1996): 530–37.

Thérond P., J. Auger, A. Legrand and P. Jouannet. "Alpha-Tocopherol in Human Spermatozoa and Seminal Plasma: Relationships With Motility, Antioxidant Enzymes, and Leukocytes." *Mol Hum Reprod* 2:10 (October 1996): 739–44.

Wallace E., H. Calvin, K. Ploetz, and G. Cooper. "Functional and Developmental Studies on the Role of Selenium in Spermatogenesis." 181–96 in G. Combs, O. Levander, J. Spallholz, and J. Oldfield, eds. *Selenium in Biology and Medicine.* Vol A. AVI, 1987.

"Why Erections Don't Happen." Mayo Clinic (20 January 1997).
http://www.mayohealth.org/mayo/9701/htm/impo–sb.htm

Zhao, X. "Antisenility Effect of Ginseng-Rhizome Saponin." *Chung Hsi I Chieh Ho Tsa Chih* 10:10 (October 1990): 586–89.

CHAPTER NINETEEN: Memory and Mental Alertness

Agus, D., S. Gambhir, W. Pardridge et al. "Vitamin C Crosses the Blood-Brain Barrier in the Oxidized Form Through the

Glucose Transporters." *Journal of Clinical Investigation* 100:11 (December 1997): 2842–48.

Allain, H., P. Raoul, A. Lieury et al. "Effect of Two Doses of Ginkgo Biloba Extract (Egb 761) on the Dual-Coding Test in Elderly Subjects." *Clin Ther 15* (1993): 549–58.

American Psychiatric Association. *Diagnostic and Statistical Manual IV.* Washington: American Psychiatric Association Press, 1994.

Banazak, D. "Difficult Dementia: Six Steps to Control Problem Behaviors." *Geriatrics* 51 (February 1996): 36–42.

Bella, R., R. Biondi, R. Raffaele and G. Pennisi. "Effect of Ace-tyl-l-carnitine on Geriatric Patients Suffering From Dys-thymic Disorders." *Int J Clin Pharmacol Res* 10 (1990): 355–60.

Bonavita, E. "Study of the Efficacy and Tolerability of L-Acetylcarnitine Therapy in the Senile Brain." *Int J Clin Pharmacol Ther Toxicol* 24 (1986): 511–16.

Calvani, M. et al. "Action of Acetyl-L-Carnitine in Neuro-degeneration and Alzheimer's Disease." *Annals of the New York Academy of Science* 663 (1992): 483–86.

Cano-Cuenca, B., J. Marco-Algarra, B. Pérez del Valle. "The Effect of Gingko Biloba on Cochleovestibulary++Pathology of Vascular Origin." *An Otorrinolaringol Ibero Am* 22:6 (1995): 619–29.

Carta A., et al. "Acetyl-l-carnitine and Alzheimer's Disease: Pharmacological Considerations Beyond the Cholinergic Sphere." *Annals of the New York Academy of Sciences* 695 (1993): 324–26.

Caso-Marasco, A., R. Vargas-Ruiz, A. Villagomez and C. Begona-Infante. "Double-Blind Study of a Multivitamin Complex Supplemented With Ginseng Extract." *Drugs Exp Clin Res* 22:6 (1996): 323–29.

Challem, J. "Acetyl-L-Carnitine Supplements Slow Progression of Alzheimer's Disease." *Nutrition Reporter* 153 (1995). http://www.thorne.com

Cipolli, C. and G. Chiari. "Effects of L-Acetylcarnitine on

Mental Deterioration in the Aged: Initial Results." *Clin Ter* 132 (1990): 479–510.

Claussen, C. "Diagnostic and Practical Value of Craniocorpography in Vertiginous Syndromes." *Presse Med* 15 (1986): 1565–68.

Debert, W. "Interaction Between Psychological and Pharmacological Treatment in Cognitive Impairment." *Life Sciences* 55:25 (1994): 2057–66.

DeFalco, F. et al. "Effect of the Chronic Treatment with L-Acetylcarnitine in Down's Syndrome." *Clin Ther* 144 (1994): 123–27.

Diamond, D., M. Fleshner, N. Ingersoll and G. Rose. "Psychological Stress Impairs Spatial Working Memory: Relevance to Electrophysiological Studies of Hippocampal Function." *Behavioral Neuroscience* 10 (August 1996): 4661–72.

Diwok, M., B. Kuklinski and B. Ernst. "Superoxide Dismutase Activity of Ginkgo Biloba Extract." *Z Gesamte Inn Med* 47:7 (July 1992): 308–11.

Dumont, E., P. D'Arbigny and A. Nouvelot. "Protection of Polyunsaturated Fatty Acids Against Iron-Dependent Lipid Peroxidation by a Ginkgo Biloba Extract (EGb 761)." *Methods Find Exp Clin Pharmacol* 17 (1995): 83–88.

Eckmann, F. "Cerebral Insufficiency—Treatment with Ginkgo-Biloba Extract. Time of Onset of Effect in a Double-Blind Study With 60 Inpatients." *Fortschr Med* 108 (1990): 557–60.

Etienne, A., F. Hecquet and F. Clostre. "Mechanism of Action of Ginkgo Biloba Extract in Experimental Cerebral Edema." *Presse Med* 15:31 (25 September 1986): 1506–10.

Gecele, M., G. Francesetti and A. Meluzzi. "Acetyl-L-Carnitine in Aged Subjects With Major Depression: Clinical Efficacy and Effects on the Circadian Rhythm of Cortisol." *Dementia* 2 (1991): 333–37.

Gerhardt, G., K. Rogalla, J. Jaeger. "Drug Therapy of Disorders of Cerebral Performance. Randomized Comparative Study of

Dihydroergotoxine and Ginkgo Biloba Extract." *Fortschritte Med* 108 (1990): 384–88.

Gessner, B., A. Voelp, M. Klasser. "Study of the Long-Term Action of a Ginkgo Biloba Extract on Vigilance and Mental Performance as Determined by Means of Quantitative Pharmaco-EEG and Psychometric Measurements." *Arzneimittelforschung* 35:1 (1985): 1459–65.

"Ginkgo Biloba." International Health News Database. http://vvv.com/healthnews/

Grassel, E. "Effect of Ginkgo-Biloba Extract on Mental Performance. Double-Blind Study Using Computerized Measurement Conditions in Patients with Cerebral Insufficiency." *Fortschritte der Medezin* 110 (1992): 73–76.

Guarnaschelli, C., G. Fugazza and C. Pistarini. "Pathological Brain Ageing: Evaluation of the Efficacy of a Pharmacological Aid." *Drugs Exp Clin Res* 14 (1988): 715–18.

Haguenauer, J., F. Cantenot, H. Koskas and H. Pierart. "Treatment of Equilibrium Disorders With Ginkgo Biloba Extract. A Multicenter Double-Blind Drug Vs. Placebo Study." *Presse Med* 15 (1986): 1569–72.

Haramaki, N., S. Aggarwal and T. Kawabata et al. "Effects of Natural Antioxidant Ginkgo Biloba Extract (EGb 761) on Myocardial Ischemia-Reperfusion Injury." *Free Radic Biol Med* 16 (1994): 789–94.

Hofferberth, B. "The Effect of Ginkgo Biloba Extract on Neurophysiological and Psychometric Measurement Results in Patients With Psychotic Organic Brain Syndrome. A Double-Blind Study Against Placebo." *Arzneimittelforschung* 39 (1989): 918–22.

Holgers, K., A. Axelsson and I. Pringle. "Ginkgo Biloba Extract for the Treatment of Tinnitus." *Audiology* 33 (1994): 85–92.

Hopfenmuller, W. "Proof of the Therapeutical Effectiveness of a Ginkgo Biloba Special Extract—Meta-Analysis of 11 Clinical Trials in Aged Patients With Cerebral Insufficiency." *Arzneim-Forsch* 44 (1994): 1005–13.

Huguet, F. and T. Tarrade. "Alpha 2-Adrenoceptor Changes

During Cerebral Ageing. The Effect of Ginkgo Biloba Extract." *J Pharm Pharmacol* 44:1 (January 1992): 24–27.

Itil, T., D. Martorano. "Natural Substances in Psychiatry (Ginkgo Biloba in Dementia)." *Psychopharmacol Bull* 31 (1995): 147–58.

Kaneto, H. "Learning/Memory Processes Under Stress Conditions." *Behav Brain Res* 83:1–2 (February 1997): 71–74.

Kanowski, S., W. Herrmann, K. Stephan et al. "Proof of Efficacy of the Ginkgo Biloba Special Extract EGb 761 in Outpatients Suffering From Mild to Moderate Primary Degenerative Dementia of the Alzheimer Type or Multi-Infarct Dementia." *Pharmacopsychiatry* 29 (1996): 47–56.

Kleijnen, J. and P. Knipschild. "Ginkgo Biloba for Cerebral Insufficiency." *British Journal of Clinical Pharmacology* 34 (1992): 352–58.

Koltringer, P., O. Eber, G. Klima et al. "Microcirculation in Parenteral Ginkgo Biloba Extract Therapy." *Wien Klin Wochenschr* 101 (1989): 198–200.

Korol, D. and P. Gold. "Glucose, Memory, and Aging." *American Journal of Clinical Nutrition* 67:4 Supplement (April 1998): 764–71.

Lawlor, B. and T. Sunderland. "Alzheimer's Disease: A Strategy for Coping With Behavioral Changes." *Consultant* 34:1 (1994): 43–46.

Le Bars, P., M. Katz, N. Berman et al. "A Placebo-Controlled, Double-Blind, Randomized Trial of an Extract of Ginkgo Biloba for Dementia. North American EGb Study Group." *Journal of the American Medical Association* 278 (1997): 1327–32.

Lupien, S., S. Gaudreau, B. Tchiteya et al. "Stress-Induced Declarative Memory Impairment in Healthy Elderly Subjects: Relationship to Cortisol Reactivity." *Journal of Clinical Endocrinology and Metabolism* 82:7 (July 1997): 2070–75.

Magarinos, A., J. Verdugo and B. McEwen. "Chronic Stress Alters Synaptic Terminal Structure in Hippocampus." Proceedings of the National Academy of Sciences of the USA 94:25 (9 December 1997): 14002–08.

Maitra, I., L. Marcocci, M. Droy-Lefaix MT and L. Packer. "Peroxyl Radical Scavenging Activity of Ginkgo Biloba Extract EGb 761." *Biochem Pharmacol* 49 (1995): 1649–55.

Marcocci, L., L. Packer, M. Droy-Lefaix MT et al. "Antioxidant Action of Ginkgo Biloba Extract EGb 761." *Methods of Enzymology* 234 (1994): 462–75.

Meyer, B. "A Multicenter Study of Tinnitus. Epidemiology and Therapy." *Ann Otolaryngol Chir Cervicofac* 103 (1986): 185–88.

———."Multicenter Randomized Double-Blind Drug Vs. Placebo Study of the Treatment of Tinnitus With Ginkgo Biloba Extract." *Presse Med* 15 (1986): 1562–64.

Oyama, Y., L. Chikahisa, T. Ueha et al. "Ginkgo Biloba Extract Protects Brain Neurons Against Oxidative Stress Induced by Hydrogen Peroxide." *Brain Research* 712:2 (18 March 1996): 349–52.

Passeri, M., D. Cucinotta, P. Bonati et al. "Acetyl-L-Carnitine in the Treatment of Mildly Demented Elderly Patients." *Int J Clin Pharmacol Res* 10:1 (1990): 75–79.

Perrig, W. et al. "The Relation Between Antioxidants and Memory Performance in the Old and Very Old." *Journal of the American Geriatrics Society* 45 (June 1997): 718–24.

Pettegrew, J., W. Klunk, K. Panchalingam et al. "Clinical and Neurochemical Effects of Acetyl-L-Carnitine in Alzheimer's Disease." *Neurobiol Aging* 16:1 (January–February 1995): 1–4.

Pietri, S., E. Maurelli, K. Drieu, M. Culcasi. "Cardioprotective and Anti-Oxidant Effects of the Terpenoid Constituents of Ginkgo Biloba Extract (EGb 761)." *J Mol Cell Cardiol* 29 (1997): 733–42.

Raabe, A., M. Raabe, P. Ihm. "Therapeutic Follow-Up Using Automatic Perimetry in Chronic Cerebroretinal Ischemia in Elderly Patients. Prospective Double-Blind Study With Graduated Dose Ginkgo Biloba Treatment." *Klin Monatsbl Augenheilkd* 199 (1991): 432–38.

Rai, G. et al. "Double-Blind, Placebo Controlled Study of Acetyl-L-Carnitine in Patients With Alzheimer's Dementia." *Curr Med Res Opin* 11 (1990): 638–47.

Rai, G., C. Shovlin and K. Wesnes. "A Double-Blind, Placebo Controlled Study of Ginkgo Biloba Extract in Elderly Out-Patients With Mild to Moderate Memory Impairment." *Curr Med Res Opin* 12 (1991): 350–55.

Ramassamy, C., Y. Christen, F. Clostre and J. Costentin. "The Ginkgo Biloba Extract, Egb761, Increases Synaptosomal Uptake of 5-Hydroxytryptamine: In-Vitro and Ex-Vivo Studies." *J Pharm Pharmacol* 44:11 (November 1992): 943–45.

Rowin, J. and S. Lewis. "Spontaneous Bilateral Subdural Hematomas Associated With Chronic Ginkgo Biloba Ingestion." *Neurology* 46 (1996): 1775–76.

Sano, M., C. Ernesto, R. Thomas et al. "A Controlled Trial of Selegiline, Alpha-Tocopherol, or Both as Treatment for Alzheimer's Disease." *New England Journal of Medicine* 336:17 (24 April 1997).

Sano, M. et al. "Double-Blind Parallel Design Pilot Study of Acetyl Levocarnitine in Patients With Alzheimer's Disease." *Arch Neurol* 49 (1992): 1137–41.

Schaffler, K. and P. Reeh. "Double Blind Study of the Hypoxia Protective Effect of Standardized Ginkgo Biloba Preparation After Repeated Administration in Healthy Subjects." *Arzneimittelforschung* 35 (1985): 1283–86.

Schneider, B. "Ginkgo Biloba Extract in Peripheral Arterial Diseases. Meta-Analysis of Controlled Clinical Studies." *Arzneim Forschung* 42 (1992): 428–36.

Schubert, H. and P. Halama. "Depressive Episode Primarily Unresponsive to Therapy in Elderly Patients: Efficacy of Ginkgo Biloba (EGb 761) in Combination With Antidepressants." *Geriatr Forsch* 3 (1993): 45–53.

Seeman, T., B. McEwen, B. Singer et al. "Increase in Urinary Cortisol Excretion and Memory Declines: Macarthur Studies of Successful Aging.'' *Journal of Clinical Endocrinology and Metabolism* 82:8 (August 1997): 2458–65.

Seif-El-Nasr, M. and A. El-Fattah. ''Lipid Peroxide, Phospholipids, Glutathione Levels and Superoxide Dismutase Activity in Rat Brain After Ischaemia: Effect of Ginkgo Biloba Extract.'' *Pharmacol Res* 32:5 (November 1995): 273–78.

Sinforiani, E., et al. ''Neuropsychological Changes in Demented Patients Treated With Acetyl-L-Carnitine.'' *Int J Clin Pharmacol Res* 10 (1990): 69–74.

Smith, P., K. Maclennan and C. Darlington. ''The Neuroprotective Properties of the Ginkgo Biloba Leaf: A Review of the Possible Relationship to Platelet-Activating Factor (Paf).'' *Journal of Ethnopharmacology* 50 (1996): 131–39.

Spagnoli A. et al. ''Long-Term Acetyl-L-Carnitine Treatment in Alzheimer's Disease.'' *Neurology* 41 (1991): 1726–32.

Taillandier, J., A. Ammar, J. Rabourdin et al. ''Treatment of Cerebral Aging Disorders With Ginkgo Biloba Extract. A Longitudinal Multicenter Double-Blind Drug Vs. Placebo Study.'' *Presse Med* 15:31 (25 September 1986): 1583–87.

Tempesta E. et al. ''Role of Acetyl-L-Carnitine in the Treatment of Cognitive Deficit in Chronic Alcoholism.'' *Int J Clin Pharmacol Res* 10 (1990): 101–07.

Thal, L., A. Carta, W. Clarke et al. ''A One-year Multicenter Placebo-Controlled Study of Acetyl-L-Carnitine in Patients With Alzheimer's Disease.'' *Neurology* 47:3 (September 1996): 705–11.

Thommessen, B. and K. Laake. ''No Identifiable Effect of Ginseng (Gericomplex) as an Adjuvant in the Treatment of Geriatric Patients.'' *Aging* 8:6 (December 1996): 417–20.

Tomlinson, B., A. Blessed and M. Roth. ''Observations on the Brains of Demented Old People.'' *J Neurol Sci* 11 (1970): 205–42.

Tyler, V. *Herbs of Choice*. Binghamton: Pharmaceutical Products Press, 1994.

Warburton, D. "Clinical Psychopharmacology of Ginkgo Biloba Extract." *Presse Med* 15:31 (25 September 1986): 1595–604.

Witte, S., I. Anadere, and E. Walitza. "Improvement of Hemorheology with Ginkgo Biloba Extract. Decreasing a Cardiovascular Risk Factor." *Fortschritte der Medizin* 110:13 (10 May 1992): 247–50.

CHAPTER TWENTY: Menopause, PMS, and Other Menstrual Problems

Abraham, G. "Nutritional Factors in the Etiology of the Premenstrual Tension Syndromes." *Journal of Reproductive Medicine* 28 (1983): 446–64.

Atkins, R. *Dr. Atkins' Vita-Nutrient Solution.* New York: Simon & Schuster, 1998.

Barber, H. "Evening Primrose Oil: A Panacea?" *Pharmaceutical Journal* 240 (1988): 723–25.

Barr, W. "Pyridoxine Supplements in the Premenstrual Syndrome." *Practitioner* 228 (1984): 425–27.

Brody, J. "Diet Linked to Menopause Complaints." *New York Times* (1997).

Brown, D. "Vitex Agnus Castus." *Quarterly Review of Natural Medicine* (Summer 1994): 111–20.

Brush, M. "Efamol (Evening Primrose Oil) in the Treatment of Premenstrual Syndrome." in D. Horrobin, ed. *Clinical Uses For Essential Fatty Acids.* Princeton: Eden Press, 1982.

Bundesanzeiger (5 January 1989).

Christy, C. "Vitamin E in Menopause." *American Journal of Obstetrics and Gynecology* 50 (1945): 84–87.

Coeugniet, E. et al. "Premenstrual Syndrome (PMS) and Its Treatment." *Arztezeitschrift für Naturhailverf* 27:9 (1986): 619–22.

Dittmar, F. et al. "Premenstrual Syndrome (PMS): Treated With a Phytopharmaceutical." *Gynäkologie* 5:1 (1992): 60–68.

Duke, J. *The Green Pharmacy.* Emmaus: Rodale Press, 1997.

Düker, E. M., L. Kopanski, H. Jarry and W. Wutke. "Effects of Extracts From Cimicifuga Racemosa on Gonadotropin Re-

lease in Menopausal Women and Ovariectomized Rats.''
Planta Medica 57 (1991): 420–24.

Elias, M. ''Aging. Mind And Menopause.'' *Harvard Health Letter* 19:1 (1993): 1–3.

Facchinetti, F. et al. ''Oral Magnesium Successfully Relieves Premenstrual Mood Changes.'' *Obstetrics and Gynecology* 78:2 (August 1991): 177–81.

Feldmann, H. et al. ''The Treatment of Corpus Luteum Insufficiency and Premenstrual Syndrome: Experience in a Multicenter Study Under Practice Conditions.'' *Hygne* 11:12 (1990): 421.

Finkler, R. ''The Effect of Vitamin E in the Menopause.'' *Journal of Clinical Endocrinology and Metabolism* 9 (1949): 89–94.

Gonzalez, E. ''Vitamin E Relieves Most Cystic Breast Disease; May Alter Lipids, Hormones.'' *Journal of the American Medical Association* 244:10 (5 September 1980): 1077.

Griffith, H. W. *Complete Guide to Symptoms, Illness and Surgery.* New York: Putnam Berkley Group, 1995.

Hirata, J., L. Swiersz, R. Small and B. Ettinger. ''Does Dong Quai Have Estrogenic Effects in Postmenopausal Women? A Double-Blind, Placebo-Controlled Trial.'' *Fertility and Sterility* 68:6 (December 1977): 981–86.

Hobbs, C. ''Black Cohosh.'' *Herbs for Health* (March/April 1998): 38–40.

———.*Vitex: The Women's Herb.* Santa Cruz: Botanica Press, 1990.

Hooper, J. ''Does Menopause Really Begin in Your 30s?'' *New Woman* 27:8 (August 1997): 118–20, 123, 142.

Houghton, P. ''Agnus Castus.'' *Pharm Journal* 253 (1994): 720–21.

Ivie, G., D. Holt and M. Ivey. *Science* 213 (1981): 909–10.

Kliejnen, J. et al. ''Vitamin B6 in the Treatment of Premenstrual Syndrome—A Review.'' *British Journal Obstetrics and Gynecology* 97 (1990): 847–52.

Lauritzen, C., H. Reuter, R. Repges et al. ''Treatment of Premenstrual Tension Syndrome With *Vitex agnus-castus.* Controlled, Double-Blind Study Versus Pyridoxene." *Phytomedicine* 4:3 (1997): 183–89.

Lawrence Review of Natural Products (April 1986).

Lawrence Review of Natural Products (March 1989).

Lehmann-Willenbrock, E. and H. Riedel. "Clinical and Endocrinological Studies of the Treatments of Ovarian Insufficiency Manifestations Following Hysterectomy With Intact Adnexa." *Zentralblatt für Gynäkologie* 110 (1988): 611–81.

Li, Wan Po. "Evening Primrose Oil." *Pharmaceutical Journal* 246 (1991): 670–76.

Mayell, M. *Off the Shelf Natural Health.* New York: Bantam, 1995.

McLaren, H. "Vitamin E in the Menopause." *British Medical Journal* ii (1945): 1378–81.

Milewicz, A. et al. *"Vitex Agnus Castus* Extract in the Treatment of Late Luteal Phase Defects Due to Latent Hyperprolactinaemia. Results of a Randomized Placebo-Controlled Double-Blind Study." *ArzneimittleForsch* 43 (1993): 752–56.

Murkies, A., C. Lombard, B. Strauss et al. "Dietary Flour Supplementation Decreases Post-Menopausal Hot Flushes: Effect of Soy And Wheat." *Maturitas* 21 (April 1995): 189–95.

Newall, C., L. Anderson and J. D. Phillipson. *Herbal Medicines: a Guide for Health-Care Professionals.* London: Pharmaceutical Press, 1996.

Perlmutter, C. "Triumph Over Menopause." *Prevention* 46:8 (August 1994): 78–87, 137, 142.

Presse, J. "Nutritional Factors in the Premenstrual Syndrome." *International Clinical Nutrition Review* 4 (1984): 54–81.

Rosenstein, D. et al. "Magnesium Measures Across the Menstrual Cycle in Premenstrual Syndrome." *Biol Psychiatr* 35 (1994): 557–61.

Rubinow, D. and P. Schmidt. "The Treatment of Premenstrual Syndrome—Forward into the Past." *New England Journal of Medicine* 332:23 (8 June 1995).

Schmidt, P., L. Nieman, M. Danaceau et al. "Differential Behavioral Effects of Gonadal Steroids in Women With and in Those Without Premenstrual Syndrome." *New England Journal of Medicine* 338:4 (22 January 1998): 209–16.

Schwingl, P., B. Hulka and S. Harlow. "Risk Factors for Menopausal Hot Flashes." *Obstetrics and Gynecology* 84:1 (July 1994): 29–34.

Slade, M. "Managing Menopause." *American Health* 13:10 (December 1994): 66–69.

Snider, B. and D. Dieteman. "Pyridoxine Therapy for Premenstrual Acne Flair." *Archives of Dermatology*: 110 (1974): 103–11.

Turner, S. and S. Mills. "A Double-Blind Clinical Trial on an Herbal Remedy for Premenstrual Syndrome: A Case Study." *Complementary Therapies in Medicine* 1 (1993): 73–77.

Tyler, V. *The Honest Herbal.* 3rd ed. Binghamton: Pharmaceutical Products Press, 1993.

———. *Herbs of Choice.* Binghamton: Pharmaceutical Products Press, 1994.

Winterhoff, H., C. Gorkow and B. Behr. *Zeitschrift für Phytotherpie* 12 (1991): 175–79.

CHAPTER TWENTY-ONE: Osteoporosis

Almustafa, M., F. Doyle, D. Gutteridge et al. "Effects of Treatments by Calcium and Sex Hormones on Vertebral Fracturing in Osteoporosis." *Q J Med* 83:300 (April 1992): 283–94.

Aloia, J., A. Vaswani, J. Yeh. "Calcium Supplementation With and Without Hormone Replacement Therapy to Prevent Postmenopausal Bone Loss." *Annals of Internal Medicine* 120:2 (15 January 1995): 97–103.

Arnaud, C. and S. Sanchez. "The Role of Calcium in Osteoporosis." *Annual Review of Nutrition* 10 (1990): 397–414.

Barger-Lux, M. and R. Heaney. "The Role of Calcium Intake in Preventing Bone Fragility, Hypertension, and Certain Cancers." *J Nutr* 124:8 Supplement (August 1994): 1406–11.

Bernstein, C., L. Seeger, P. Anton et al. "A Randomized, Placebo-Controlled Trial of Calcium Supplementation for Decreased Bone Density in Corticosteroid-Using Patients With Inflammatory Bowel Disease: A Pilot Study.'' *Aliment Pharmacol Ther* 10:5 (October 1996): 777–86.

Bronner, F. ''Calcium and Osteoporosis.'' *American Journal of Clinical Nutrition* 60:6 (December 1994): 831–36.

Dawson-Hughes, B., G. Dallal, E. Krall et al. ''A Controlled Trial of the Effect of Calcium Supplementation on Bone Density in Postmenopausal Women.'' *New England Journal of Medicine* 323:13 (27 September 1990): 878–83.

Devine, A., I. Dick, S. Heal et al. ''A Four-Year Follow-Up Study of the Effects of Calcium Supplementation on Bone Density in Elderly Postmenopausal Women.'' *Osteoporos Int* 7:1 (1997): 23–28.

Fujita, T., Y. Fujii, R. Kitagawa and M. Fukase. ''Calcium Supplementation in Osteoporosis.'' *Osteoporos Int* 3 Supplement 1 (1993): 159–62.

Heaney, R., J. Gallagher, C. Johnston et al. ''Calcium Nutrition and Bone Health in the Elderly.'' *American Journal of Clinical Nutrition* 36:5 Supplement (November 1982): 986–1013.

Kaufman, J. ''Role of Calcium and Vitamin D in the Prevention and the Treatment of Postmenopausal Osteoporosis: An Overview.'' *Clinical Rheumatology* Supplement 3 (14 September 1995): 9–13.

Masi, L. and J. Bilezikian. ''Osteoporosis: New Hope for the Future.'' *Int J Fertile Women's Med* 42:4 (July–August 1997): 245–54.

Need, A., H. Morris and M. Horowitz. ''Intestinal Calcium Absorption in Men With Spinal Osteoporosis.'' *Clinical Endocrinology* 48:2 (February 1998): 163–68.

Nordin, B. ''Calcium and Osteoporosis.'' *Nutrition* 13:7–8 (July–August 1997): 664–86.

O'Brien, K. ''Combined Calcium and Vitamin D Supplementation Reduces Bone Loss and Fracture Incidence in Older Men and Women.'' *Nutrition Reviews* 56 (May 1998): 148–58.

O'Brien K., S. Abrams, L. Liang et al. ''Bone Turnover Response to Changes in Calcium Intake Is Altered in Girls and Adult Women in Families With Histories of Osteoporosis." *J Bone Miner Res* 13:3 (March 1998): 491–99.

Prince, R., A. Devine, I. Dick, A. Criddle. "The Effects of Calcium Supplementation (Milk Powder or Tablets) and Exercise on Bone Density in Postmenopausal Women." *J Bone Miner Res* 10:7 (July 1995): 1068–75.

Recker, R. "Prevention of Osteoporosis: Calcium Nutrition." *Osteoporos Int* 3 Supplement 1 (1993): 163–65.

Reid, I., R. Ames, M. Evans et al. "Effect of Calcium Supplementation on Bone Loss in Postmenopausal Women." *New England Journal of Medicine* 328:7 (18 February 1993): 460–64.

Slovik, D. "The Vitamin D Endocrine System, Calcium Metabolism, and Osteoporosis." *Spec Top Endocrinol Metab* 5 (1983): 83–148.

Spencer, H. and L. Kramer. "Osteoporosis, Calcium Requirement, and Factors Causing Calcium Loss." *Clinical Geriatric Medicine* 3:2 (May 1987): 389–402.

Uitterlinden A., H. Burger, Q. Huang. "Relation of Alleles of the Collagen Type Ialpha1 Gene to Bone Density and the Risk of Osteoporotic Fractures in Postmenopausal Women." *New England Journal of Medicine* 338:15 (9 April 1998): 1016–21.

Walden, O. "The Relationship of Dietary and Supplemental Calcium Intake to Bone Loss and Osteoporosis." *Journal of the American Dietetic Association* 89:3 (March 1989): 397–400.

CHAPTER TWENTY-TWO: Enlarged Prostate (BPH)

Braeckman, J. "The Extract of Serenoa Repens in the Treatment of Benign Prostatic Hyperplasia: A Multicenter Open Study." *Current Therapeutic Research* 55 (1994): 776–85.

Breu, W., F. Stadler, M. Hagenlocher and H. Wagner. *Zeitschrift für Phytotherapie* 13 (1992): 107–15.

Boccafoshi, C. "Confronto Fra Estratto di Serenoa Repens e Placebo Mediate Prove Clinical Controllata in Pazienti con Adenomatosi Prostatica." *Urologia* 50 (1983): 1257–68.

Bundesanzeiger (23 April 1987).

Bundesanzeiger (5 January 1989).

Bundesanzeiger (1 February 1990).

Bundesanzeiger (6 March 1990).

Carilla, E. et al. "Binding of Permixon, a New Treatment for Prostatic Benign Hyperplasia, to the Cytosolic Androgen Receptor in the Rat Prostate." *Journal of Steroid Biochemistry* 20 (1984): 521–23.

Casarosa, C. M. Di Coscio and M. Fratta. "Lack of Effects of a Lyposterolic Extract of Serenoa Repens on Plasma Levels of Testosterone, Follicle-stimulating Hormone, and Luteinizing Hormone." *Clinical Therapeutics* 10 (1988): 585–88.

Champault, G. et al. "Double-Blind Trial of an Extract of the Plant Serenoa Repens in Benign Prostate Hyperplasia." *British Journal of Clinical Pharmacology* 18 (1984): 461–62.

Duke, J. *Handbook of Medicinal Herbs.* Boca Raton: CRC, 1985.

El Sheikh, M., M. Dakkak and A. Saddique. "The Effect of Permixon on Androgen Receptors." *Acta Obstetrica and Gynecologica Scandinavica* 67 (1988): 397–99.

Glanze, W., ed. *The Signet/Mosby Medical Encyclopedia.* Signet, 1987.

Goetz, P. *Zeitschrift für Phytotherapie* 10 (1989): 175–78.

Hansel, R. and H. Haas. *Therapie mit Phytopharmaka.* Springer-Verlag, 1984.

Harnischfeger, G. and H. Stolze. *Zeitschrift für Phytotherapie* 10 (1989): 71–76.

Hirano, T., M. Homma and K. Oka. "Effects of Stinging Nettle Root Extracts and Their Steroidal Components on the Na+, K(+)-ATPase of the Benign Prostatic Hyperplasia." *Planta Medica* 60:1 (February 1994): 30–33.

Lichius, J. and C. Muth. "The Inhibiting Effects of Urtica Dioica Root Extracts on Experimentally Induced Prostatic Hyperplasia in the Mouse." *Planta Medica* 63:4 (August 1997): 307–10.

Mittman, P. "Randomized, Double-Blind Study of Freeze-Dried

Urtica Dioica in the Treatment of Allergic Rhinitis." *Planta Medica* 56:1 (February 1990): 44–47.

Murray, M. "Saw Palmetto Extract Vs. Proscar." *American Journal of Natural Medicine* 1:1 (1994): 8–9.

Newall, C., L. Anderson and J. D. Phillipson. *Herbal Medicines: A Guide for Health-Care Professionals.* London: Pharmaceutical Press, 1996.

"Prostate Enlargement: Benign Prostatic Hyperplasia." http://www.niddk.nih.gov/health/urolog/pubs/prsenlrg/prsenlrg.htm #aging.

Steinman, D. "Treating Prostate Troubles." *Natural Health* 23:6 (November/December 1993): 56–59.

Strauch, G. et al. "Comparison of Finasteride (Proscar) and Serenoa Repens (Permixon) in the Inhibition of 5-alpha Reductase in Healthy Male Volunteers." *European Urology* 26 (1994): 247–52.

Sultan, C. et al. "Inhibition of Androgen Metabolism and Binding by a Liposterolic Extract of 'Serenoa repens B' In Human Foreskin Fibroblasts." *Journal of Steroid Biochemistry* 20 (1984): 515–19.

Swanston-Flatt, S., C. Day, P. Flatt et al. "Glycemic Effects of Traditional European Plant Treatments for Diabetes. Studies in Normal and Streptozotocin Diabetic Mice." *Diabetes Research* 10:2 (1989): 69–73.

Tasca, A. et al. "Treatment of Obstruction in Prostatic Adenoma Using an Extract of Serenoa Repens: A Double-Blind Clinical Test Vs. Placebo." *Minn Urol Nefrol* 37 (1985): 87–91.

Twelves, C. "Folinic Acid Rescue and Methotrexate Toxicity." *The Lancet* (29 March 1986): 773.

Tyler, V. *Herbs of Choice.* Binghamton: Pharmaceutical Products Press, 1994.

———.*The Honest Herbal.* Binghamton: Pharmaceutical Products Press, 1994.

Vahlensieck, W., Jr. "Benigne Prostatahyperplasie: Behandlung mit Sabalfruchtestrakt." *Frotschrittle der Medezin* 111 (1993): 323–26.

Wagner, H. and H. Flachsbarth. "A New Antiphlogistic Principle From *Sabal serrulata*, I." *Planta Medica* 41 (1981): 244–51.

Wagner, H. et al. "A New Antiphlogistic Principle From *Sabal serrulata*, II." *Planta Medica* 41 (1981): 252–58.

Werbach, M. and M. Murray. *Botanical Influences on Illness.* Third Line Press, 1994.

CHAPTER TWENTY-THREE: Skin and Scalp

Afifi, A. et al. "High Dose Ascorbic Acid in the Management of Thalassemia Leg Ulcers—a Pilot Study." *British Journal of Dermatology* 92 (1975): 339.

Ardire, L. "Necrotizing Fasciitis: Case Study of a Nursing Dilemma." *Ostomy Wound Management* 43:5 (June 1997): 30–34, 36, 38–40.

Bassett, I., D. Pannowitz and R. Barnetson. "A Comparative Study of Tea Tree Oil Versus Benzoylperoxide in the Treatment of Acne." *Medical Journal of Austria* 153:8 (15 October 1990): 455–58.

Bhushan, M. and M. Beck. "Allergic Contact Dermatitis From Tea Tree Oil in a Wart Paint." *Contact Dermatitis* 36:2 (February 1997): 117–18.

Buck, D., D. Nidorf and J. Addino. "Comparison of Two Topical Preparations for the Treatment of Onychomycosis: Melaleuca Alternifolia (Tea Tree) Oil and Clotrimazole." *Journal Family Practice* 38:6 (June 1994): 601–05.

Carson, C. and T. Riley. "Antimicrobial Activity of the Major Components of the Essential Oil of Melaleuca Alternifolia." *J Appl Bacteriol* (March 1995): 264–69.

———. "Toxicity of the Essential Oil of Melaleuca Alternifolia or Tea Tree Oil." *J Toxicol Clin Toxicol* 33:2 (1995): 193–94.

Chithra, P., G. Sajithlal and G. Chandrakasan. "Influence of Aloe Vera on the Glycosaminoglycans in the Matrix of Healing Dermal Wounds in Rats." *Journal of Ethnopharmacology* 59:3 (January 1998): 179–86.

———. "Influence of Aloe Vera on the Healing of Dermal

Wounds in Diabetic Rats." *Journal of Ethnopharmacology* 59:3 (January 1998): 195–201.

Davis, R., J. Kabbani, and N. Maro. "Aloe Vera and Wound Healing." *J Am Pod Med Assoc* 77 (1987): 165–69.

Davis, R., W. Parker, R. Samson and D. Murdoch. "Isolation of a Stimulatory System in an Aloe Extract." *J Am Podiatr Med Assoc* 81:9 (September 1991): 473–78.

Del Beccaro, M. "Melaleuca Oil Poisoning in a Seventeen-Month-Old." *Vet Hum Toxicol* 37:6 (December 1995): 557–58.

DeNavarre, M. *The Chemistry and Manufacture of Cosmetics,* Vol. III, Carol Stream: Allured Publishing Corp., 1988.

Egger, S., G. Brown, L. Kelsey et al. "Studies on Optimal Dose and Administration Schedule of a Hematopoietic Stimulatory Beta-(1,4)-Linked Mannan." *International Journal of Immunopharmacology* 18:2 (February 1996): 113–26.

Faoagali, J., N. George and J. Leditscke. "Does Tea Tree Oil Have a Place in the Topical Treatment of Burns?" *Burns* 23:4 (23 June 1997): 349–51.

Foster, S. "Aloe Vera: The Succulent With Skin-Soothing, Cell-Protecting Properties." *Herbs for Health Magazine* http://www.healthy.net/hfh/articlesHFH/Aloe.htm

Fulton, J. "The Stimulation of Postdermabrasion Wound Healing With Stabilized Aloe Vera Gel-Polyethylene Oxide Dressing." *J Dermatol Surg Oncol* 16:5 (May 1990): 460–67.

Grindley, D. and T. Reynolds. "The Aloe Vera Phenomenon: A Review of the Properties and Modern Uses of the Leaf Parenchyma Gel." *Journal of Ethnopharmacology* 16 (1986): 117–51.

Gustafson, J., Y. Liew, S. Chew et al. "Effects of Tea Tree Oil on Escherichia Coli." *Lett Appl Microbiol* 26:3 (March 1998): 194–98.

Hackzell-Bradley, M., T. Bradley and T. Fischer. "A Case Report. Contact Allergy Caused by Tea Tree Oil." *Lakartidningen* 94:47 (November 1997): 4359–61.

Hammer, K., C. Carson, T. Riley. "Susceptibility of Transient and Commensal Skin Flora to the Essential Oil of Melaleuca Alternifolia (Tea Tree Oil)." *Am J Infect Control* 24:3 (June 1996): 186–89.

Heggers, J., A. Kucukcelebi, D. Listengarten et al. "Beneficial Effect of Aloe on Wound Healing in an Excisional Wound Model." *Journal of Alternative and Complementary Medicine* 2:2 (Summer 1996): 271–77.

Howe, M. "Nature's Cure-All." *Country Living* 19 (July 1996): 34ff.

Jacobs, M. and C. Hornfeldt. "Melaleuca Oil Poisoning." 32:4 *J Toxicol Clin Toxicol* (1994): 461–64.

Johnston, C. et al. *Journal of the American College of Nutrition* 17 (1998): 366–70.

Kaufman, T., N. Kalderon, Y. Ullmann and J. Berger. "Aloe Vera Gel Hindered Wound Healing of Experimental Second-Degree Burns: A Quantitative Controlled Study." *Journal of Burn Care and Rehabilitation* 9:2 (March–April 1988): 156–59.

Knight, T. and B. Hausen. "Melaleuca Oil (Tea Tree Oil) Dermatitis." *Journal of the American Academy of Dermatology* 30:3 (March 1994): 423–27.

Lantin, B. "Tea Tree Oil: The Old Healer." *The Daily Telegraph* (1 August 1997): 19.

————."Red Faces For Career Women." *The Daily Telegraph* (6 February 1998).

Nenoff, P., U. Haustein and W. Brandt. "Antifungal Activity of the Essential Oil of Melaleuca Alternifolia (Tea Tree Oil)." *Skin Pharmacol* 9:6 (1996): 388–94.

Plemons, J. et al. "Evaluation of Acemennan in the Treatment of Aphthous Stomatitis." *Wounds* 6 (1994): 40–45.

Raman, A., U. Weir and S. Bloomfield. "Antimicrobial Effects of Tea-tree Oil and Its Major Components on Staphylococcus Aureus, Staph. Epidermidis and Propionibacterium Acnes." *Lett Appl Microbiol* 21:4 (October 1995): 242–45.

Rodríguez-Bigas, M., N. Cruz and A. Suárez. "Comparative Evaluation of Aloe Vera in the Management of Burn Wounds in Guinea Pigs." *Plast Reconstr Surg* 81:3 (March 1988): 386–89.

Schmidt, J. and J. Greenspoon. "Aloe Vera Dermal Wound Gel Is Associated With a Delay in Wound Healing." *Obstetrics and Gynecology* 78:1 (July 1991): 115–17.

Schorah, C. et al. "The Effect of Vitamin C Supplements on Body Weight, Serum Proteins, and General Health of an Elderly Population." *American Journal of Clinical Nutrition* 34 (May 1981): 871.

Shapiro, S., A. Meier and B. Guggenheim. "The Antimicrobial Activity of Essential Oils and Essential Oil Components Toward Oral Bacteria." *Oral Microbiol Immunol* 9:4 (August 1994): 202–08.

Stenson, J. "Runners Should Take Steps to Prevent Toenail Fungus." *Medical Tribune News Service* (1996). http://pharmacy-web.com/WHP/InfoService/MedTribune/Abstract/M960321d. html

Strickland, F., R. Pelley and M. Kripke. "Prevention of Ultraviolet Radiation-Induced Suppression of Contact and Delayed Hypersensitivity by Aloe Barbadensis Gel Extract." *Journal of Investigative Dermatology* 102:2 (February 1994): 197–204.

Taylor, T. et al. "Ascorbic Acid Supplementation in the Treatment of Pressure-Sores." *Lancet* II (1974): 544.

Tyler, V. "Aloe: Nature's Skin Soother." *Prevention* 50 (April 1998): 94ff.

———."Create Your Own Herbal First-Aid Kit." *Prevention* 50 (August 1998): 93ff.

Van der Valk, P., A. de Groot, D. Bruynzeel et al. "Allergic Contact Eczema Due to 'Tea Tree' Oil." *Ned Tijdschr Geneeskd* 138:16 (16 April 1994): 823–25.

Villar, D., M. Knight, S. Hansen and W. Buck. "Toxicity of Melaleuca Oil and Related Essential Oils Applied Topically on Dogs And Cats." *Vet Hum Toxicol* 36:2 (April 1994): 139–42.

Visuthikosol, V., B. Chowchuen, Y. Sukwanarat et al. "Effect of

Aloe Vera Gel to Healing of Burn Wound. A Clinical and Histologic Study." *Journal of the Medical Association of Thailand* 78:8 (August 1995): 403–09.

Welford, H. "The Perfect Remedy? Ask an Aborigine." *Independent* (6 August 1997): 7.

CHAPTER TWENTY-FOUR: Varicose Veins

Bisler, H. et al. "Wirkung von Rosskastaniensamenextrakt auf die Transkapillare Filtration bei Chronischer Venoser Insuffizienz." *Deutsche Med Wochenschr* 111 (1986): 1321–29.

Bundesanzeiger (5 December 1984).

Cebo, B., et al. "Pharmacological Properties of Saponin Fractions in Polish Crude Drugs: Saponaria Officinalis, Primula Officinalis, and Aesculus Hippocastanum." *Herba Pol* 22 (1976): 154–62.

Delacroix, P. "A Double-Blind Study of Endotelon in Chronic Venous Insufficiency." *La Revue de Médicine* (August 31–7 September 1981): 27–28.

Diehm, C., H. Trampisch, S. Lange and C. Schmidt. "Comparison of Leg Compression Stocking and Oral Horse-Chestnut Seed Extract Therapy in Patients With Chronic Venous Insufficiency." *Lancet* 347:8997 (3 February 1996): 292–94.

Duke, J. *The Green Pharmacy*. Emmans, Pa.: Rodale Press, 1997.

Greeske, K. and B. Pohlmann. "Horse Chestnut Seed Extract—An Effective Therapy Principle in General Practice. Drug Therapy of Chronic Venous Insufficiency." *Frotschrittle der Medezin* 114:15 (30 May 1996): 196–200.

Guillaume, M. and F. Padioleau. "Veinotonic Effect, Vascular Protection, Anti-inflammatory and Free Radical Scavenging Properties of Horse Chestnut Extract." *Arzneimittelforschung* 44:1 (January 1994): 25–35.

Haas, H. Arzneipflanzenkunde (1991).

Johnson, E. *American Journal of Pharmacology* 118 (1946): 164.

Kreysal, H. et al. "A Possible Role of Lysosomal Enzymes in the

Pathogenesis of Varicosis and the Reduction in Their Serum Activity with Venostatin.®'' *Vasa* 12 (1983): 377–82.

Masquelier, J. "Stabilisation du Collagene par les Oligomeres Procyanidiques." *Acta Therpeutica* 7 (1981): 101–05.

McEwan, A. et al. "Effect of Hydroxyethylrutosides on Blood Oxygen Levels and Venous Insufficiency Symptoms in Varicose Veins." *British Medical Journal* 2 (1971): 138.

Newall, C., L. Anderson and J. D. Phillipson. *Herbal Medicines: A Guide for Healthcare Professionals.* London: Pharmaceutical Press, 1996.

Prosperio, G. et al. "Cosmetic Uses of Horse Chestnut (Aesculus Hippocastanum) Extracts, of Escin and of the Cholesterol/Escin Complex." *Fitoterapia* 51 (1980): 113–28.

Rao, S. and K. Cochran. "Antiviral Activity of Triterpinoid Saponins Containing Acylated β-Amyrin Agylcones." *Journal of Pharmacological Science* 63 (1974): 471.

Rehn, D., M. Unkauf, P. Klein et al. "Comparative Clinical Efficacy and Tolerability of Oxerutins and Horse Chestnut Extract in Patients With Chronic Venous Insufficiency." *Arzneimittelforschung* 46:5 (May 1996): 483–87.

Rudofsky, G. et al. "Odemprotektive Wirkung und Klinische Wirksamkeit von Rosskastaniensamenextrakt im Doppelblindversuch." *Phlebol Proktol* 15 (1986): 47–53.

Thebaut, J. "A Study of Endotelon on the Functional Manifestations of Venous Insufficiency. A Double-Blind Study of 92 Patients." *Gazette Medicale* 92:12 (1985).

Tierney, L. and M. Erskine. "Chapter Nine." In S. Schroeder, M. Krupp, L. Tierney and S. McPhee, eds. *Current Medical Diagnosis and Treatment 1990.* Norwalk: Appleton & Lange, 1990.

Tstsumi, S. and S. Ishizuka. "Anti-Inflammatory Effects of the Extract Aesculus Hippocastanum and Seed." 67 Shikwa Gakutto (1967): 1324–28.

Tyler, V. *Herbs of Choice.* Binghamton: Pharmaceuticals Products Press, 1994.

Weiss, R. *Herbal Medicine.* Gothenburg: AB Arcanum, 1988.

INDEX